Intro

D0906423

Quacks

Fakers & Charlatans in English Medicine

to W.F.B.

Quacks

Fakers & Charlatans in English Medicine

Roy Porter

TEMPUS

Illustrated edition published 2000

PUBLISHED IN THE UNITED KINGDOM BY:

Tempus Publishing Ltd
The Mill, Brimscombe Port
Stroud, Gloucestershire GL5 2QG

PUBLISHED IN THE UNITED STATES OF AMERICA BY:

Tempus Publishing Inc.
2A Cumberland Street
Charleston, SC 29401

Tempus books are available in France, Germany and Belgium
from the following addresses:

Tempus Publishing Group	Tempus Publishing Group	Tempus Publishing Group
21 Avenue de la République	Gustav-Adolf-Straße 3	Place de L'Alma 4/5
37300 Joué-lès-Tours	99084 Erfurt	1200 Brussels
FRANCE	GERMANY	BELGIUM

British Library Cataloguing in Publication Data.
A catalogue record for this book is available from the British Library.

ISBN 0 7524 1776 2

Typesetting and origination by Tempus Publishing.
PRINTED AND BOUND IN GREAT BRITAIN.

Contents

List of illustrations

Colour Section

Acknowledgements

This book has emerged from an, I trust, fruitful interplay between two different areas of investigation. It stems, first, from a long-term engagement with the history of unorthodox medicine, which I explored in sundry papers delivered, and essays published, during the 1980s. I am very grateful to all who have commented on these, and offered much-needed criticism. Certain chapters of this book draw upon some of these previous writings; I have, however, incorporated new material throughout, and made considerable alterations in interpretation and emphasis. Insofar as there is a degree of restatement of argument and information, it has been demanded by the need to articulate the analysis as part of a wider whole.

Second, this work has developed out of a broader endeavour to investigate the socio-cultural history of illness and medicine in England, from around the mid-seventeenth century to the early Victorian age, using as evidence the letters, diaries, journals, and autobiographies of people as patients. This project has been jointly undertaken with Dorothy Porter. We have elsewhere published two co-authored volumes arising out of that study: *In Sickness and in Health* (Fourth Estate, 1988), which looks at popular experience of illness; and *Patient's Progress* (Polity Press, 1989), a study of the relations between the sick and their (regular) doctors. Without Dorothy's immense stimulus and labour in that collaboration, the present book would lack its essential contextual framework.

For, though this work is entirely self-standing, the account of the health culture of pre-modern England developed in those earlier volumes informs the present text. Such arguments can hardly be spelt out again in detail here – it would have been intolerably space-consuming. The reader who finds some of the assertions about pre-modern medical culture made below tendentious or obscure is therefore respectfully asked to refer to the two other volumes for further elucidation and supporting evidence.

This study would not have been brought to completion without the uniquely pleasant working conditions provided by the Wellcome Institute for the History of Medicine; for which Steve Emberton is especially to be thanked I am pleased, as ever, to acknowledge my debts to the Wellcome Trustees. Andy Foley at the Institute has gallantly manned the xerox machines, and Sally Bragg and Marika Antoniw have typed portions of the manuscript with their never-failing cheerfulness and accuracy. Without Sally's vast eleventh-hour aid, the book would probably not have appeared at all: I am specially grateful to her. As always, Jean Runciman has proved the perfect copy-editor and indexer: learned, accurate and ever-smiling. An anonymous referee read the typescript with speed and charity, and John Banks saw the book through the press with great care. My thanks to both. The dedication to this book is but a small token of gratitude for the tremendous kindness, tolerance, friendship and support which Bill Bynum has given me over the years.

RSP August 1988
Wellcome Institute for the History of Medicine, London

Note to Illustrated Edition

I am delighted to have an opportunity to see this book once more in print, especially in a handsomely illustrated version. After all, the culture of quackery hinged heavily on visual appeal.

I have pondered long whether to undertake major revisions to the text (published *as Health for Sale: Quackery in England 1650-1850* by Manchester University Press back in 1989) and have decided against it. Much water has flowed under the history of medicine bridge during the last decade, but there has been surprisingly little work published on British quack medicine in the long eighteenth century; while I could modify my views here and there, and add new pieces of information, I do not feel minded, as of now, to change my overall reading of the subject.

I would, however, like to take this opportunity of giving my warmest thanks to Andrea Meyer Ludowisy, of the Iconographic Collection at the Wellcome Trust, for her invaluable help in finding and reproducing the illustrations.

Roy Porter
January 2000

Preface

> The history of quackery, as practised in England, I remember hearing old Mr.
> Sheridan say, would make a useful and no less amusing book.
> Henry Angelo, *Reminiscences*

To prevent confusion, or to sharpen controversy, I must clarify at the outset the force of the term 'quack' as it will be habitually used, as a term of historical analysis, throughout this book (henceforth, the intrusive inverted commas will disappear). I do not believe that the historian should start off from a hard-and-fast, timeless, moralizing definition of the quack. In early modern England, the term was polemically tossed around as an accusation: used to brand someone supposedly practising medicine in bad faith. But the historian – or, at least, this historian – is scarcely qualified to open such windows on to men's souls (though, if pushed, I would judge that many of those 'medicasters' and 'charlatans' commonly arraigned as tricksters were less cheats than zealots: if we are to speak of delusion, it is primarily self-delusion). I am, in this respect, glad to follow W.F. Bynum's wise dictum that 'quack is as quack does': our criteria for applying the category must be not essentialist but behavioural. Certain characteristic sorts of activities and self-presentations, pursued by certain medical operators, set them aside as that particular variety of medicine man we may heuristically call the quack.

Hence, endorsing what my colleague, Christopher Lawrence, has dubbed 'the poverty of essentialism', I disclaim any absolute, Platonic meaning for my application of the term. I shall take as quacks the broad spectrum of those operators who were typically pilloried as such; and in doing so, this being a work of history, the term will convey neither blame nor praise. He (or she) was called a quack who transgressed what those in the saddle defined as true, orthodox, regular, 'good' medicine. He who chose to operate as a quack, or had no alternative but so to do, thus became, willy-nilly, something of an abnormal, and had to adopt the behaviour that best enabled him to survive and thrive as an outsider. To be more specific, quacks will be my shorthand (and morally neutral) term of art for those who drummed up custom largely through self-orchestrated publicity; who operated as individual entrepreneurs rather than as cogs in the machine of the medical community; whose dealings with their clients were largely one-off; and who depended heavily upon vending secret nostrums. The list of their typical attributes could obviously be extended, refined, and disputed.

Critics may retort that my rough-and-ready definitions entail the inclusion of figures who were not 'really' quacks, and vice versa. This is, however, as it should be, for the resultant sense of blurred and contested boundaries is surely a useful index of how things really were. Altruistic doctors did not confront thievish quacks like white meeting black (only the most dyed-in-the-wool Whig history still polarizes the past in terms of confrontations between saints and sinners, heroes and villains). Rather, the panorama presents individual medical practitioners of many stripes, some more, some less engaged in quackish activities. Look at the typical pamphlet published by the most respectable physician enumerating the virtues of his local spa or medicinal waters, suggested Thomas Beddoes around the turn of the nineteenth century: were not such works for all the world just like barely camouflaged quack bills? Many perfectly reputable Georgian physicians engaged without a blush in commercial activities that would have resulted in their names being struck off the Register in the straitlaced world of late-Victorian professional medicine.

Others may argue that the term quack is so hopelessly emotive that it is best jettisoned entirely as a term of historical analysis. Perhaps. Yet, for reasons explained in chapter 8, I have grave doubts about substituting phrases such as 'fringe doctors', since I believe their connotations are misleadingly anachronistic. I might have resorted to such circumlocutions as 'those operating at the hard commercial end of medicine', but these introduce cumbersomeness without clarity. On the whole, the familiar term, used in a slightly unfamiliar sense, has seemed best.

Regular doctors have often been the heroes of historians, and fringe and folk medicine have had their followers; but few scholars have chosen to champion the quacks, and the result is that we know little about them. In terms of rectifying such ignorance, the present book is more a palliative than a panacea; it may, at least, purge some of the ancient errors that plague the subject. No reading of quackery could, in any case, hope to be definitive until some of the gaping gaps in our grasp of orthodox medicine are eliminated. Not least, we still have nothing approaching a wide-ranging, well-researched economic history of medicine, in all its branches, as practised in the first industrial, the first consumer society. We equally lack proper studies of the cultural meanings of medicine – the place of the doctor, and the resonances of the healing arts, in society. In default of such accounts of regular medicine, what will be said below about quackery may well prove premature.

Moreover, I am well aware of the unevenness of the coverage of this book. Many facets of quackery are barely discussed, if mentioned at all. Ignorance and lack of space have between them much to do with this. There are abundant aspects of quackery upon which neither I, nor anyone else, has yet undertaken the necessary research. Thus, I have personally sampled Georgian provincial newspapers for signs of the promotion of quack preparations and of their itinerant activities, and I have made grateful use of admirable local studies – above all, those of P.S. Brown for Bath and Bristol, and J.J. Looney for Yorkshire. But no one has yet undertaken systematic research upon the press's role in the fortunes of quack medicine. Similarly, recent work by Jonathan Barry and Hilary Marland suggests it would be particularly fruitful to research the function of quacks within the total medical economy of particular neighbourhoods; I regret I have not carried out such an in-depth local study. I trust, however, that this present survey at least makes a start, and highlights, if only by its shadows and shortcomings, what work remains to be done.

Moreover, the patchy coverage of the subject offered here is also the product of the destructive hand of time; unsurprisingly, original documentation about quacks survives more precariously than hospital records or professorial lecture notes. I know, for instance, of no substantial extant business records of any seventeenth- or eighteenth-century mountebank (did they keep them in the first place?). For want of the kinds of cash-books that have survived in some quantity for regular doctors, we remain tantalizingly ignorant as to whether common-or-garden quacks made a decent living, or whether 'superquacks' such as James Graham ever gained the great fortunes which the talk of the town bestowed upon them. Likewise, the British Library boasts a magnificent collection of metropolitan quack handbills dating from the late seventeenth century but no archive, so far as I am aware, possesses the equivalent bills for, say, a century later. Is this just an accident of survival? Or does this gap tell us about some genuine historical change (for example, a decline in certain modes of quack business activity, or the rising role of the newspaper, replacing the handbill as the engine of publicity)?

Despite these lacunae in materials and deficiencies in research, the time seemed ripe for a provisional overview and interpretation: something useful, amusing even. I have not attempted to explore all facets of quackery. I have said next to nothing about the manufacture, ingredients, and efficacy of their electuaries and essences, balms, boluses and bitters. Nor have I made any attempt to evaluate their healing skills, or want of them, though this would be fruitful in the light of the Regency social commentator Henry Angelo's comment that quacks were men of 'much ingenuity… who, though not of regular practice, yet introduced many new and beneficial modes of alleviating and even curing diseases'. Rather, the question this book chiefly tackles concerns the changing public identity and standing of the quack, as the branch of the medical profession openly, and sometimes unashamedly, making a living out of what Beddoes called 'the sick-trade'.

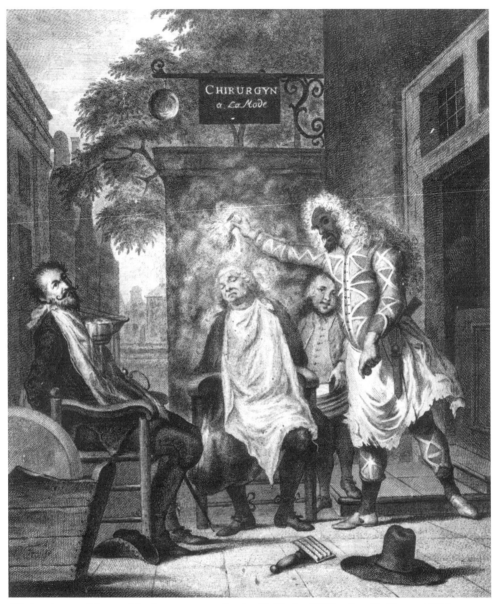

Harlequin, magician and barber: an engraving by P. Tanje, 1758, after C. Troost, 1738, showing the mystery and showmanship of such itinerant tradesmen.

1 Quackery

Quackery was a bad thing, as everybody in pre-modern England knew, and the quack was a wretch – a 'turdy-facy, nasty-paty, lousy fartical rogue', in Ben Jonson's definitive phrase.[1] The journalist Ned Ward went on to elaborate the 'Character of a Quack' more effusively:

> A Shame to Art, to Learning, and to Sense,
> A Foe to Virtue, Friend to Impudence,
> Wanting in Nature's Gift and Heaven's Grace,
> An Object Scandalous to the Human Race;
> A Spurious Breed by some Jack Adams got,
> Born of some Common Monstrous God-knows-what;
> Into the World no Woman sure could bring
> So vile a Birth, such an un-man-like thing.[2]

Quacks, mountebanks, charlatans, and the like were the sweepings of the gutter, mere scum 'bred up to a Mechanic Employment', as Daniel Turner commented – illiterate, ignorant, often foreign, commonly Jews. They possessed no medical abilities. Their much-trumpeted arts and arcana, pills and potions, were at best worthless, and, all too often, positively deadly draughts. They laid claims to miraculous powers, encyclopaedic learning, wonder cures, stupendous successes, the patronage of popes, princes and people, and universal applause. But all this was utter bunkum. For they were nothing but liars, cheats, and impostors. Above all, quacks were other people. Everybody felt happy in execrating the quack, because, everybody could agree, the quack was someone else.

Nobody ever called himself a quack. Unlike the (in some ways comparable) terms 'witch' or 'heretic', the label 'quack' was never pinned upon oneself, but always hurled against others. It always conveyed insult and abuse, always meant a bad, base doctor – indeed, in Thomas Beddoes's apt phrase, the 'bastard brethren' of the healing profession. Most commonly, of course, the acction of quackery issued from the mouths of those blessed with the attributes – or at least the reputation – of being regular doctors, and was targeted against those lacking them. But by no means always. All manner of itinerants and nostrum-vendors – precisely those themselves accustomed to being lashed as quacks – energetically returned the compliment, calling each other names, ferreting out quacks from amongst their own ranks, or detecting charlatanism in high places. And even the very scions of the profession felt few inhibitions about occasionally accusing each other of gross quackery.

Thus, when in 1788 the esteemed West Midlands practitioner William Withering – pioneer of digitalis therapy – seemed to Dr Erasmus Darwin to be poaching clients from

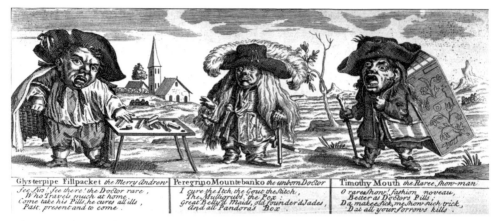

Three travelling tradesmen, including the itinerant medicine vendors Glysterpipe Fillpacket and Peregrino Mountebanko.

his son, Robert Waring Darwin, the senior physician indicted Withering of the 'solemn quackery of large serious promises of a cure'.[3] Similarly, when Darwin's friend Dr Thomas Beddoes promoted the use of artificial gases to treat consumption, Beddoes reflected that he was bound to be accused of quackery by his own tribe. Therein lay a delicious irony, since Beddoes had set himself up as the Grand Inquisitor of the quacks, whom he was eager to suppress by law (would he have ended up hoist on his own petard?). For much of the nineteenth century, doctors introducing new diagnostic technology, such as the ophthalmoscope, always ran the risk of being accused by old-guard senior brethren of stooping to 'quackery'.

'Quack' was thus the ubiquitous swearword of an occupation many of whose terms were smeared with dubious connotations (consider the verb 'to doctor'). The quack was to the physician what the hack was to the poet, and the pretender to the king. But as well as being a multipurpose idiom of abuse, the label of quack was also, with some consistency, pinned upon a particular genre of medical operator – those who cried up their goods in the market, surrounded by zanies and monkeys, jokes and buffoonery, those who pasted bills upon walls, who puffed their wares in newspapers, who circuited the nation, who mass-marketed cure-alls and catholicons. What exactly was wrong with such operators?

Certain fusillades fired off against them – for example, aspersions against their social origins – were part of the common coin of insult in a society eager to right itself, after having just been turned upside-down in the Civil War. Visions of bad men creeping up through the floorboards have a timeless quality. Who were these quacks, a late-Elizabethan writer had asked, but a pack of:

> runnagate Jews, the Cut-throats and robbers of christians, slow-bellyed monkes who have made their escape from their cloysters, simoniacall and perjured shavelings, shifting and out cast Pettifoggers, Trasonial Chymists, light-headed and trivial Druggers and Apothecaries, sun-shunning

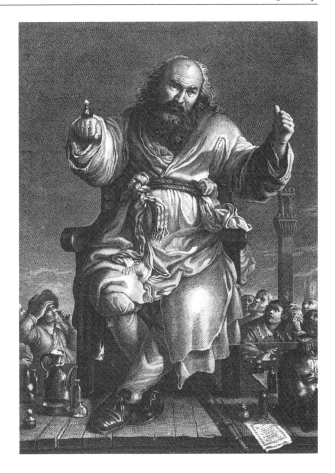

A charlatan performing with props before a crowd in Sienna. Engraving by G.B. Polanzani after S. Pacini after G. Mei.

nightbirds and corner-creepers, dull-pated and base Mechanickes, Stage players, Juglers, Pedlers, Prittle-pratling barbers, filthie Grasiers, curious bath keepers, common shifters, cogging cavaliers, lazy clowns, toothless and tatling old wives, chattering char-women, long-tongued midwives, Dog leeches and such like baggage.[4]

'You shal sooner finde a black Swan than an honest man in this Bunch', the author concluded. Such vilification echoes down the centuries.

But the specifically medical capacities of the quacks were impugned, too. For one thing, they were not qualified to practise. They had not been to university, or even undergone proper apprenticeship. They had no medical degrees, diplomas, or certificates; they were not enrolled in medical colleges or corporations, or licensed to practise.

For another – and this followed as the night the day – quacks were know-nothings; they had, judged the surgeon Daniel Turner, but a 'pitiful stock of knowledge'. They had mastered none of those approved continents of learning, from Greek and Latin to botany and anatomy, which every erudite practitioner required. Their books, bills, and patents bulged with grotesque blunders – of grammar, pharmacology, and diagnosis – which exposed them as arrant sciolists. How (thundered James Makittrick Adair, self-appointed late eighteenth-century Quack-Finder General) could Godbold's nostrum possibly be sovereign (as claimed) both for asthma and for consumption? – anyone but a blithering idiot knew these were utterly diverse disorders requiring clean contrary therapeutics.

The consequence of this ignorance (the charge continued) must be that quacks were peddlers not of panaceas but of poisons. Worse still, they revelled in the unethical trick of marketing their nostrums as secrets, so the public could not even tell what dross they were swallowing. In claiming spectacular cures, quacks made a great hullabaloo about testimonials, reporting the miraculous recovery of Lady A and the Revd Z; but all of these were bogus. It was lucky for quacks, claimed the good Dr Adair, that 'dead men tell no tales'.

These ignoramus empirics further attempted to mask their ineptitude behind a rhetorical phantasmagoria, trading upon esoteric words and pretentious pseudo-technicalities. They were thus all mouth, slick-talking, smart operators, adepts in sleight-of-hand and showmanship, spouters of what Ned Ward called 'senseless cant'.

Most damning of all, it was said that these masters of mendacity were callous conmen, cruelly fleecing the public, exploiting illness and trust. Indeed, for many contemporaries, imposture was the heart of the matter. In his *Dictionary* (1755), Samuel Johnson was to build a fraud charge into the very definition of the quack, regarding the creature as

1. A boastful pretender to arts which he does not understand.
2. A vain boastful pretender to physic, one who proclaims his own Medical abilities in public places.
3. An artful, tricking practitioner in Physic.

In short, the appellation 'quack' marked out a man as Mr False Pretences.

Public opinion during the 'long eighteenth century' was especially nauseated by the odour of deceit. In the mood of reaction triumphant after the Restoration, particular store was set by preserving the social order, so easily threatened by the seductive wiles of spellbinding rabble-rousers and zealot false prophets. Apologists warned of extremists and subversives and the spread of such evils as fashion, paper money, newspapers, the masquerade; novelty in religion, in taste, in natural philosophy; and the machinations of projectors, jobbers, bubblers, speculators, prophets, enthusiasts, etc. – all of which between them were creating a crazy fantasy world of false appearances, tinsel illusion, and Mandevillian hypocrisy. Medical quacks were not the least villains in this assault on four-square truth, reason, and common sense launched by the forces of fiction and trumpery, illusion and delusion. The triumph of quackery seemed as imminent as the empire of Dullness.

May the historian then assume, as a working definition, that the quack may thus be told apart from the authentic doctor by virtue of such attributes – by his being an ill-bred, uneducated, ignorant, inept impostor? The answer, quite obviously, is no – and for all the good reasons that contemporary quacks themselves never tired of pointing out. For one thing, the various elements in the Identikit definition do not, in fact, perfectly tally with those operators who were habitually branded as quacks. For instance, so-called quacks not infrequently possessed some authentic, formal medical or academic qualification, or an official diploma that licensed practice. In post-Restoration London, John Pechey, for example, was widely accused of quackish practices. He advertised his cures by handbills, through which he offered his services cut-price: 1s a consultation, 2s 6d a visit, the parish poor free. Yet he was a graduate of Oxford University, who, after receiving a medical apprenticeship from his father, became a licentiate of the College of Physicians. He dismissed the accusations of quackery levelled against him as nothing but sour grapes, contending how 'Many Men make it their business to ridicule the Public Way of Practice, because it thwarts their Private Interest'. In Pechey's polemic – one destined to run and run – self-publicizing, far from being arrant quackery (which, of course, he abominated with all his heart) was the very apex of public spirit.

Numerous other practitioners widely denounced as quacks had similarly received a regular education or sported a degree. James Graham, a century later, had studied at Edinburgh under Cullen and Black – what finer medical training was there? Theodor Myersbach, the fashionable uroscopist, had acquired a degree from Erfurt. And, like scores of regular practitioners, many quacks, such as William Brodum, Samuel Soloman, and Ebenezer Sibly, had bought their MDs from St Andrews or Aberdeen. In a world where academic honours could legitimately be purchased, possession of a medical degree cannot of itself be taken as proof positive of competence. And the reverse is equally true: are we automatically to deny that men such as Nicholas Culpeper or Dr Johnson's friend Robert Levet were competent practitioners, solely for want of ever having undergone formal medical training?

Quacks who had never paced the quadrangles of a college were condemned for their unlettered 'empiricism', that is, practice by trial and error, with no formal theoretical grounding. But they had their answer. What value were the arid doctrines of the schools when compared to the university of life? They had travelled, sat at the feet of the famous adepts, winkled out medical secrets, if not from China to Peru at least from Turkey to Italy and Muscovy to France. In many of the authentic arts of medicine – not least such surgical techniques as tooth-drawing or bone-manipulation, which formed the staple of many an itinerant's livelihood – it was practice, not theory, which made perfect. Who dared belittle empiricism in physic, when, from Bacon to Locke, the empirical philosophy was being celebrated as the key to progress in scholarship and science? Indeed, precisely because they set such store by experience, rather than hide-bound authority, quacks often laid claim to pioneering innovation and experiment in therapeutics. Many of the most prominent late seventeenth-century quacks, such as John Case, boasted of their skills in 'spagyrick chemistry', rather as eighteenth-century operators championed medical electricity.

Quacks further denied the charge that their therapeutics were rash, dangerous, and outlandish. It hardly held water. Even Dr Adair, in the end, decided that the worst that could be said against most quack remedies was that they were 'pilfered… from regular practice', being the standard materia medica of the pharmacopoeia – above all, opiates, mercurials and antimoniacs – dolled up in fancy dress.[5] Likewise, a glance at quack pamphlets shows that they typically shared the *Weltanschauung* of regular physic, embracing its disease language and its doctrines of solids and fluids, humours and complexions, as will be investigated in chapter 5. Novel disease categories (for example, the idea of 'nervous' conditions), and innovations in treatments (for example, the use of medical electricity) were shared by faculty and quacks alike. One index of this

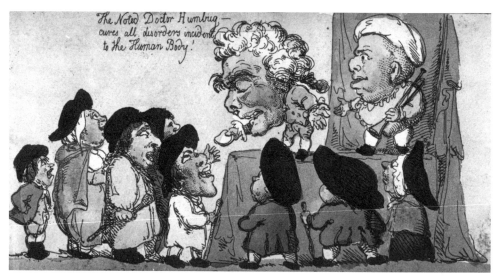

The Noted Doctor Humbug — cures all disorders incident to the Human Body!

Doctor Humbug, an itinerant medicine vendor, selling his wares from a stage with the aid of an assistant. Coloured etching, 1799.

convergence is the fact that it was regular doctors, such as David Hartley, who sanctioned the parliamentary purchase (at a cost of £5000) of the secret of Mrs Joanna Stephens's empiric stone-dissolving medicine.

Thus, most of the litmus tests that might be proposed to divide quacks from pukka doctors in the event confuse rather than clarify the issues. This applies, above all, to the charge that quacks were incompetent impostors, cynically intent from mercenary motives upon rooking the public. But who is to judge their motives? And what criteria would one use? The question is as sterile – and irrelevant – as asking whether late medieval pardoners believed in the efficacy of relics, or (that long-running Enlightenment debate) whether Mahomet, or Moses, was an impostor. Some empirics, we may surmise, merely plied a trade in pills; others, such as the pioneer sex therapist, James Graham, were – so far as one can judge from their careers and writings – obsessional enthusiasts, hooked on their own ideas.

In any case, if historians are to put quacks under the microscope and scrutinize their credentials, should not we do the same for the regulars? Thus ran, of course, the thrust of the quacks' counter-accusations. The faculty excoriated quacks for their patter, showmanship, and egoism. But who could match the princes of the profession in ostentatious ritual and self-advertisement? Augustan satire teems with caricatures of pompous physicians, mumbling their dog-Latin mumbo jumbo, garbling tags from Hippocrates and Galen, swanking around in their grand carriages decked out with running-footman ('a travelling sign post', snarled Smollett, 'to draw in customers') – and all to drum up custom and amaze the world. Of course, when a scion of the faculty relieved a patient by his skill with soothing words, that was not quackery but a good bedside manner. Or when a regular larded his speech with polyglottal polysyllabics unintelligible to his patients, this was not quackish mystification, but science (*we* might say it was blinding the sick with science).

Likewise with therapeutics. Regulars praised their own treatments as safe and successful. As Dr Walter Harris contended, towards the close of the seventeenth century:

> The difference between a *Real Physician*, and a *Quack-Pretender*, does commonly appear in this, that the first is *Cautious*, *Deliberate*, and *Prudently Timorous* in all *Doubtful* cases, or *Dangerous* circumstances, generally to others, in their several degrees, as he would be content to be dealt withall himself under the same circumstances; the *Latter* is *Rash*, *Inconsiderate*, and stifly *heady* in every thing he does, his *Ignorance* makes him *Daring*, and he always ventures to Promise *Infallible success*, from the *nicest, most uncertain, and most Desperate Remedies* that are known in *Nature*, or contrived by *Art*.[6]

But what did this really mean? After all, quacks themselves (as we shall see chapter 5) often accused regulars of reckless recourse to desperate remedies – for example, excessive dosing with mercurials in venereal cases. Likewise, what the likes of Harris would laud as 'prudently timorous' procedures, might, from another viewpoint, be condemned as culpably timid. Were not what Harris damned as the 'daring' and 'desperate remedies' of the irregulars the very lifeblood of innovation and improvement? 'In physic, all changes… have been forced on the regulars by the quacks', opined Isaac Swainson late in the eighteenth century: 'and all the great and powerful medicines are the discoveries of quacks. The introduction and improvements of inoculation: the use of mercury, antimony, opium, and the bark; like all the bold innovations in religion and policy, are owing to quacks. Benefits produce the bitterest ingratitude. The regulars adopted the discoveries, and persecuted their benefactors.' Swainson thus countered the standard charge: 'In the administration of remedies, there is this difference between the regulars and irregulars. The latter always attempt a cure, sometimes desperately. The former perpetuate diseases, to perpetuate a profitable attendance. This is the general fact, to which there are honourable exceptions.'[7] Swainson's notion that 'quackery' was the engine of invaluable innovation, was grudgingly accepted even by Dr Adair.

Thus the quacks' critics seemed guilty of the very atrocities they blamed on others. The point was not lost on the public. Indeed, a genre of works exposing the 'quackery of the medical profession' cascaded from the press, some written by empirics, others by journalists and critics, all accusing the medical profession itself of the vices and vanities it anathematized in others. Many noted that it was not only itinerants and tradesmen who were involved with nostrums. Scores of perfectly orthodox practitioners also cashed in on patent medicines or even proprietary pills prepared to secret formulae. Nehemiah Grew, MD, FRS, patented 'Epsom Salts'; a century later, Dr Thomas Henry, the eminent Manchester chemist and founder member of the Manchester Literary and Philosophical Society, patented antacids and medicines for nervous diseases. Most famously (or notoriously) of all, Dr Robert James, with his Oxford MD, became a public celebrity with those best-selling febrifuge powders, for which Horace Walpole had such a 'superstitious veneration', but which may have hastened the deaths of Dr Oliver Goldsmith, John Howard, and Laurence Sterne, among others, for they were amongst the most potent antimonial preparations of the day. James, it was widely alleged by his fellow doctors, had

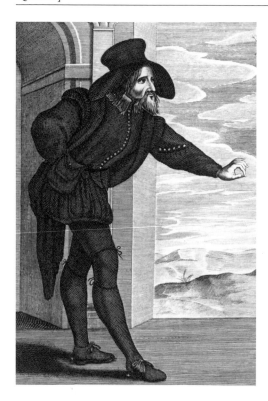

A theatrical representation of a doctor. Line engraving.

knowingly fudged the formula of his patent – to maximize secrecy – with the result that the unpredictable mixture of ingredients would readily prove a health hazard.

Many other leading regulars attached their names to cures in such a way that, even if they did not directly profit from their sales, their public fame was blazoned forth. Thus that giant of the Augustan faculty, Dr Richard Mead, had his name attached to a rabies powder, Mead's 'Pulvis Antylisus'; Dr Hans Sloane promoted medicinal chocolate; Dr Paul Chamberlain, FRCP, marketed teething necklaces; and so forth. Making money out of nostrums and engaging in self-publicizing, activities the Victorians deemed obnoxious to professional ethics, were regarded as marks of a good business nose – rational self-interest – by the Georgians. When Edward Jenner developed his own stomach medicine, John Hunter exuberantly wrote to him: 'Dear Jenner, I am puffing of your tartar as the tartar of all tartars, and have given it to several physicians to make trial, but have had no account yet of the success. Had you not better let a book-seller have it to sell, as Glass of Oxford did his magnesia? Let it be called Jenner's Tartar Emetic, or anybody's else that you please. If that mode will do, I will speak to some, viz, Newberry, &c.'[8] (John Newbery was, of course, the leading wholesale distributor of proprietary medicines.) Jenner also put his name to indigestion lozenges, which proved highly popular, being sold by Savory at Piccadilly. It was in reaction to such activities that nineteenth-century anti-vaccination campaigners (who branded vaccination itself as quackery) portrayed Jenner as a man consumed by greed. All in all, it was two-faced, argued Jeremiah Jenkins, for regulars to engage in character-assassinating quacks, when they themselves drew upon their nostrums, and even fraternized with them: 'Do not many of them [he asked] prescribe

James's Fever Powders; which do not possess any advantage whatever over the antimonial powder – Have not members of the College dined at Dr. Brodum's table? Are not many apothecaries licenciates in quackery, and expose nostrums for sale?'[9]

Not surprisingly, therefore, for every anti-quack tirade (penned by 'Misoquackus' and the like), a squib was fired against collegiate imposture – works such as *Medicina Flagellata, or the Doctor Scarify'd* (1721), or the pseudonymous Gregory Glyster's *A Dose for the Doctor* (1759), which launched a scathing 'analisation of such Aesculapian imposition' as 'large sounds with little meaning' and 'medical mystery'. Of course, such works argued, quacks were guilty of sharp practice; but who was not? Early modern commentators were sceptical about the professions in general; from Ben Jonson, through Butler, Gay, Swift, and Pope to Henry Fielding and Tobias Smollett, it was 'a world of quacks', in which all professions were conspiracies against the laity. 'How flourishes *Health* and *Peace*?', inquired a correspondent in the *Tory Tatler* for Friday 8 December 1710:

> All's one, I answer'd; *Never a Barrel the better Herring*. Poor *Health* must needs be in a fine Condition, when so many Physicians, Quacks, Surgeons, and Apothecaries are her sworn Enemies, and whole Magazines of Pills and Drugs lie in wait for her Destruction. It is indeed often ask'd, what Disease a Man died of, Fever, Pleurisie, or the like; but properly speaking, the Question should be, not what Distemper, but what Doctor did he die of: Distempers seize Men, but the Physicians execute 'em…. For my part, I never hear an Apothecary's Mortar ringing, but I think the Bell's a tolling; nor read a Doctor's Prescription, but I take it for a Passport into the next World…

In short, the Georgian public was inclined to hear the faculty arraign quackery and retort, 'if the cap fits, wear it'. When quacks accused regulars of pursuing a quackery of their own, and public spokesmen hinted that irregulars and regulars were like as two peas in a pod, the constitution of a quack was far from a cut-and-dried matter.

Thus many of the demarcation criteria commandeered by contemporaries to diagnose a quack – ignorance, ineptitude, mercenariness – cannot be taken at face value for historical analysis. Does the category of quacks then simply crumble in our hands? Are we perhaps dealing, as with the proverbial 'reds under the bed', with an entirely phantom group – rather as Professor Davis tells us that there never were any 'Ranters' in the seventeenth century except in the lurid imaginations of scare-mongering reactionary ideologues and modem Marxist historians.[10]

Should we then not be concerned with the history of quacks at all, but only with 'quacks' as a label – or rather a libel? Thomas Szasz, Sander Gilman and others have recently drawn attention to stereotyping as a device whereby 'normal' society – the 'moral majority' – defines and defends itself by conjuring up wild images of dangerous outsiders, deviants, delinquents, and monsters.[11] Over the centuries, Jews, witches, homosexuals, blacks, *femmes fatales*, the insane, and so forth, have all been subjected to such mythical misrepresentation as being the Other, leading to stigmatization and, frequently, persecution. Should we therefore be concentrating exclusively on the history of such scapegoating? Upon the demonic image of the quack, and the Humpty-Dumpty power to command the use of words exercised by medical orthodoxy?

Clearly, this story of stigmatization is critically important. But I also wish, in the succeeding chapters, to go beyond images and examine the history of quacks, taking them as a real-life scatter of operators – who worked, of course, within the fields of force and the lexicon of meanings stipulated by orthodoxy. I intend to explore them not just as bogeymen but as businessmen. For there were swarms of dealers in medicine, just as there were traders in trinkets and chapbooks, in victuals and drink, in lodgings and entertainment; quacks were regular tradesmen if they were irregular doctors.

Contemporaries vilified individual quacks. But they also deplored their epidemic nature. The nation was running alive with them, *O tempora*! Their existence was inexcusable, their success scandalous. Scores thronged London; many more were peripatetics, wreaking havoc round the country, often on regular circuits, pulling teeth, fitting trusses, selling drugs and drops. Tavern walls were plastered with their bills; people pored over them in coffee-houses; their advertisements screamed out from the newspapers. And an elite of quacks rose to fame, fortune, and even title. How could all that be, given the charlatans were such obvious sharks and that true medicine was established by authority, reason and law, and organized into colleges, corporations, and companies?

The answer – or at least the common rationalization – lay in an ingrained, if largely unarticulated, psycho-sociology of deception and delusion, which treated most of mankind as knaves and fools. On the one hand, quacks were portrayed as malicious, machinating manipulators – henchmen of the Devil almost. On the other, the populace (above all, the plebs) were dismissed as congenitally gullible and gormless, dupes of their own lumpenproletarian passions. If the herd were victims, they were certainly willing victims, for they were prey to a credulity that ensnared them in whatever captivated their foolish fancy, excited their greed, or inflamed their enthusiasm.

To us, this oft-articulated psychopathology of quackery seems hopelessly glib, reductionist and question-begging. But it should be clear why it exercised a powerful contemporary appeal, for it offered a comprehensive explanation of the hold exerted not just by 'medicasters' but by a corps of crooks and criminals. A typical mid-century blast, *The Cheats of London Exposed: or, the TRICKS of the TOWN Laid Open to Both Sexes. Being A clear Discovery of all the various Frauds and Villainies that are daily practised in in that great City*, denounced the confraternity of partners-in-crime, viz:

Highwaymen	Duffers	Bawds
Scamps	Setters	Whores
Sharpers	Pretended friends	Pimps
Gamblers	Mock Auctions	Jilts
Kidnappers	Register Offices	Gossips
Waggon-hunters	Bullies	Fortune-tellers
Money-droppers		

All such pests and plagues were guilty, alongside the quacks, each in his own special way, of that offence so scandalous to the Augustan mind: fraud.

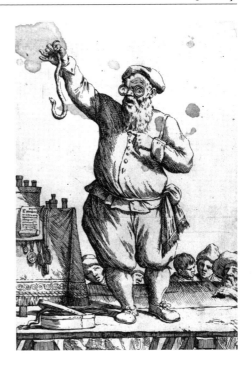

A travelling medicine peddler performing with a snake. Etching by G.M. Mitelli.

Thus the masses were taken in by quackery, much as they had traditionally been duped by magic, by alchemy, superstition, and popery, and had recently been mesmerized by puritan prophets, mechanic preachers, and the saints. The sway of princes and populist demagogues alike continued to haunt the critical spirits of the Enlightenment – as did all those other ideologues and charismatic individuals that the post-Restoration ruling elite found it comforting to lump together dismissively as the 'irrational'. Indeed, those who denounced medical quackery often contended (partly to establish guilt by association) that it was but one symptom of a grand conspiracy of chicanery and delusion. Wesley and the Methodists were slated as religious quacks, and Wilkite rabble-rousing as political quackery. In similar vein, Gillray portrayed Charles James Fox as the 'Westminster Mountebank'. 'There are also not a few instances of regal quacks,' Dr Adair argued, 'of which MASSINELLO, OLIVER CROMWELL, and the late PRETENDER to the British throne, may be adduced as examples',[12] while Tobias Smollett assured readers of *Launcelot Greaves* that 'we have quacks in religion, quacks in physic, quacks in law, quacks in politics, quacks in patriotism, quacks in government'.[13]

This empire of knaves over fools was a sad law of human nature. Thus Erasmus Darwin, whose Enlightenment optimism was punctured by popular folly, thought 'Ignorance and credulity have ever been companions, and have misled and enslaved mankind'. The human race had always been duped by the 'fictions of fancy, of witchcraft, hobgoblins, apparitions, vampires, fairies, of the influences of stars on human actions, miracles wrought by the bones of saints, the flights of ominous birds, the predictions from the bowels of dying animals, expounders of dreams, fortune tellers, conjurers, modern prophets, necromancy, cheiromancy, animal magnetism, metallic tractors, with endless variety of folly'.[14] In this context, *si populus vult decipere, decipiatur* ('if the people want to be deceived, let them') became one of the prime platitudes of the century. Yet in reality, the public mind was not so loftily blasé. For it was far from being only the *canaille* who were flocking to the quacks. The Georgian century in particular saw the emergence of ultra-chic quacks courted by clients from the *beau monde*; some, such as the oculist William Read, were even knighted. What was the world coming to?

And, more shocking still, quacks were not merely successful at courting custom but were also, against all reason, science and nature, actually working cures. Of course, the world might agree that almost all the cures claimed by quacks were jiggery-pokery, supported by spurious testimonials. But candid doctors also admitted that sometimes quacks really did heal – not, of course, because of any real grasp of medical science, therapeutic innovation, or surgical skill, but merely – and, it was implied, rather disgracefully – by enlisting the patient's imagination. A few physicians took this healing power of the imagination – what we now call the 'placebo effect' – in their stride. It was to be expected. Given that, as Dr John Moore noted, so many patients in those halcyon days of hypochondria were sick solely by fancy, it was only proper that they should be cured equally by suggestion, by grace of the hocus-pocus ministrations of quacks. Quacks thus enjoyed their successes, remarked William Wadd, 'because, like drowning men, when honest practitioners give no hope, they catch at every twig. Thus, the love of life on the one hand, and the love of gain on the other, create a tolerably good correspondence between the quack and the public.'[15]

This was the typical hypochondriac's progress, as plotted by Dr John Moore. The sick man initially consulted a regular. Failing to find a cure, he worked his way through 'the whole tribe'. He subsequently moved on to quacks, receiving from them an 'appearance of sympathy which the rest of his acquaintance refuse'... 'and they possibly relieve or palliate the cositiveness, the flatulency, the acidities, and other symptoms which are brought on by the anxiety attendant of this complaint.' What such quacks could never achieve (argued Moore, speaking as a regular physician) was the eradication of the disease: 'the original cause... continuing in spite of all their bitters, and their stomachies, and their purgatives, and analeptics, the same symptoms constantly recur. The wretched patient growing every hour more irritable, remedies hurry on the bad symptoms with double rapidity.' So what happens finally? – anything and everything gets tried, until, out of sheer desperation:

> he returns to physicians, goes back to quacks, and occasionally tries the family nostrums of many an old lady. His constitution being worn by fretfulness and by drugs, he at length despairs of relief, and either sinks into a fixed melancholy, or roused by indignation, his good genius having whispered in his ear, *fuge medicos et medicamina*, he abandons the seat of his disappointments, tries to dissipate his misery by new objects and a different climate, consults no practitioners of any country, sex, or denomination; and forms a fixed resolution to swallow no more drugs.[16]

Despair, one might think. Yet from the depths comes relief: 'from which happy epoch, if the case be not quite desperate, he has the best chance of dating his recovery.' If Moore

*A man in the costume of a theatrical caricature of a
doctor. Coloured etching by A.G*

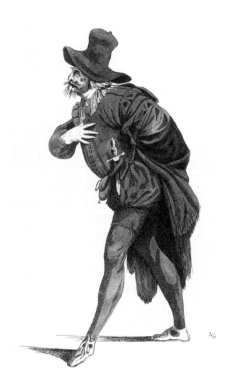

could thus see the grim humour of regulars, quacks, and the sick all being each other's
dupes in turn, other spokesmen were hardly amused, waxing indignant against the
possibility that such quackery and medicine should be reduced to a level.

Thus, scandalously, quackery seemed to be succeeding – at least doing well if not doing
good. Contemporary intellectuals, bristling with disdain for the masses, viewed this
absurdity *de haut en bas* with a certain resignation: it was a cameo in the perennial human
comedy. 'Man is a dupeable animal', pondered Southey: 'Quacks in medicine, quacks in
religion and quacks in politics know this and act upon that knowledge. The credulity of
man is unfortunately too strong to resist the impudent assertions of the quack.' Those
falling foul of medical quackery deserved marginally more sympathy than the victims of
other sorts, judged Southey, for, in their case, it was a consequence of the desperation born
of pain and disease. 'Sickness humbles the pride of man', he argued: 'it forces upon him a
sense of his own weakness, and teaches him to feel his dependence upon unseen Powers:
that therefore which makes wise men devout, makes the ignorant superstitious. Among
savages the physician and the conjuror are always the same. The operations of sickness and
of healing are alike mysterious, and hence arises the predilection of many enthusiasts for
quackery, and the ostentation which all quacks make of religion, or of some extraordinary
power in themselves.' But if the gullibility of the sick was the more excusable, the guilt of
the medical quack was consequently the greater, for he swindled people not only of their
money, but their health, and even their lives: 'They pretend to a knowledge in physick and
surgery, on the meer foundation, perhaps, of having done the menial offices of gentlemen
of the faculties; or perhaps a few receipts from some of their own vile fraternity. They have

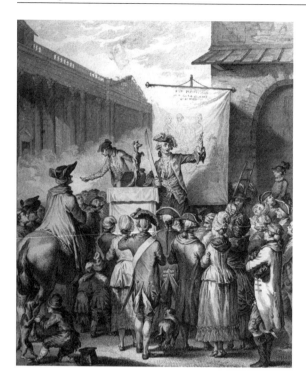

An intinerant medicine vendor performing on stage. Engraving by I. Helman, 1777, after J. Bertaux, 1776.

nothing to recommend them but a consummate effrontery; and no other means of palming their pestiferous compounds upon the unwary, than groundless assurances, and insolent detraction.'[17]

Contemporaries thus explained the fortunes of quackery largely in terms of human nature, the eternal dialectic of knaves and fools. It is distressing that historians have so uncritically taken over this explanatory model. On the one hand, many historians of quackery have regarded it as their right or duty to vent their anger against quacks, as targets of legitimate wrath. Opening a scholarly article evaluating seventeenth-century quackery, L.R.C. Agnew writes in high dudgeon:

> Having spent several years in such quack-infested fields as cancer research and nutrition, I find it difficult to be objective about quackery, even quackery in seventeenth-century England. I do not like quacks; indeed, I despise them, and while I recognise that an occasional quack remedy or relief has been imported into orthodox medicine, I cannot evince the least sympathy for the breed, those crab lice that have feasted parasitically on the body medical since the very beginning of recorded medical history.[18]

Exposing the evils of past quackery has often been made to serve as an object lesson for the present. James Harvey Young's superb deflations of American healer-dealers, in *The Toadstool Millionaires* and elsewhere, have had as their hidden agenda the evils of irregular medicine in America today. Similarly, Grete de Francesco's *Die Macht des Charlatans*, written in Germany under the Third Reich – a well-researched and still informative volume – lays bare the techniques pre-modern charlatans deployed to hold the masses as a moral fable against Nazi demagogy.

Another genre of the history of quackery substitutes amusement for anger, treating quacks, in bantering terms, with droll condescension, as bizarre eccentrics, their audacity scarcely less funny than the gulls' credulity. This tradition trivializes heterodox medicine into a familiar string of apocryphal anecdotes – stories of the colourful Katterfelto and his talking black cats, or of James Graham 'discovering' the damsel who later became Emma Hamilton, and exploiting her sex appeal through having her pose as his 'Goddess of Health'. Quackery is thereby reduced to a freak-show, a chapter in The History of Popular Delusions, a standing satire upon human nature. Neither of these approaches thus integrates the history of quackery into the history of society or the history of medicine.

A more serious move to confront the specificity of quackery lies in the attempt, recently made by a few historians, to assimilate it within the prehistory of 'fringe' medicine, regarded as an expression of an 'alternative' tradition. From the sixteenth century, Paracelsus and his followers repudiated mainline scholastic and humanistic medicine and pioneered an alternative healing incorporating elements both newly 'scientific' and popular, including herbal lore, and making an appeal to Nature. During the nineteenth century, a host of radical medical cosmologies blossomed – homoeopathy, Thomsonianism, Coffinism, medical botany, naturopathy and the like. Were not the quacks, then, the baton-carriers in the seventeenth and eighteenth centuries, bridge-figures in this great relay race of anti-establishment, populist, alternative medicine?

Such attempts to historicize the quacks – rather than to denounce or deflate them – are welcome; nevertheless, I shall argue, particularly in the next chapter, that it is not primarily as part of a long-running struggle between orthodoxy and fringe, centre and periphery, establishment and radicals, corporatism and populism, that we should best situate the history of the quacks.

What *prima facie* gives this vision of the battle of orthodoxy versus heterodoxy its particular attractiveness (aside from the opportunities it affords for taking sides) is the stress that medical sociology and the historical sociology of medicine have placed upon the consolidation of medicine as a profession. Idealists cast the triumph of medical professionalism as the protection of vulnerable clients from the *laissez-faire* jungle; cynics, or realists, regard it rather as the raising of a monopolistic, self-serving oligarchy upon the backs of the sick. But in all such readings, the enormous influence of professionalization models for framing our image of the organization of past medicine has encouraged a polarized vision, in which the division between insider and outsider is depicted as relatively sharp, and as hinging upon ethical (or pseudo-ethical) grounds. The history of quack medicine is thereby implicitly viewed as fundamentally distinct from (even the polar opposite of) the history of professional medicine.

This perhaps makes sense in respect of the last century and a half. From the early Victorian period in particular, liberal and progressive campaigners within the medical profession, orchestrated by Wakley's *Lancet*, used the assault on the many-headed hydra of quackery as the rallying call for the reformation and purification of the medical profession. And the cumulative effect of this reformist tide was that series of changes, embodied in legislation stretching from the Apothecaries' Act (1815) through the Medical Registration

Act (1858) and beyond, which elevated medicine on to a more professional, more ethical plane, in part through erecting a tighter *cordon sanitaire* between it and what it abhorred as money-mongering quackery. But to transplant these modern demarcations between orthodoxy and heterodoxy back into earlier times involves serious risk of anachronism, of reading the present back into the past.

In my view, these professionalization models, which presuppose primary distinctions between orthodoxy and heterodoxy, can be a positive hindrance when confronting the problem of understanding the economy of pre-modern medicine. We would do better to pay more attention, as Margaret Pelling has so rightly emphasized, to medicine as an occupation rather than as a vocation. Medical men of all sorts were competing for custom, recognition, and reward. Each in his own way – top physician, humble general practitioner, empiric, folk healer – made his bid to seize the moral high ground in a medical arena in which the law was acknowledged to be dog-eat-dog. It is revealing that most of the anecdotes passed down to us about pre-modern practitioners centre, admiringly, on their love of lucre and their success in gaining it. In lectures to students delivered at his private anatomy school, William Hunter made no bones about the fact that medicine was a cut-throat business, in which only the most ambitious would enjoy 'the happiness of riches'.[19] With such cash-conscious competition (the ambience against which Victorian professional medicine reacted), it is the similarities rather than the differences between quacks and regulars that deserve to be highlighted.

In early modern England, different occupations offered diverse pathways to prosperity: some opted for rugged individualism, others for the collective security of corporate status, still others for the leg-up, but possibly humiliating deference, provided by patronage networks. Medicine was no exception. Many doctors – the regulars – tended to consolidate stable practices with familiar clients, relying upon face-to-face contact and personal recommendations. They carved out steady careers, solid incomes, and safe reputations. Quacks were those seeking custom from the anonymous consumer – the faceless crowd, the nameless reader – through the media of advertising, publicity, and the sale of standardized commodities. In professional terms, they were the wild men of the trade; in entrepreneurial terms, they were its frontiersmen.

Fully to understand these divergent paths to the same goals of fame and fortune, we need to introduce a further factor into the discussion: the customer. The sick have always been ignored in histories of quackery, caricatured as gaping fools and mindless morons. In place of this image of passive dupes, let us substitute a different model. Early modern England was full of sick people seeking medical services and faced with agonizingly complex choices as to which sorts of practitioners to prefer: learned or folk, cheap or dear, general or specialist, regular or quack. All kinds of patients – not just the poor or ignorant – ended up, at least sometimes, calling on the services of quacks. Their decisions were neither worse nor better informed than their choices of regular practitioners. We shall grasp the business of quack medicine – as of regular – only by taking due account of the highly intricate, shifting, often mistrustful relations between supply and demand, dealer and customer. We shall understand both better when we see how far medical history is part and parcel of economic and social history as a whole. This is the agenda to be explored in the succeeding chapters.

2 Medical entrepreneurship in the consumer society

We cannot thus wave aside the presence of quacks as the product of psychological aberration, a monster of mass delusion. We need rather to account for the features of irregular medicine by invoking precisely the same causal clusters – social, economic, political, administrative, cultural – that explain its regular counterpart. It would be unhistorical to analyse the fortunes of quackery as if it were *sui generis*, a world apart from all the other modes of medicine jostling for their place in the sun in a disease-riddled society. We must hence survey the total demand for medical aid and the aggregate supply of healers, within the economy as a whole, seeing how 'demand' was segmented into distinct components, partly through conventional divisions of labour (for example, the distinction between internal and external medicine, the territories respectively of physicians and surgeons), and partly by dint of competition.

In a magnificent survey of medical provision in eighteenth- and nineteenth-century France, Matthew Ramsey has laid bare the complex equilibrium of forces that assured quacks a certain place, though a rather circumscribed one, in that society. Folk and popular healers continued to meet most of the medical needs of the peasant masses 'below': their proverbial and religious lore exerted a powerful appeal, and often they performed their services gratis. Regularly qualified physician-surgeons usually catered, by contrast, for the polite and the propertied. But there remained plenty of ordinary people, typically situated at neither pole of the social spectrum – those for whom a regular's services might be too expensive, or intimidating, but for whom a *maige* might seem too vulgar – who would, occasionally at least, pay for the skills of the itinerant bone-setter, oculist or tooth-drawer, or would buy a bottle of never-failing quack venereal disease medicine, hair restorer, purgative cordial, or blood cleanser. Yet the French itinerant or nostrum-vendor typically remained rather small beer. Especially from the 1780s, a licensing system, run by royal mandate through the Société Royale de Médecine, checked the legal circulation of nostrums. Later, in the nineteenth century, national and local legislation formally outlawed unlicensed medicine, thereby clipping the wings of fly-by-night quacks. French commercial healers hardly rose to become captains of industry. In assessing the distribution of medical enterprise in England, comparison with France should be kept in mind.

A naively 'progressivist' view of the development of medicine might assume that the farther back in time one looks, the fewer recognized providers of health care populate the map (always excepting folk healers, witches, and the like). This inference may, however, be dubious. Seventeenth- and eighteenth-century commentators commonly remarked what a well-stocked trade medicine was (if by that term we include all those grinding a living wholly or partly out of providing medical services). Like lawyers, doctors seemed to be springing up like weeds, and this was judged no cause for pride. For what was it but a mark of general malaise, the exploitation of misfortune, and the degeneracy of the times? Prominent among those swarms of medical men (and women) were a ragtag-and-bobtail army of quacks and empirics; early in the seventeenth century, Robert Burton celebratedly remarked, if with some exaggeration, that 'there are in every village so many Mountebanks, Empiricks, Quacksalvers, Paracelsians', elbow to elbow with the ranks of the regulars. A late seventeenth-century bill announcing 'The Sick May Have Advice for Nothing' informs readers that the 'world is daily pester'd by unskilful Pretenders to Physick, who infatuate the People with their Printed Papers, wherein they pretend to perform Matters beyond Reason' – clearly the author did not rank himself amongst them, for he proceeded to reassure his readers that not all one read in handbills was rubbish.[1]

There were, of course, excellent grounds for this proliferation, for pre-modern England was racked by chronic and acute diseases, all too commonly terminating in premature death. Numerous fine works of scholarship have documented in depth this parlous state of morbidity and mortality. There is no need to rehearse in detail here how the English nation was prey to decimating epidemics of Bubonic plague (up to 1665), of smallpox, and many other fevers and infections such as typhus, diphtheria, scarlatina and measles; how levels of maternal and infant mortality remained tragically high (sepsis and gastro-enteric conditions were largely responsible); and how chronic (and often ultimately fatal) maladies such as consumption, scurvy, and venereal diseases grew more troublesome and prevalent during the long eighteenth century. Poverty, dearth, ill-balanced diet, environmental hazards, poor personal hygiene, and squalid living conditions all left people ultra-susceptible to the micro-organisms that invaded them without their existence even being known. All the evidence – experiential and statistical, official and private – converges to prove that people suffered from debilitating and often death-dealing diseases far more than nowadays, as low life-expectancy figures abundantly demonstrate. Contemporaries were fully aware of such dangers, and they looked to medicine for protection and counterattack.

But pre-modern medicine was (even according to the most charitable reading) at best only very partially successful in defying, or vanquishing, disease. The healing arts of two or three centuries ago – before bacteriology, diagnostic technology, pharmaceutical research laboratories, sterile operating-theatres, and so forth – were, and were perceived to be, at best only sporadically effectual in overcoming the major lethal and crippling diseases. Today's nuisances, like measles, were killers in the 'world we have lost'. The limitations of traditional therapeutics and pharmacy form a familiar story, which does not need to be repeated. Of the great fatal diseases, medical skill unambiguously conquered only one, smallpox, before the present century. Plague disappeared, of course, though that was no triumph of medicine, but there is little sign that any of the other commonly fatal diseases – except perhaps ague, or malaria – was undoubtedly in retreat much before the mid-nineteenth century. Thereafter, the decline of infectious disease owed more to general improvements in living conditions than to therapeutic breakthroughs. If someone developed bloody flux or 'putrid sore throat', grew asthmatic or started spitting up blood, in 1650, 1750, or even in 1850, there was no medical procedure to be initiated that would assuredly rectify the condition and restore the sick person to the pink of health. Things were different by 1950, thanks to 'magic bullets' such as penicillin, but that is merely a measure of how recently surgery and scientific pharmacology have rescued mankind from lethal diseases.

Likewise, there were scores of sickness states rampant through the seventeenth, eighteenth, and nineteenth centuries, which were painful, disabling, debilitating, or disfiguring, and from which vast numbers suffered: gout, dropsy, worms, rickets, spinal deformities, skin ulcerations, scurvy, repeated miscarriages, deteriorating sight and hearing, gonorrhoea, depression, and so forth – illnesses that did not, in the short run, terminate people's lives, but which often put an end to their active, working, or enjoyable existences, and made living more or less burdensome. Once again, contemporary medicine had no sure-fire prophylactics or cures for such conditions.

Hypothetically, such a situation might have discredited medicine altogether. Finding that doctors, treatments, and drugs proved dubiously successful in curing their ills, the sick (one could suggest) might have despaired of medicine altogether, abandoning themselves into the hands of God, providence, prayers, and priests, or perhaps trusting to the healing power of Nature or some other Stoical recourse. Some obviously did. But what the sick typically did was, above all, to sample more and more sorts of doctors and medicine, even indulging in a 'try anything' approach, which might be dignified with the appellation of the 'experimental method', or, more honestly, be viewed as the triumph of hope over experience.

Those who could afford to do so frequently drew upon a wide range of regular physicians, seeking second, third, and fourth opinions, and showing no compunction about also sampling the therapies and drugs of empirics. In terms of practical efficacy, the sick probably experienced little measurable difference between the rather mixed benefits of physician-prescribed, apothecary-supplied medication, and the patent and proprietary concoctions of the nostrum-mongers. For regular and irregular medicaments shared a common stockpot of active and effective ingredients, pre-eminently mercury as a purge and specific against venereal infections; antimony as a febrifuge (the staple of Dr James's evergreen Fever Powders): opium as a general analgesic, sedative, decongestant and bowel-settler; and aloes, senna, rhubarb, etc., as purgatives.

One of the main grouses, after all, of the faculty against proprietary medicines was that so many had been filched from the *Pharmacopoeia Londiniensis*, the official recipe book published under the imprimatur of the College of Physicians – sometimes with the addition of some fancy, but useless, cosmetic ingredients (frequently an extra nip of alcohol in tonics and restoratives) – and, it was alleged, generally at a high mark-up. Empirics retaliated, however, by pointing out that their mass-produced nostrums, costing a shilling or two per bottle or tin, ran out cheaper than a physician's visit and the subsequent pelican-sized apothecary's bill. Early in the nineteenth century, the medical author Jeremiah Jenkins alleged that an apothecary, dispensing for a fashionable patient, would expect to net ten shillings a day in bills.

High sickness levels led to high medical demand and to shoals of practitioners. And, most relevantly for the present discussion, they also sustained a proliferation of types of healer. Evidence from literate lay people shows that, when well, they tried to keep themselves well-informed about all manner of remedies and regimes, and the successes and failures of local practitioners, and that, when sick, they eagerly threw themselves into such healing options as were available. They would (as opportunities and pockets permitted) go in for self-dosing, try family remedies, seek the advice of friends, use trusted local regular practitioners, inquire about new arrivals, perhaps travel up to a large city, a spa, or even London, to call upon a famous expert, or alternatively seek to persuade an eminent physician to diagnose and treat by post. But the sick – and not just the sick poor – would commonly also try out folk remedies, buy proprietary nostrums, visit some local adept of name or fame, sample the elixirs of a passing quack or do anything and everything else to satisfy that right and duty of self-help which counted so much in the culture of Protestant and Enlightened England. So long as disease remained powerful, so did all forms of healing. 'My Wife took a Doce of Phisick by Advice of Betty Morice', wrote the Lancashire gentleman Nicholas Blundell in 1713, 'tis the 3rd time she has taken from her'.[2] No shame was attached to going beyond the magic circle of the regular medical profession in search of relief. If some resorted to quack medicines out of a genuine experimentalism, or even a perverse vanity, most did so from desperation, having already tried everything else in vain. Recourse to such a variety of cures could be seriatim, or all might be tried out more or less at once. Whichever way, the empire of disease, and the relative inefficacy of medicine, jointly paved the way for lively medical pluralism.

Limited regulation

I have argued that traditional medicine was, and was widely seen to be, a 'dad's army' in the face of invasions of epidemic sickness. Desperation created an insatiable demand for a multiplicity of healers; amongst these were quacks. Of course, such a demand would have been inoperative if the right of all and sundry to practise medicine, or the access of consumers to drugs, had been effectively curtailed by law. Throughout early modern Europe, the freedom of people to practise trades and of consumers to purchase goods and services was widely – and often increasingly – limited (as, of course, were freedoms of speech, publication and worship). Restrictions took various forms, usually including the privileging of incorporated guilds limiting entry into a closed craft, while authorizing specific manufactures to be sold at official prices, and also the conferral of monopoly rights (for example, to vend soap or glass) upon individual entrepreneurs and courtiers. Such regulations were always cloaked in an ideology of public benefit: both consumer and craftsman were professedly being 'protected' against exploitation, national interests were being upheld, and proper social order maintained. Behind this rhetoric there invariably lay, however, the self-serving monopolistic interests of commercial and occupational cliques, and the opportunism of the prince in milking industry for fiscal advantage and patronage.

Healing was among the skills in which, throughout Europe, the regulation of practice was extended as part of the mercantilistic policies of the 'new monarchies' from the Renaissance onwards and the *Cameralwissenschaft* of enlightened absolutism. In most European states, guilds, regulated by city governments, defined the right to practise medicine – no more, and no less, than, say, tanning, painting, or silk-weaving – limiting it to those 'free' of their corporation. In England, various corporate cities had their medical guilds. Above all, the Tudors formalized corporate regulation of medicine in London, where the pickings were undoubtedly richest. The Barber-Surgeons Company (founded in 1540, under Henry VIII), and the Society of Apothecaries (founded in 1617), were

A group of doctors and medical students surround a dying patient. Watercolour painting.

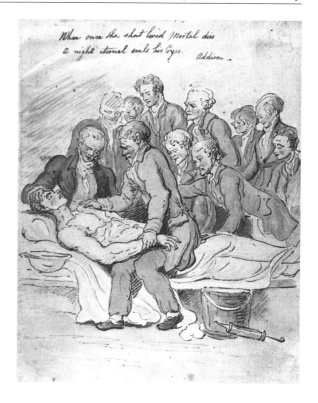

granted royal privileges to admit duly qualified operators, blessed with exclusive rights to practise in the metropolis.

Most weighty were the powers conferred by royal charter upon the College of Physicians of London. Power in the College was restricted to a privileged elite (fellows forming the governing body standardly had to be graduates of Oxford and Cambridge), who, in turn, were granted generous powers to license and oversee medical practice within the capital. Unlicensed practitioners could be summoned to answer charges before its court, and even barred from practice and punished; its royal charter also granted to the College rights to police other branches of medicine (for example, to inspect apothecaries' shops for adulteration). In the event, as the outcry of radicals from the seventeenth century onward makes plain, both the Surgeons' Company and the College of Physicians became entrenched oligarchies, dominated by self-perpetuating cliques.

In theory, this bestowal of jurisdictions upon self-selecting corporations could have entailed a dramatic restriction upon the practice of medicine in the metropolis – could have silenced the quacks. Indeed, as Cook has argued, leading elements within the College of Physicians under the early Stuarts were eager to serve as agents of regulation within a paternalistic, divine right state, implementing Laud's policy of 'Thorough': idealism and opportunism piped the same tune. Under Elizabeth, James I, and Charles I, the College energetically ferreted out and prosecuted pirate practitioners.

Judicial power might thus have drastically curtailed the activities of unorthodox healers in England, as happened across the Channel. Take for instance the *cause célèbre* in which Franz Anton Mesmer, pioneer of therapeutic hypnotism, was in effect driven out of practice in Vienna (despite his impeccable credentials) by pincer pressure from the medical faculty and imperial authority, only to undergo equivalent ostracism from Paris some years later, thanks to a comparable alliance. A similar fate befell Samuel Hahnemann, the founder of homoeopathy, who was drummed out of practice in Germany. At a more humdrum level, the Société Royale de Médecine denied licences to most of the nostrum-mongers whose panaceas it tested.

In the event, no such stringent policing became normal in England. There were various reasons. It was partly because, at bottom, the English monarchy did not consistently possess the power, during the seventeenth century and even more so throughout the eighteenth, to uphold Colbertian mercantilism. The Civil War dealt the regulationist ambitions of the College a sharp blow. From the Restoration, both Parliament and public opinion inveighed against the pretensions of chartered companies dubbed as creatures of the court. From gutter journalism to classical Smithian political economy, privileged corporations got an increasingly bad press.

In any case, the English Crown had no special will to back the ambitions of the medical colleges – Charles II gave his half-hearted and fickle favour more to the Royal Society and to cliques of medical chemists than to the College of Physicians. Moreover, he and his successors were shameless opportunists in deploying medical licensing. Monarchs did a trade in licensing the practice of foreign mountebanks in England. They also promoted the privilege of patenting. Anyone was entitled to patent a medicine. The preparation had to be a novel formula (there was no need to prove that it worked). Its specifications were to be revealed to the Patent Office, where patents were open to public inspection. In return, the patentee acquired legal monopoly over the product (and access to the courts to prosecute pirates). The benefit to the Crown and its servants (beyond a rather nebulous exercise of protection) amounted to some £150. Around one hundred medical patents were taken out during the eighteenth century, for ownership of a formal patent probably brought some prestige to a nostrum.

Through its opportunistic deployment of these devices, the Crown drastically undermined the prospects for regular medicine to enjoy a normalizing role, authorized to slay the dragon of quackery. Kings perversely seemed to be conferring special favour upon the quacks. The practice, restored at the Restoration, of touching for the king's evil (scrofula) formed a further instance – amounting to direct royal quackery, though physicians were too tactful to say so. The foreign mountebank's licence and the medical patent were both – or so it seemed – the royal seal of approval. Aside from court physicians and surgeons, which regulars could boast similar favours from on high?

Quacks were naturally not slow to exploit their windfall. They blazoned forth the trappings of their royal patents – seals, crests, and coats of arms – as though they were proofs positive of personal royal blessing. At a later stage, payment of stamp duty upon proprietary medicines was similarly exploited by dealers pleased to adorn their publicity with slogans such as 'by Royal Authority'. Guardians of orthodoxy were, of course, incensed by this royal habit of playing ducks and drakes with the doctors, for patent-toting quacks were thereby, as John Corry complained, 'licensed to kill'.[3]

The eighteenth century – the high noon of Continental 'medical police' – saw a further eclipse of prospects for stamping out unorthodox healing in England. In London, the College

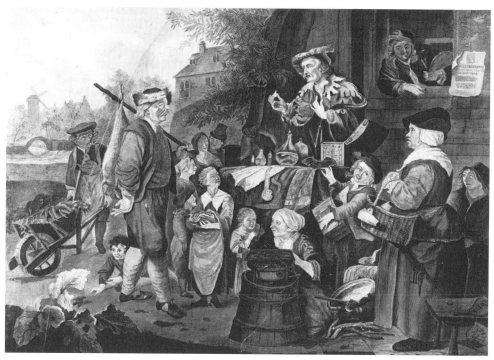

A medicine vendor selling his wares in a village square with the assistance of a monkey. Pen drawing.

of Physicians, perhaps sensing its own impotence and unpopularity, largely abandoned its former crusade against unlicensed practice and retreated into its shell. Its energies were directed more at internal demarcation disputes within the profession – the legacy of its war against the apothecaries – and with maintaining its own elitist ethos, the atmosphere of an exclusive gentlemen's club, against those campaigning to have its fellowship thrown open – especially to graduates of the Scottish universities. The consequence was that many of the leading lights of London medicine, such as the Quaker John Fothergill and the royal obstetrician, William Hunter, were excluded from the College's fellowship, while empirics such as Joshua Ward could flourish beyond the clutches of the College.

Not surprisingly, perhaps, the practice of medicine proceeded with even less regulation in the provinces, where socio-economic transformation was at its most rapid. In the absence of legislation specifying minimum requirements for general practice, no hurdles stood in the way of setting up in medicine, and the notional divide between the regular and the quack might matter little to the public as contrasted to such factors as reputation, personality, and experience. In medicine, as in manufacture, the fastest-growing centres of population – the industrial North and Midlands – generally lacked even the ground plan of guild organization (characteristic of older cities such as Norwich) which would have regulated entry into the profession and the power to practise.

A free market thus in effect became the norm, in which, as Irvine Loudon in particular has documented, even regular practitioners (those who had completed formal apprenticeship or a university education) often found themselves competing for custom

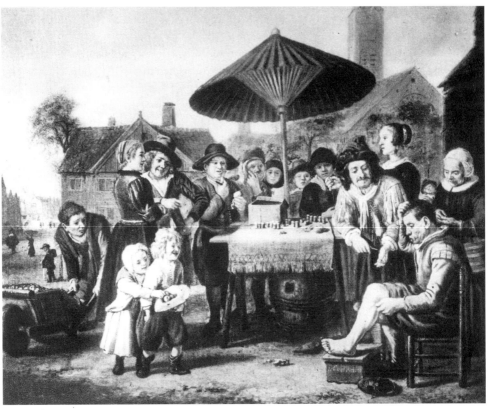

A travelling medicine vendor demonstrating his wares on a puzzled man in front of an audience. In the background, the man's wife is counting out the fee. Process print, 1931, after J. Victors.

with their colleagues. One of the profound anxieties expressed in the Manchester physician Thomas Percival's *Medical Ethics* (1803) was that, pressed by the iron logic of the cash nexus, practitioners themselves would resort to such quackish practices as undercutting, price wars, gimmicks, nostrum-mongering, and client-poaching: overt competition induced quackery. Percival, however, did not see the solution in corporate regulation, say on the French model (which he presumably regarded as obsolete), but in engendering an informal *esprit de corps*.

Such a spirit may have arisen in some areas, perhaps sustained by the camaraderie of a local medical society. Nevertheless, the complaint crescendoed, particularly in the late eighteenth and early nineteenth centuries, from regular doctors that the jungle law governing marketplace medicine inevitably worked to their own disadvantage (and thereby against honest practice) in face of rivalry from cowboys of all kinds – not least, mere chemists and druggists, unscrupulously extending their operations from sale of medicaments to the practice of medicine itself. Mounting dissatisfaction amongst surgeon-apothecaries played a major part in the reformist campaign culminating in the Apothecaries' Act of 1815, which defined the legal qualifications for what we may call general practice. Yet, to the disgust of reformers, the Act (like subsequent ones) signally did not prohibit irregular practice – surely a concession to realism, because, in the *laissez-faire* atmosphere of the early nineteenth century, fresh curbs upon free trade would have been hard to rationalize and impossible to enforce. Regulation had become a dirty word in political circles. As the physician Thomas Hodgkin argued in the 1830s, quackery ought to disappear, but 'it cannot be put down by law'; rather, he continued in pious vein, 'the public may be so enlightened as greatly to diminish [their] appetite' for 'the marvellous... confidently promising... treatment of disease'. The idea of killing quackery through coercion was politically a non-starter in Peelite England.

The same applies to the use of the courts. The law, civil and criminal, proved next to useless for those campaigning against quack practice. Judges deemed that *caveat emptor* should apply no less in medicine than in other fields of contract. Juries resented the occasional attempts of physicians to manipulate the courts to uphold their privileges. When, after one of his patients had died, physicians launched a prosecution against John St John Long, the irregular specializing in consumption 'cures', Long had no difficulty in calling eminent lay witnesses to testify to his skills and integrity, and the judge and jury were disposed to acquit. If anything, the law courts acted in favour of quacks. When the eminent physician John Coakley Lettsom printed certain defamatory remarks against the nostrum-vendor William Brodum, the threat of legal action triggered an out-of-court settlement and a retraction. The public saw more need to be protected against the medical oligarchy than against individual quacks.

Georgian England is often represented as the apogee of privilege, patronage, and jobbery established through Walpole's 'Robinocracy'. Victorians, in particular, liked to think they had destroyed 'old corruption' in medicine no less than in government, thanks to their new-broom reforming liberalism, replacing it with a career open to the talents. But the dichotomy between the two centuries, and the heroic story of progress, are equally phony – indeed, in some ways the mirror-opposite of the truth. In medicine, at least, it is the eighteenth century, not the nineteenth, that presents relatively open practice in which regulation was lax and multiple paths to practice were available. This situation was superseded in the Victorian age by the tightening of professional controls and the rational-bureaucratic goal (which in other contexts would be called a restrictive practice) of a 'single portal' into the profession. The eighteenth century saw few obstacles placed by the state in the way of medical entrepreneurship.

Lay power

Quack medicine may be outlawed, or at least harassed, by legislation, though this, I have argued, did not occur under the Georges. Alternatively, its credibility can be overshadowed by the towering intellectual authority possessed by regular medicine. In certain situations, the orthodox can command assent, thanks to their acknowledged ethical superiority and indisputable scientific stature. If all agree that medical science is necessarily esoteric, lying far beyond the powers of any but experts who have undergone intense professional training, then not only is the empiric discomfited, but – more important – the sick person himself can have no leverage. Arguably, it is this situation that

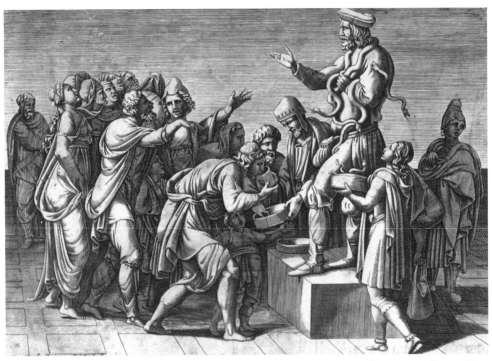

Draped with live snakes, a medicine seller promotes hus wares to an enthusiastic audience. Line engraving after G. Romano.

has emerged during the course of the last century. The medical establishment has visibly grown so mighty, so unified, so scientific, so successful, that the sick have increasingly acquiesced (albeit with much grumbling) in its procedures and authority; patients have become passive. (The very authority of the medical establishment has, of course, sparked counter-currents in favour of alternative medicine.)

But the passive patient, accustomed to place implicit trust in medicine, was a rare bird in pre-modern times. Scrutiny of the letters and diaries of the sick reveals that they exercised acute vigilance in monitoring their own illnesses, actively picking and choosing amongst practitioners, and eager to participate in their own treatment (which often thus included a large element of self-treatment). Such active patient involvement in husbanding health creates a fertile breeding-ground for quackery. The hard-bitten physician would contend this is because the meddlesome, know-all patient is easy game to the exploitative quack. A less cynical formula would suggest that in a medical milieu in which sure-fire cures were few, there was correspondingly greater scope for varied interpersonal rapport between the sick and their doctors: the heterodox operator might have something special to offer. To grasp precisely how the activity of the patient in pre-modern medicine was conducive to quackery, it is necessary to address the wider question of lay medical culture as a whole.

We have already noted one stimulus: the fact that people were so vulnerable to illness, and that no single magic bullet or therapeutic regime could be guaranteed to cure. In this

A busy London street scene, full of people selling their wares. A man is holding a placard advertising Doctor Rock, a famous nostrum-merchant. Engraving

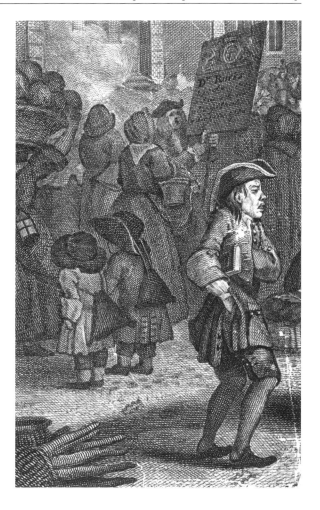

context, the long eighteenth century constitutes a crossroads in health. Sickness continued unabated, yet the long march of 'secularization' (however defined) was conferring a relatively enhanced value upon physical well-being, or at least, survival, in the here-and-now, and setting rather less store by the salvation of the immortal soul. Physical health thus grew more highly prized, though no less elusive. Living life 'in the body' in a world of sickness, people took steps actively to supervise their own health care.

Another reason – or matrix of reasons – has been advanced by the medical sociologist Nicholas Jewson. In the dialogue of power between the patient and the regular medical profession, argues Jewson, it was the layman (he clearly had wealthy patients primarily in mind) who paid the piper and called the tune. Jewson contends that we should analyse Georgian medicine in terms homologous to Namier's now-classic account of Georgian power politics. Namier showed how the political strings of Georgian England were pulled by grandees, whose wealth was translated into political influence through the exercise of bribery, corruption and patronage; to a large degree, career politicians themselves were in aristocratic pockets and had to be duly deferential. Hence, suggests Jewson, the key to Georgian medicine lies, in a parallel way, in grasping how physicians, like politicians, could not help but move in the force-field of lay patronage, influenced by the sway, and tied to the purse-strings of fee-paying patients.

For reward and authority, status and advancement, physicians looked not to the plaudits of the profession – as they would later – but to the favour of the fashionable. *Au fond*, it counted far more to be Pitt the Younger's physician than President of the Royal College of Physicians. Moreover, in matters of clinical knowledge and judgement respecting diagnosis, prognosis, regimen, and therapy, practitioners learned to listen to polite society. Social weakness here played its part. The prudent doctor knew when and how to ingratiate himself to patients' whims.

Remarking that the medical 'profession is overrun with quacks', Beddoes detailed the intellectual and vocational prostitution that followed from doctors being more concerned to make money than make whole. He offered an anecdote:

> One of the princesses being taken ill, and Dr. Gisborne in attendance, her royal highness enquired of the doctor if she might not indulge in the use of a little ice cream, as she thought it would greatly refresh her. D. G. who never contradicted his royal patients, answered that he 'entirely agreed with her royal highness;' and the ice was accordingly provided. His Majesty, visiting the chamber and observing the glass, with some of the ice still remaining in it, seemed alarmed, on the supposition that it might be improper; but her royal highness assured him that she had the doctor's permission for what she had done. His Majesty ordered the doctor into his presence, and observing to him that he had never heard of ice being recommended in such cases before, expressed his apprehension that it was on some new system. The doctor seemed at first a little confounded, but quickly recovering himself, replied, 'Oh no, please your Majesty, it may well be allowed provided it be taken warm' – 'Oh well, well, doctor, very well, very warm ice, warm ice.'[4]

But eighteenth-century practitioners were intellectually as well as socially vulnerable. For understanding disease before the stethoscope, the X-ray, the pathological laboratory, and the exploratory operation depended first and foremost upon the patient's account of his symptoms rather than the clinician's ability to use the techniques of his trade to ascertain for himself. To that degree, the patient's own 'history' commanded a privileged status.

This (pre-professionalized) situation, in which regular doctors were both expected, and obliged, to take their cues from the patient – indeed, to kowtow to patients' whims – was resented by leading physicians. What is striking, however, in the present context, is that they explicitly characterized that implicit deference demanded by the Quality patient of his doctor as a source of quackery. Thomas Beddoes thus deplored the flattery, equivocations, sycophancy, and white lies often resorted to, perforce, by the private practitioner in an exchange in which he acted as a kind of superior flunkey to the wealthy patient. By acquiescing in such intellectual prostitution, the practitioner reduced himself to a quasi-quack. Thus the implication of Jewson's analysis is that, with the protocols of lay patronage defining relations between purchasers and performers, *all* medical

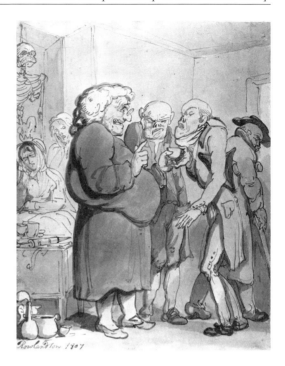

Patients consulting an obese quack.
Watercolour painting by T. Rowlandson,
1807.

interchanges – including those with regulars – would smack of quackery. Such a situation could not fade until professionalization gained power.

Furthermore, Jewson has argued that the patient's purse power, coupled with an enduring ignorance of internal physiological processes, combined to encourage a proliferation of speculative medical systems: the sick expected to be told what was wrong in explanatory formulations that made sense. Humoral medicine retained its hold, alongside the newer chemical and mechanical models. Some medical theories privileged the heart, some the blood, others the nerves. Thus regular medicine itself, aided by ignorance and pressurized by patients shopping around between rival philosophies, produced a cacophony of explanatory systems – each equally vacuous, argued Bernard Mandeville in his *Treatise on the Hypochondriack and Hysterick Diseases* (1730).

Above all, this was a situation suggestively prefigurative of the theoretical superabundance of nineteenth-century *alternative* medicine. The thrust of Jewson's argument is thus that patient power was able during the long eighteenth century to impose upon *regular* medicine those terms of existence we nowadays view as typical of *quackery*.

Thus, in clinical interactions where the patient's voice carries some clout, distinctions between so-called quacks and regulars need to be viewed in a different light, or, more specifically, assume a reduced significance – at least, to the patient! Educated Georgians believed it was their positive duty to know enough about medicine to evaluate and collaborate with their physicians. As we shall see below, there were many organs through which such medical knowledge circulated to the laity. The vast expansion of the press proved a particularly good medium for public information and discussion.

Georgian public opinion was, of course, like everyone else, against quackery, but it did not always see eye-to-eye with the College as to who the quacks were. The medical coverage offered by that quintessential repository of educated lay opinion, the *Gentleman's Magazine*, founded in 1731, is here revealing. The *Magazine*'s contributors and correspondents deplored charlatanism, but they were not automatically hostile to the practitioners usually identified as the prime quacks of the age, such as Joanna Stephens, Sally Mapp, Joshua Ward, or John ('Chevalier') Taylor. Sally Mapp, the bone-setter, had a good press. One set of verses exploits her success to ridicule the regulars:

> YOU Surgeons of London, who puzzle your Pates,
> To ride in your Coaches, and purchase Estates,
> Give over, for Shame, for your Pride has a Fall,
> And Doctress of Epsom has out-done you all.

Lay opinion, as crystallized in the *Gentleman's Magazine* and similar periodicals, did not view medical practice in terms of any 'great divide' between practitioners proper and improper, official and marginal, legal and twilight, elite and vulgar. As Jewson's model would predict, it assessed practitioners individually, on their own merits. The *Magazine* showed no animus against irregular practice *per se*. The target of anti-quack feeling was rather faddery (seen as vain, absurd affectation), and, perhaps above all, secret practice. Private interest promoted the general good. Public opinion as expressed in the *Magazine* condemned the puffing of proprietary medicines by those who refused to divulge their composition to the public. Such naked self-serving, sanctimoniously masquerading under the cloak of humanity, raised hackles, as is shown in a review of *Medical Advice to the Consumptive and Asthmatick People of England; wherein the present method of treating disorders of the lungs is shewn to be futile and fundamentally wrong, and a new and easy method of cure, a short book by Philip Stern, MD*. The review alleges of Stern's performance that:

> The purpose of this advice is to recommend a nostrum invented by the author… He conceals his medicine, he says, for no other reason than because if he was to discover it so as that it might be prepared by every apothecary, it would be neglected…. However, it is much to be regretted, that medicines thus offered to the publick are not by appointment of the legislature examined by persons properly qualified to ascertain their inefficacy or utility. That on one hand, a useful discovery might not be disregarded as the imposition of a quack; and on the other, that the weak and credulous might not be defrauded of their money for some thing that is useless, if not hurtful to their health.[5]

The real point here, as so often, is that the party guilty of quackery signed himself as an 'MD'. In other words the lay public would here have perceived the real divide as being not between regulars and empirics *per se* but between practitioners opening their knowledge to the public and those concealing it for private gain, whoever they might be. One of the most constructive projects launched in the *Gentleman's Magazine* was significantly a tabulation of some two hundred nostrums, noting their applications, their London sales-points, and their cost. What the lay public valued was access to information about all available medicines. Many orthodox practitioners, by contrast, viewed lay medical involvement as a health threat, because a little learning was a dangerous thing.

Quackery thus found eager ears in a culture in which lay people expected to exercise some sway over their physicians, much as they would hire a hairdresser or fire a cook. And the sick could plausibly exert such control, confident that no unbridgeable knowledge gap divided the attentive layman from the practising medico. People from all walks of life and strata of society were deeply involved in medical self-care. The kitchen garden and the hedgerow provided raw materials for hundreds of herbal remedies; grocers' shops and general stores sold the ingredients for others – notably Eastern spices, such as cumin, nutmeg, and cinnamon, which were becoming more widely and cheaply available. Wet-nurses, maids, stable-hands, cooks, and so forth all fancied their skills at mixing special preparations, applying a poultice, 'breathing a vein' (that is, letting blood) or drawing teeth. Adages about health and sickness and data about regimes and remedies circulated throughout society, passed round and handed down by word of mouth. They also appeared in family recipe collections, in magazines and newspapers and in self-care books and pamphlets.

The self-dosing habit – stemming from choice no less than economy – was crucial to the viability of quackery. It meant that resort to the regular practitioner did not become an automatic reflex, universally the done thing. It could heighten the attractions of applying to the quack doctor or of using proprietary medicines. For people accustomed to sturdy self-medicating might sometimes feel uncomfortable with the ministrations of their regular general practitioner – a man who would, perhaps, apply moral pressure upon the patient to abandon his own pet therapies and obey doctors' orders. By contrast, the sick could readily buy the preparations of quacks with anonymity and impunity, incorporating their use, however they chose, into their self-dosing regimes. Thus deployed, popular medical self-help and irregular medicine were far from being mutually exclusive, rather feeding off each other. Thus one of the more important early self-instruction manuals, *Every Man His Own Doctor* (1672), was issued by a practitioner, John Archer, who also published a quack bill not only puffing his own volume, but giving notice of his availability at his chambers in the Haymarket, London, both to see patients and to sell a slate of nostrums, viz:

> elixir proprietatis
> tincture of saffron
> elixir guaici
> aqua cordialis
> tobacco
> sternutatory or sneeze powder
> pills and drops
> cordial diet drink
> morbus pill
> corroborating pill
> astringent or stichback pill
> cordial pill
> purging bolus[6]

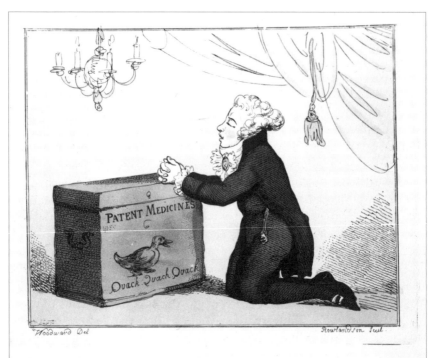

THE QUACK DOCTOR'S PRAYER!!

ILLUSTRIOUS fhade of the renowned *Doctor Rock*, ftill continue, I befeech thee, to pour down thy Influence on the Endeavours of thy modern Reprefentative, *Doctor Botherem*; thou knoweft the regular Gradations of the Profeffion, from a Show Box at a Country Fair, to the luxury of a Chariot rattling down Pall-Mall; it would, therefore, be vain and idle to attempt Difguife before thy penetrating Wifdom.

I'm the Eyes of the Undifcerning, my miraculous *cure-all-able* Vegetable Drops, called *Never-failibus Infallialibus*, appear the Wonder of the prefent Age, the Ingredients are fuppofed to Iffue from the Laboratory of ESCULAPIUS himfelf beyond the Power of Mortal Analization; but thou well knoweft how the World is deceived; to thee it appears nothing more than a Decoction of Beet-root, Lump-Sugar, Spring-Water, the beft Coniac Brandy, and a Dafh of Hollands Gin.— Thou, alfo, knoweft its great Reputation was firft aquired by curing *Lady Dun-Dizzle* of Indigeftion, by throwing her into a temporary State of foothing Intoxication, fince which Time the old Lady reforts as regularly to her Drops, as her Dram Bottle.

To deceive thee is impoffible, thou knoweft we are not infallible, but are all liable to little Accidents in the Exercife of our Calling, that are not altogether fo pleafing on Reflection; but what grieves me moft, is the Recollection of the fudden Demife of *Alderman Marrowfat*, even on the firft Experiment of my *Anti-Gorgean Pills*, and at the very Inftant he was about to recommend their wonderful Effects to the Mayor, and the whole Body Corporate.

Yet notwithftanding the Sweets of the Profeffion amply compenfates for the Bitters, therefore deign to continue to me my Carriages and Equipage, my Town and Country Refidence, and all other good Things of this Life, and thy humble Petitioner fhall ever praife thee.

PRINTED BY E. SPRAGG, NO. 27, BOW-STREET, COVENT-GARDEN.

'The Quack Doctor's Prayer'. A practitioner invokes the name of Doctor Rock, while kneeling beside his medicines. Coloured etching by T. Rowlandson, 1801, after G. Woodward.

Critics were in no doubts that lay auto-medication was the fifth column of quackery (it is no accident that the verb for self-dosing was to 'quack' oneself: Horace Walpole spoke of his father, Sir Robert, having 'quacked his life away'). Puffed up with a few ideas derived from 'dispensatories and practical compilations' and from their peers, fashionable amateurs were in danger – they plied such powers of patronage – of subverting independent medical judgement and of poisoning their servants and retainers withal.

Worst of all, physic itself was being reduced from a sober science to that ultimate quackery, fashion. It was an age of fashion, claimed Dr Adair, not just in designs and decor but in disease. Time was when the malady à la mode was the vapours. Then the newfangled idea of nervous disease caught on, though nowadays, Dr Adair contended, towards the close of the eighteenth century, nerves were decidedly *démodé* and biliousness was all the rage. Adair found those lay know-alls who usurped the physician's prerogative of diagnosis quite insufferable: 'instead of my patients giving me a detail of their symptoms, by which I might judge of the nature of the disease, the answer generally was, "Doctor, I am bilious;" and, on enquiry, I found that they had generally been in the habit of taking medicines to carry off the supposed offensive bile.'[7]

Yet if (as many doctors claimed) lay self-dosing opened the floodgates to quackery, what was this but the profession's own chickens coming home to roost? For the medical profession itself was filling the bookshops with writings, from penny pamphlets to weighty tomes, aimed at a health-conscious lay readership. Dozens of books hit the market claiming to be *The Family Physician* (1807), or *The Poor Man's Medicine Chest* (1791), offering *Physick for Families* (1674), or *Domestic Medicine* (1769), many of them going through multiple editions. Mirroring such books, popular journals, from John Dunton's *Athenian Mercury* onwards, acted as exchanges of medical information between laymen and laymen and from doctors to laymen. Many were penned by orthodox doctors. Most influential of all was William Buchan's *Domestic Medicine*, which first appeared in 1769 and continued in print for almost a century (every Scottish cottage, it was claimed, had its copy of Buchan and the Bible). This genre notionally professed to teach every man to guard his own health. Yet did not their authors also expect that readers would, once thereby better informed, henceforth also draw more heavily upon the services, and products, of practitioners? To that extent, no matter who the author was, the genre collectively served in effect as a 'quack's bill'.

Indeed, such self-care works commonly recommended materia medica and nostrums by name. John Theobald's *Every Man his own Physician* (1766) praised Richard Mead's preparation against rabies, Joanna Stephens's powders against the stone, and Sir Hans Sloane's ointment; Hugh *Smithson's Complete Family Physician* (1781) advised Daffy's Elixir for stomach complaints and Anderson's Pills as a 'rough but safe' purge. The dangers of such collusion between commercial doctors and enthusiastic auto-medicators were pointed out in Southey's mordant observation that such books ought to be entitled 'Every Man his Own Poisoner'.

Not least, home physic publications extolled the benefits of keeping ready stocked medicine chests. Today's bathroom cabinet, with its pain-killers, cough mixtures, and antiseptics, hardly bears comparison to the medicine chests – one for gentlemen, one for ladies, one for horses – containing well over a hundred different preparations which

Richard Reece was advertising in his *Domestic Medical Guide* at the beginning of the nineteenth century. Reece's chests included laudanum, calomel, antimony, guiacum and extract of lead: the most potent drugs available. William Buchan, for his part – despite his dread of excess drugging – recommended that every well-equipped home should have supplies of:

> Adhesive Plaster, Agaric of Oak, Ash coloured Ground liverwort, Burgundy pitch, Cinnamon water, Crabs claw prepared, Cream of Tartar, Elixir of vitriol, Flowers of sulphur, Gentian root, Glauber's salts, Gum ammoniac, Gum arabic, Gum asafoetida, Gum Camphor, Ipecacuanha, Jalap, Jesuit's Bark, Liquid laudanum, Liquorice root, Magnesia alba, Manna, Nitre or Salt peter, Oil of almonds, Olive oil, Pennyroyal water, Peppermint water, Rhubarb, Sal ammoniac, Sal prunell, Seneka root, Senna, Snake root, Spirits of hartshorn, Spirits of wine, Sweet spirits of nitrate, Sweet spirits of vitriol, Syrup of lemons, Syrup of oranges, Syrup of poppies, Tamarind, Turner's cerate, Vinegar of squills, Wax plaster, White ointment, Wild Valerian root, and Yellow basilicum ointment.

The Enlightenment's dream of perfecting health and prolonging life thus turned into a dilemma. Progressive doctors such as Buchan argued that the greater the popular diffusion of medical know-how, the more successfully the quack peril would be overcome, since charlatanism fed off ignorance. Whether practitioners liked it or not, sick people would inevitably medicate themselves: the urge – or the necessity – was ineradicable. Kept ignorant, Buchan warned, they would do this badly, falling victim to foolish wise women, quacks, and nostrum-mongers. For 'while men are kept in the dark, and told that they are not to use their own understanding, in matters that concern their health, they will be the dupes of designing knaves'. By contrast, enlightened citizens, receiving responsible medical advice, would treasure their health effectively, and so puncture the specious promises of the quacks.

Here lay a rousing, populist, Enlightenment ideology: the diffusion of knowledge would deal death-blows to quackery no less than to magic, witchcraft, and popery. The argument was often adduced. Back in 1653, John Finch had informed his sister, Anne, that in Italy 'Mountebankes are more numerous and rich' than anywhere else in Europe, precisely 'because the common country people are the most ignorant under heaven'.[8] Such a view perfectly pandered to Protestant prejudices about progress.

Arguably, however, it constituted the reverse of the truth. Was it not primarily the medically alerted laity, rendered anxious about hazards to their health and their duties of health care, who resorted most eagerly to the commercial quacks? Nostrum-mongers were openly angling for the self-care addicts. Thus John Badger vended his 'OLBION or The Cordial Antidote' as: 'a Noble and Generous Medicine, confirmed by the Experience of above Twenty Years private practice, and now publish'd at the Request of several Persons for a general Good, that every one may be his own Physician at an Easie and Cheap Rate.' The preparation (which, Badger claimed, 'comforts and strengthens the viscera, Liver and Spleen, and opens all Obstructions thereof) was, ostensibly at least,

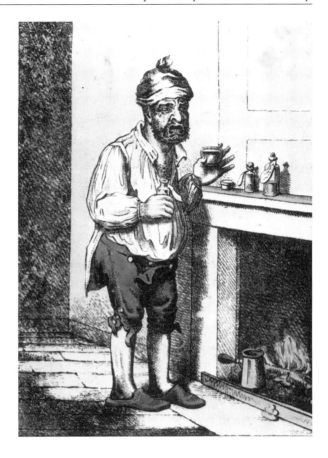

A man stands by a fireplace and pulls a peculiar face after taking some medicine. Coloured etching by J. Gillray, 1800.

pitched at a rather superior public, since his bill flourished several untranslated quotations from Hippocrates.

The Georgian public thus clung to its right to medicate itself, not least through buying manuals and stocking up with proprietary potions. Behaviour of this kind was not unique to health care, but was integral, as Lorna Weatherill has recently documented, to wider patterns of consumer behaviour within the market economy, and hence needs to be understood in its broader context. The extension of domestic commodity exchange was a fundamentally crucial growth sector in the English economy during the century and a half after the Restoration, the period Maxine Berg has termed the 'age of manufactures'. The growing availability and acquisition of everyday goods defined the cultural ambience of the emergent 'consumer society'. Following Holland's 'golden century', English society became characterized by a growing availability of, and involvement in, material objects, the property not just of a rich elite but of a wide midriff of the social spectrum. Affluence, social emulation, and ownership went together.

Some of the belongings forming backdrops to the lives of Georgian families were objects unknown within more traditional domestic economies: newspapers, iron bedsteads, tablecloths, china cups or cheap Hogarth prints, for instance. In addition, those with surplus cash now found it more convenient, or prestigious, to purchase ready-made certain items traditionally made up in the kitchen, still-room, stables, or backyard: beer, candles, soap, starch, dyes, paints, ink, ironmongery, and so forth. Moreover, the affluent increasingly drew upon professionals to perform expert services previously carried out by household members: tutors, music teachers, hairdressers, milliners, rat-catchers, house-painters, face-painters and the like – all newly found entrée into multitudes of Georgian homes. Affluence, convenience, and prestige played their parts in spreading the pleasures of participating in a consumer culture – previously reserved for gentry conspicuous consumption – to the average bourgeois household.

Increasing resort to buying medicines and related items such as cosmetics in commodity form must be understood as part of this surge in material goods. Recourse to paid professional tooth-drawers, accoucheurs, oculists and so forth likewise reflects the parallel move to purchasing services from outsiders. Obviously, both these trends were good news for quacks. The eighteenth century, as often observed, was the golden age of the apothecary, because he was particularly well placed to cash in upon the 'pudding time' in dispensing medicines – in his twin role as emergent general practitioner, he was also prescribing them. But nostrum-mongers had opportunities to do better still, because they, unlike mere apothecaries, were adept at pitching for the mass-market, using novel commercial devices to be explored later in this chapter.

As burgeoning bourgeois culture set more store by the ownership of things, a fetishism of goods developed the tendency to endow material objects with extraordinary powers. Among other things, this meant that medicaments assumed greater status in the healing process. Orthodox humanistic medicine had traditionally privileged healing through regimen, diet and pursuit of the non-naturals: drugs were subsidiary. During the long eighteenth century, focus arguably switched from these lengthy and elaborate processes of medical management to the investment of greater faith in the power of the pill – healing power thus becoming crystallized, through some imaginative alchemy, into tangible commodities. Regular medicine itself leant more heavily upon drugs (patients apparently expected them to be prescribed, and surgeon-apothecaries derived their profit from them). And empirics cashed in all the more, appealing to the conceit that in a paper of powders or a jar of ointment there lay some sort of quasi-magical virtue – 'charm' was Buchan's derisory term.

Enshrined therein was a further myth of commercial capitalism, purchaser power, expressed in the idea that relief and health were things that money could buy – and also in the more down-to-earth concept of value for money. Quack medicines thus very commonly sold at precisely a penny a pill, in packs of twelve or twenty-four. The sick were more prepared to fork out for medicines than for advice. For drugs possessed a reassuring tangibility – solid and substantial, they could be swallowed, applied, or rubbed in. They also suggested speed and convenience – it was less trouble to gulp a pill than to follow an exacting regimen or diet over many months. Not least, when taking shop-bought nostrums, the patient was the master.

But this reification of healing into commodity form also, in the event, conveyed quite perturbing implications in Georgian England. For its implicit message that health was a need that could be satisfied by consumption of medicines became intertwined with that quintessentially bourgeois anxiety: hypochondria.

The eighteenth century grew preoccupied with *malades imaginaires*. Up to the late seventeenth century, hypochondriasis had been classed as an organic disorder of the lower abdomen. By the nineteenth century, by contrast, it had migrated to become the mental state – indeed, the psychiatric condition – of morbid anxiety about health. This transformation had many precipitants, amongst them the pursuit of sensibility, the vogue of fashionable disorders and the emergence of 'psychiatry' itself. But it also had much to do with Georgian medical self-help. In a milieu in which individual self-care remained a prime duty, sufferers were exposed as never before to medical cautions, and the sick had unprecedented access to an arsenal of potent drugs. Pain and sickness were on people's minds, and hopes raised that treatments were available to overcome them.

Physicians, of course, dismissed hypochondriacs – those, mocked Adair, 'who are sick by way of amusement and melancholy to keep up their spirits' But the hypochondriac, though the bane of the doctors, was equally the victim of (over-)attention from the collective voice of the medicos. Worse still, hypochondria was a malaise in a destructively compulsive vortex with doctors for, as Dr Robert James observed, the patient, while ostensibly seeking a cure, insensibly wanted his clinical relationship to be interminable. 'No disease is more troublesome, either to the Patient or Physician, than hypochondriac Disorders', he explained: 'and it often happens, that, thro' the Fault of both, the Cure is either unnecessarily protracted, or totally frustrated; for the Patients are so delighted, not only with a Variety of Medicines, but also of Physicians.'

Hypochondria is thus a symptom of a fearsome syndrome which contains a clue to quackery. On the one hand, bourgeois man, pursuing 'possessive individualism' within the acquisitive society, thought of himself as the ultimate proprietor of his body, which political economy deemed the source of labour and thereby value (unlike the aristocrat, bourgeois man could not rely upon the mystique of 'blood' and stock). The efficient running of the animal machine therefore assumed critical importance, requiring attentive psychosomatic maintenance. Georgian consciousness was thus encouraged to look inwards, introspecting upon the painful perturbations of the self.

Yet the culture required that the anxious self expressed itself, by conversion, in the idiom of physical malaise, and this, in turn, was to be assuaged not (as was traditional) through religion or philosophy but therapeutically, via the consolations of medicine. The market promised ever more alluring medicines to soothe away the hypochondriac's pains. But, as was widely recognized, morbid introspection was bound to be worsened through indulgence in medicines. Swallowing further drugs merely concentrated attention upon bodily states, while the nostrums to which hypochondriacs commonly resorted – above all, nerve tonics and specifics against venereal disease – proved ineffectual, or further undermined health.

Not least, many such medicines – analysed more fully in chapter 5 – were habit-forming, containing opiates and alcohol. Contemporaries recognized that hypochondria and addiction were kin. Critics berated the emergent consumer society for its degenerate reliance upon an unprecedented range of stimulants – tea, coffee, tobacco, spirits, alcohol, and medical and recreational drugs. Medical moralists dissecting the 'English malady', from George Cheyne early in the Georgian era to Thomas Trotter at its close, depicted the descending spiral whereby items initially consumed for the pleasures of the palate or the relief of pain, in time created cravings for themselves, which further consumption could never gratify, or at least not without appalling side-

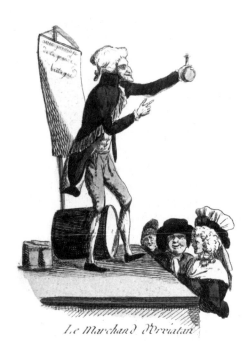

A nostrum-vendor performs his pitch on stage before a small audience. Coloured etching.

Le Marchand d'Orvietan

effects and withdrawal symptoms. Georgian England was becoming a medicated society, drunk on self-drugging.

Hypochondria, quackery, and addiction thus formed a vicious circle. Frankenstein-like, the consumer society was giving birth to a new personality type: man the consumer, pained by deprivation and craving commodities. He thus grew addicted to 'consumption'; it was his disease. Sickness, and the response to it through medicines in commodity form, were integral to this process. Quackery was the capitalist mode of production in its medical face.

The marketplace

The ubiquity of sickness and the tenacity of a lay, self-help consumer culture combined to create a demand for commercial medicine which, in England, unlike most Continental nations, the state and the medical colleges could not, or would not, arrest. What emerged in England was an unusually spectacular blossoming of commercial medicine, thanks to the particularly propitious conflux of economic opportunities.

Medical practitioners of all types capitalized on the economic buoyancy of the home market in England during the long eighteenth century. As Holmes, Loudon and others have shown, the emergent common-or-garden general practitioner notably improved his practice, income, and status, and an elite of London physicians and surgeons grew rich beyond the dreams of their forebears. Regulars were not embarrassed to crave profit and preferment, nor did they conceal their success behind the decent fig-leaf of professional respectability donned by their Victorian successors. In 1695, John Radcliffe thus wrote to Mr Colbatch, Surgeon General to the Army, congratulating him upon his 'new

Acquisition of Fame, by the help of your renowned Styptick'.

Practitioners profited in various ways from economic improvements. Improved roads – this was the age of the turnpike – facilitated paying calls in rural areas. Advanced carriage design and coach-building took the bumps out of life for affluent physicians such as Erasmus Darwin. Better postal and carriage networks, credit supply (due to country banks) and other infrastructural advances made it easier for provincial practitioners to obtain regular supplies of medicaments from London wholesalers and to practice postal diagnosis.

The standard private practice of the regular doctor depended upon building up and maintaining a core of faithful patients. Their satisfaction would broadcast his fame, but his visibility could be enhanced in other ways too, such as by obtaining an honorary position at a hospital, or, perhaps, through publishing. His income would accrue from consultation fees (if he were a physician) or billing for drugs (in the case of an apothecary).

But certain practitioners – regularly trained or not – took extra advantage of the special opportunities afforded by the marketplace to sell their names and wares more widely, some of them acting as what Oliver Goldsmith called 'advertising physicians', and marketing nostrums.

Advertising held the key. It would be simplistic to imply that quacks advertised and regulars set their face against it. All practitioners advertised; some simply did it more nakedly, more aggressively, more forthrightly, than others. The scrupulous doctor, suggested the Quaker practitioner Thomas Hodgkin, should nail a small brass plaque to his door; if too large, it would reek of quackery. The distinction between the quack and the regular, in this matter as in so many others, was thus a code of convention. Quack doctors took eager advantage of the new prospects for reaching a mass audience through advertising.

The traditional quack drummed up custom by face-to-face contact, as a mountebank (literally one who stood upon a bench) or a charlatan (the Italian *ciarlare* means to chatter). It was a limited, though effective, way of spreading the gospel. The Restoration epoch then proved the halcyon age of the handbill and the wall-poster. 'It is incredible, and scarce to be imagin'd', Defoe looked back at 1655 in his *Journal of the Plague Year*,

> how the Posts of Houses, and Comers of Streets were plaster'd over with Doctors Bills, and Papers of ignorant Fellows; quacking and tampering in Physick, and inviting the People to come to them for Remedies; which was generally set off, with such flourishes as these, (viz.) INFALLIBLE preventive Pills against the Plague. NEVER FAILING Preservatives against Infection. SOVERAIGN Cordials against the Corruption of the Air. EXACT Regulation for the Conduct of the Body, in Case of an Infection: Antipestilential Pills.INCOMPARABLE Drink against the Plague, never found out before. An UNIVERSAL Remedy for the Plague. The ONLY-TRUE Plague-Water. The ROYAL-ANTIDOTE against Kinds of Infection; and such a Number more that I cannot reckon.

Such bills directed customers to the services or stocks of the practitioner, whose address they gave. Their effectiveness was local and limited. Bills stuffed into the hands of passers-by might meet only one pair of eyes.

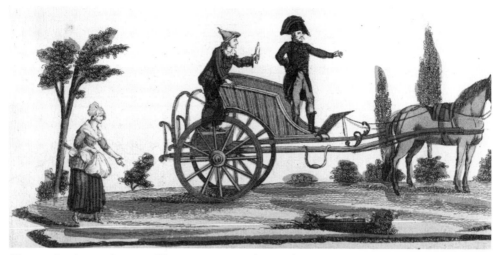

*Two performing medicine peddlers in costume rehearse their speeches on a horse-drawn carriage.
Coloured etching*

It was the eighteenth century that revolutionized marketing, by vastly extending the
means of both communicating information to the public (publicity) and of supplying
goods to them (distribution). The growing sophistication of advertising and promotion
stunts made brand-name goods – a concept virtually unknown before – familiar to the
public. Impressive improvements in communications, in wholesale chains and retail
outlets, created national markets for manufactured products for the first time. From small
fry such as the strop-maker George Packwood, right up to whales such as Josiah
Wedgwood, whose ambition was to be 'vase-maker to the universe', manfacturers seized
the new openings for their wares.

The advent of the standardized, brand-name commodity forms the great growth area of
non-regular medicine in the Georgian era. Scores of brand-name medicaments emerged
– Dr James's Powders, Anderson's Scots Pills, Hooper's Female Pills, Dr Radcliffe's
Famous Purging Elixir, Turlington's Pills, Bateman's Pectoral Drops, Daffy's Elixir,
Stoughton's Great Cordial Elixir (advertised as approved by about twenty Eminent
Physicians of the College), Godfrey's Cordial, Friar's Balsam, Ward's Pill and Drop,
Velno's Vegetable Syrup, to name just a few – whose sales rocketed to astronomical levels.
In twenty years, some 1,612,800 doses of James's Powders were sold.[9]

To attain such sales, nationwide advertising had to be pioneered. To some degree,
quacks attempted this by printing bills that could be simply adapted (by filling in blanks
in longhand) for use in any market or city. But medicine proprietors made superb use of
the new medium of the newspaper to promote their wares and signpost retail outlets.
Newspapers were particularly significant as mouthpieces for proprietary medicines
because their owners and agents doubled as the principal distributors for the medicines.
Bookshops and circulating libraries also served as medicine stockists. In 1784, the *Coventry
Mercury* begged to inform readers that an entire alphabet of nostrums – over a hundred in
all – could be purchased at the local bookstore, coming to a climax with:

Radcliffe's Purging Elixir
Ruston's Pills for the Rheumatism
Royon's Ointment for the Itch
Spilsbury's Drops
Stoughton's Elixir
Swinfen's Electuary for the Stone and Gravel
Spirits of Scurvy Grass
Sans Pareille Powder
Storey's Worm Cakes
Smyth's Scouring Drops
Steel Preservative
Specific Purging Remedy for Venereal Diseases, by Wessels
Tasteless Ague and Fever Drops
Turlington's Balsam
Tincture of Centaury
Tincture of Valerian
Vandour's Pills, for Nervous Complaints
Velno's Vegetable Syrup
West's Elixir

...and, last but certainly not least, for they were among the most popular, Ward's White Drops.

The Georgian medicine consumer was thus brought face-to-face, especially when poring over his newspaper, with no less a range of shop-counter medicines than is available nowadays, many of them, in those unregulated times before the Food and Drugs Acts and the advent of prescription-only medicines, extremely potent brews. In the history of the mass promotion and distribution of manufactures in the early Industrial Revolution, an innovatory role was played by proprietary medicine vendors. Quack medicines were among the very first standardized, nationally marketed, brand-name products.

Various other publicizing gimmicks were exploited by the inventive eighteenth-century business projector. Not least was the puff, or concealed advertisement, the most notorious instance of which is embedded right at the beginning of that favourite children's story *Goody Two-Shoes*, possibly written by Dr Oliver Goldsmith, and distributed by the proprietor of newspapers and nostrum-owner John Newbery:

CHAP.1.

How and about Little Margery and
her Brother.

CARE and Discontent shortened the Days of Little Margery's Father.
– He was forced from his Family, and seized with a violent Fever in a Place where Dr. James's Powder was not to be had, and where he died miserably

As these publicity initiatives suggest, nostrum-vendors took full advantage of the commercial opportunities afforded by a buoyant market. They were not (despite persistent stereotypes) appealing primarily to the *hoi polloi*, who could afford nothing better. The calculus of eighteenth-century commercialism did not aim for the mass market, catering to the lowest common denominator: that would hardly have been economically feasible or profitable. Rather, nostrum-mongers pitched at those sufficiently literate, urban, in-touch and affluent to be reading newspapers or visiting bookshops and circulating libraries.

Indeed, as the Georgian century wore on, many operators addressed themselves more assiduously to richer market openings, moving up-market in their cultural appeal and capitalizing upon those powerful forces of emulation, snobbery and fashion that leading entrepreneurs in other sectors, such as Wedgwood, manipulated so adroitly. As chapter 4 will show, this attempt to win custom amongst the genteel, or at least the aspirant, is evident in the tags, catchphrases, body-copy and by-lines associated with nostrums. Empirics selected their brand names to chime with the fashionable, elitist, progressive aspirations of Enlightenment high society, evoking the reputations of top scientists, the cosmopolitanism of exotic wisdom, the philanthropic associations of ecumenical religion, the benevolence of the Great ('Cordials Angelical, Royal, Golden, Imperial', as one critic complained).[10] Above all, quack medicines were commonly named (legitimately or not) after famous orthodox physicians, such as Mead, Sloane, or Fothergill.

Many nineteenth-century irregular medical movements, as chapter 8 will discuss, boldly declared their outright opposition to commercialism, fashion and the corruption of orthodox medicine, advocating instead a 'return to Nature'. In total contrast, however, the eighteenth-century empiric basked in the glories of the mode, and in the culture and even the medicine of the age. Quackery did not set itself up as the great god, 'Alternative', replete with a radical medical ontology and distinctive therapies. Rather, marketplace medicine pirated, plagiarized, and popularized the practices of the establishment, seeking to render them more accessible, cheaper, and more palatable to the buyers (and more profitable to the projectors!), by economies of scale and the perfection of salesmanship. Eighteenth-century quackery colluded rather than collided with regular medicine.

This absorption of quack medicine within the mores of the market is of great cultural significance. Craving the attention of opinion-making fashion-setters and media controllers, quacks were ultimately doomed to sycophancy, even more than most tradesmen. For this reason quack medicine – offensive, bizarre, and distasteful though many found it – could be socially contained because it was a safe project, confining itself within the conventions of a market society thriving on events, exhibitions, and exhibitionism. Enthusiastic religion and radical politics spelt danger in post-Restoration England because they presented alternative, critical metaphysics that rocked the boat of oligarchic consensus. Not so with quack medicine. The 'Enthusiast in Physick' was not a schismatic or a revolutionary but an entertainer; radical, if radical at all, only as radical chic. Precisely because it thus posed no real social threat, at least till the mid-nineteenth century, quackery remained highly socially acceptable.

Indeed, quackery elevated itself to provide decent entertainment for the leisured, polite society of the Enlightenment. Sixteenth- and seventeenth-century quackery had a strong plebeian tang, often using vulgarisms for disorders and diseases. Take, for example, the Bill of the 'Infallible Mountbanke' (1685), which listed complaints such as

> The Cramp, the Stitch
> The Squirt, the Itch
> The Gout, the Stone, the Pox
> The Mulligrubs
> The Bonny Scrubs
> And all Pandora's Box.

or a bill headed *The Woman's Prophecy or the Rare and Wonderful Doctrines* (1677), which offered to cure 'the Glimmering of the Gizzard, the Quavering of the Kidneys, and the Wambling Trot'. Such patter obviously goes with the traditional mountebank's ambience of street-corner buffoonery, clowning, and Jack Puddings. But in the politer ambience of the eighteenth century all this was being supplanted by refinement and decorum in presentation. Take, for example, the elevated tone used by James Graham, the pioneer sexologist of the 1780s, in the 'Lecture on Generation' which he delivered to polite society. Touching upon the role of sperm in conception:

> Nor is it a little whimsical, or even ridiculous, to suppose [he told his auditors] that all those animalcula, are *homunculi*, little men and little ladies striking and playing about in the male seed, each of them endeavouring to get first into the ovarium, and from thence into the womb, so that in time they may become fine ladies and gentlemen, princes, prime ministers, lawyers, heroes, proud, lazy, luxurious parsons, duellers, and other modern men of honour, idiot magistrates, theatrical buffoons, desperate gamblers, rascally tumblers, divine and moral philosophers, and even (if you allow me to descend so very low) electrical quack-doctors.

The act, as can be seen, is elevated, allusive, idealized. Following the strategy of *ars celare artem*, it is a salesmanship that hides its own salesmanship. Quacks had traditionally sold pills; but Graham was selling dreams, even wet dreams. And such etherealization of quackery in the Enlightenment was not unique to Graham, but was paralleled by performers such as Cagliostro and Katterfelto, and by the sublime style of John ('Chevalier') Taylor's 'Ciceronian' lectures on the eye. Indeed, Taylor characteristically announced on the title-page of his autobiography (forsooth! which seventeenth-century empiric wrote a three-decker autobiography?) that it contained a 'Dissertation on the Art of Pleasing'. Georgian quackery was thus gentrifying its pitch, rather as Grub Street hacks were increasingly putting on airs and graces as critics, and one-time barnstorming strolling players were becoming performing theatrical stars. Surplus wealth, market mobilization, the newly ubiquitous voice of the media, the tyranny of fashion, improvements in communications, the commercialization of leisure – all these made England during the long eighteenth century a time of golden opportunity for performers willing to chance their arm at manipulating the media. The Georgian age turned quackery into style, thus emphasizing the affinity between the healing and the performing arts, both presided over by Apollo.

Of course, these arguments must not be overstated. Precisely because quack advertising was trading in fantasy, one must not take its own claims literally; we must not let it gull us. Indeed, we might be tempted to demur, and suggest that though the tone was elevated, in reality the quack vendors were small-time higglers and their buyers mainly confined to the masses. Yet there seems much counter-evidence to adduce against these propositions. For one thing, many of the leading quacks of the Georgian age undoubtedly became rich and famous. If we associate Victorian fringe medicine with provincial, dissenting worthies, the cream of the eighteenth-century empirics are a very different kettle of fish. Through therapeutic success, business acumen and drive, many Georgian medicine-mongers made their pile – the uroscopist Myersbach allegedly gained 'a fortune equal to that of a German prince' and succeeded in hobnobbing in high society. Nathaniel Godbold, promoter of a successful Vegetable Balsam, mainly intended as a venereal disease treatment, started life as a baker, but eventually cleared £10,000 a year from the sale of his medicine, investing in a country house near Godalming for £30,000. Isaac Swainson, who acquired Velno's Vegetable Syrup, designed to counter consumption, was originally a woollen-draper, but he won respect as a scholar and bought a fine house with grounds at Twickenham, where he laid out a scientific botanical garden. Swainson claimed to sell 20,000 bottles of the mixture a year (two-thirds, he alleged, were ordered directly or indirectly by the faculty), securing him, according to Joseph Farington, an income of £5,000 per annum.

Yet there were even bigger fish. William Read, 'the most laborious advertiser of his time', according to Joseph Addison, began life as a tailor, turned himself into a successful oculist, made a fortune, treated Queen Anne (for which he was knighted in 1705) and became friend and host to the literati of his day. His fellow oculist John Taylor rose from a modest start as a Norwich surgeon's son to become the most feted operator in Europe, a sort of Casanova of the eye. From the profits of his Pill and Drop, Joshua ('Spot') Ward was able to turn himself into a respected philanthropist, endowing at least four London 'hospitals' for the sick poor; his pharmaceuticals became designated regulation issue for the navy; he gained the friendship of the great; and, having successfully manipulated George II's dislocated thumb (the royal physicians had diagnosed gout), he won entrée at Court. A report – doubtless self-inserted but presumably true – in the *Daily Advertiser* for 10 June 1736 informed readers that: 'By the Queen's appointment, Joshua Ward Esq., attended at Kensington Palace with eight or ten persons, who in extraordinary cases had received a great benefit by taking his remedies. Her Majesty was accompanied by three surgeons, and several persons of quality, the patients were examined, money was distributed to them and Mr Ward was congratulated on his success.' In turn, Ward's royal connections won him special privileges, including the much-trumpeted right to drive his coach-and-six through St James's Park. He was also (partly because he cured Sir Joseph Jekyll, the Master of the Rolls) uniquely given personal exemption from legislation empowering the College of Physicians to inspect medicines.

The quacks were not, thus, all small men. Over the centuries, the most parroted accusation against quacks was that they were utterly plebeian – 'some painters, some

Joshua Ward. Line engraving, 1820, after T. Bardwell.

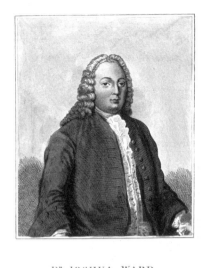

Dr JOSHUA WARD.

glaziers, some tailors, some weavers, some joiners, some cutlers, some cooks, some bakers, and some chandlers', ran William Clowes's tirade in the Elizabethan era.[11] But eighteenth-century irregular medicine shows the emergence of something different, the growth of marketplace medicine as big business.

Finally, is this conclusion borne out when we scrutinize the buyers of quack medicine? Obviously market research is almost impossible: for quacks, we do not even possess the lists of clients which regulars' cash-books sometimes afford us. The overwhelming majority of transactions between quacks and their clients have left not the slightest mark upon the archives. A few remarks may, however, be made with some confidence. For one thing, so many proprietary and patent medicines could not have continued on the market – in some cases from early in the eighteenth century right through to the twentieth – without sizeable and steady sales. Certain products, like many itinerants, were admittedly here today and gone tomorrow; but others had endurance. London empirics such as John Case advertised profusely for decades. This bespeaks a substantial body of buyers, many probably regular buyers.

Further indirect evidence that the clientele for quacks and their products was stable and sophisticated lies in the fact that many advertisements were specifically pitched at female buyers. 'Most Dear and Highly Esteemed Women', opens Stephen Draper's late seventeenth-century bill, in which he mainly offered his services as a man-midwife ('I will keep your secrets as my own life', he promised, while appealing to women 'to be no longer ashamed to apply themselves to men').[12] Because women had lower average rates of literacy, probably less spending money, and perhaps less freedom to consult a quack, we may assume that it was worthwhile specializing in medicines for women only if a reasonably secure middle-class buyership could be anticipated.

Pricing policy probably also affords further evidence of who the buyers were. Had they been targeted primarily upon the dregs – the 'poor innocent wretches', and the 'Brainless

Multitude' singled out by the journalist Ned Ward – quack medicines would have had to be sold dirt cheap. But the advertised prices were certainly not rock-bottom. One shilling – something approaching a day's wages for a labourer or a dozen pints of ale – was the cheapest price typically fixed upon a nostrum such as the Elixir Magnum Stomachum; and, even in the seventeenth century, they were not infrequently advertised at two or three shillings a bottle or jar, and occasionally more. John Case's Saffold's Cordial Elixir went for 2s for a half-pint, hardly a give-away price, and James's Powders were positively expensive at 2s 6d for two. Kennedy's Lisbon Diet Drink – a venereal disease cure – sold at half a guinea per bottle, and patients were advised to drink two a day: clearly only for affluent lechers.

These are pointers to the probability that many buyers of commercial medicines came from what we may very broadly call the middle bands of English society, including craftsmen, artisans, and those members of the petit bourgeoisie who might be leafing through a newspaper in a tavern or making purchases in a general store. This seems to be confirmed by the observation of 'Poplicola', who, prefacing the list of empirical remedies published in the *Gentleman's Magazine*, explains that:

> the rich and the great (generally speaking) will seek relief, secundum artem, from the regular physician, and true bred apothecary, for whom provision is made in the college dispensatory. But the majority of mankind (in hopes of saving charges, and on a presumption of surer help) are apt to resort to the men of experience, as they are called, whose remedies they are induced to think, from their advertisements (so often repeated, and at so great expense) have been successful in the cure of the several distempers for which they are calculated.[13]

The implication here that the buyers of quack medicines were of roughly the same class as the quacks themselves may well be shrewd.

Quack advertising depended heavily upon testimonials. For obvious reasons, those whose miracle recoveries were dramatized were members of the respectable classes – the occasional gentleman or titled lady, clergyman, Justices of the Peace, church-wardens, merchants, provincial mayors, and so forth. Cornelius à Tilbourg printed testimonials claiming to emanate from people such as Richard Greenaway (cured of stone), Lady Ann Seymore (recovered in seven weeks from a lameness in her limbs) and Sir John Andrews (cured of a 'cancerated' lip). Critics warned that no credence should be vested in these testimonials. Possibly. Yet many members of polite, fashionable, and literary society not only used such doctors and remedies (albeit lethally: Horace Walpole tells us that both his father and Lord Bolingbroke were 'killed by empirics') but quite spontaneously publicized their own attachment to them. Lord Chesterfield, for instance, after making use of Joshua Ward's medicines, noted that: 'I very early took Mr Ward's drop… reaped great benefit from it, and recommended it to so many of my friends that I question whether the author of that great specifick is more obliged to any one man in the kingdom than myself excepting one.'[14] It would be hard to imagine a more glowing accolade – though, of course, Gibbon's father, to ingratiate his second wife with his outraged son, informed Edward that she was the 'Lady that saved your life at Westminster by recommending Dr Ward when you was given over by the regular Physicians'.[15] Henry Fielding was another vocal advocate of Ward's medicines. When his health gave way in the 1740s and dropsy set in, he found no relief from the Duke of Portland's Medicine, as recommended to him by Ranby, the king's surgeon. Judged a 'Bath case', he tried the waters, but equally to no avail. Berkeley's Tar-Water did not help either. In desperation, he became the patient of Dr Ward, who largely helped him recover.

One could multiply examples of attachment to quack doctors and their medicines. Horace Walpole, Joseph Farington, and Fanny Burney all swore by the virtues of Dr Robert James's famed fever powders. Byron was a great believer in Acton's Corn-rubbers and in the virtues of Opodeldoc ointment for easing rheumatism (through it he had 'fought off the flannels for this time').[16] Cowper also used it.

Of course, Georgian table talk rings with warnings against the perils of quackery. 'Let me beg you not to have anything to say or do with the Magnetizers', warned Lady Bessborough in 1787:

> If they can do nothing it can be of no use, & if they can really affect the human frame it may as well do it harm as good. I am not at all sure that your sister's being so subject to these cramps & spasms may not have been a consequence of that if there is anything in it. At all events I have some reasons, which I cannot well explain by letter, why I wish you to avoid, in as quiet a way as you can, going or even conversing, if you can help it, with any of them.[17]

But people were no more ambivalent about quack medicines than they were about orthodox ones. When his wife, Margaret, was wasting with consumption, Boswell shopped around the different regular London doctors, including the ultra-fashionable Richard Warren and Sir George Baker. But he also called on the nostrum-vendor Nathaniel Godbold 'and got a pint of bottle of his vegetable balsam' for her; alas, the disappointed Boswell records, 'she would not try it as yet'. Boswell had a try-anything attitude with medicines (as is evident from the mix of quack nostrums and regular physic he took for gonorrhoea). It upset him that his wife was offended by his buying her patent medicines: 'I was very miserable. She seemed hurt from a notion that I grudged the expense of a physician because I talked of the difficulty of getting free of them. This distressed me deeply.' Unable to decide between fringe and orthodoxy, the Boswell family descended into chaos: 'I was sending for Sir George Baker again, but she stopped me I was for calling Dr. Warren'.[18]

Respectable, educated people tended to think quack medicines at least worth a try, without necessarily investing any particular faith in them. In 1767, Sylas Neville had a 'return of the toothache', and drew upon a proprietary medicine, with no luck: 'Mack's Anodyne fluid has done me no good'.[19] Some were rather more ashamed of dabbling in the unorthodox – in the Victorian era, Charles Darwin, testing out hydropathy, told his friend, Hooker, 'I feel certain that the water-cure is no quackery'.[20] Others were bold as brass – 'Rose at seven', wrote Dudley Ryder, 'Began to take my quack medicine again in order to take it quite out to see whether it will do me any good or no.'[21]

The Revd Edmund Pyle shared a similar spirit of adventure, enjoying dosing himself and reporting the results to his friends. 'When I took Mrs Stephens' medicines', he noted, 'I swallowed two ounces of soap a day, for six months together. Besides the oyster shell, or egg shell powder, in small beer, to the quantity that will lie on a half-crown with each dose of soap; I think the doses were 3 or 4 in a day.' Presumably he was taking Mrs Stephens's medicine for the stone – though maybe he was simply testing what effects it would have. He also experimented with 'some tricks for the gout', including 'The Duke of Portland's Powder', which disagreed with him violently ('thanks to my constitution, am not killed'). Indeed, he concluded, gout was best left alone: 'He that is subject to it, had better bear the fits, as nature throws them out than strive to put her out of her way, which if you do furca licet, usq recurret.'[22] Quackery was widely execrated. The anonymous versifier of 'On the Prevailing Taste for Quack Medicine', warned:

> For Heaven's and for your own sakes,
> Beware, my friends, beware of quacks!…
> Think how egregiously they fools us,
> Who vaunt, the same specific Bolus,
> Or fam'd Elixir, can root out
> A fever, dropsy, stone or gout!…
> Too sure I am, these boasted nostrums
> Like those dispensed from country rostrums
> More mortal men deprive of breath
> Than Battle, Murder, Suddain Death […][23]

The foregoing chapter has attempted to explain the tenacity of quackery despite such execrations and contemporary hopes that it was a throwback bound to disappear with progress. Far from disappearing, it flourished, and it did so because of the specific orientation of a commercial capitalist, spectacle-loving, consumer-oriented society, in which the very goal of the quacks – to persuade the public to consume medicine – was expedited by the same forces that explain why the society became more heavily medicine-consuming at large. The parallels, not the antitheses, between quackery and orthodoxy stand out.

3   The career of quacks

In a traditional face-to-face society, most goods, if not home-made, are manufactured by local craftsmen – cobblers, blacksmiths, gunsmiths, milliners, etc. The transactions are usually personal, the goods usually made up to individual order. The tradesman is known in person, and his long tenure in his job is the earnest of his skill and trustworthiness. The relationship between customer and supplier generates a certain mutual confidence.

Take such intimacy away and the hazards of the transaction multiply for all parties. Early in the nineteenth century, Anne Lister, a Halifax lady, saw an advertisement inserted by a London tailor, Radford of Piccadilly, promising to make greatcoats 'cheap'. She sent her order, with her measurements, through the post. The garment arrived late, and the quality of the cloth and workmanship were inferior. Miss Lister was angry. Such an 'open market' transaction promised mutual advantage. The tailor would enlarge his business, the buyer get clothes cheap and fast. In the event, the outcome was mutual aggravation: 'determined never to trouble Radford or any such advertising cheap person again'.[1]

This cameo exemplifies the problems and prospects facing the quack doctor and his clients. In pre-modern times, business opportunities were probably not propitious – outside the metropolis at least – for the medical quack with a mind to set himself up as the equivalent of the local blacksmith or corn-chandler, as a permanent tradesman with roots in the community. The quack specializing in manual dexterity – dealing with eye complaints, treating deafness, fitting trusses, or pulling teeth – would not have found the average market town alone provided him with trade enough. Or, if he were basically a nostrum-monger, he would come into competition with the local apothecary, the druggist, and probably the general store. Hence it made better sense for the irregular doctor to be an itinerant (mobility additionally gave the unscrupulous the advantage of being able to make himself scarce before his failures became obvious to all). With the relatively restricted demand levels of the traditional economy, the prudent quack took his services direct to a geographically wider clientele. There was nothing intrinsically disreputable about so doing. After all, it was an economy in which much of the workforce was constantly on the tramp, in search of seasonal labour; and a host of specialists – actors, musicians, entertainers, scientific lecturers, recruiting officers – spent their lives on the road. (So too, in a slightly different way, did regular doctors: Erasmus Darwin reckoned he travelled some 10,000 miles a year seeing patients.)

Itinerant healers came in many shapes and sizes. Some were two-bit operators doubling as packmen, peddlers, and hucksters, and selling as they strolled or setting up their stages at markets and booths at fairs. Others were altogether more substantial. The flamboyant Prussian Gustavus Katterfelto toured the provinces in great style in the 1780s with his special influenza cures. Similarly, once his 'Temple of Health' had collapsed in London in

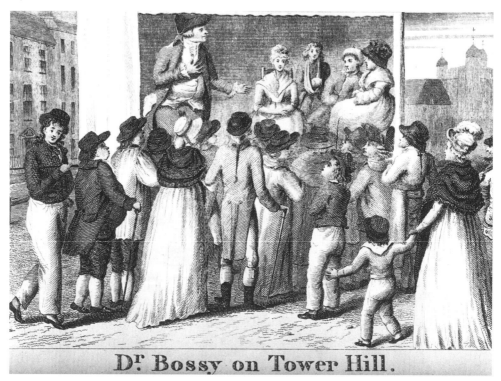

Dr Bossy on Tower Hill.

Doctor Bossy, an infamous medicine vendor, performing on stage to a crowd at Tower Hill. Etching.

the early 1780s – had he grossly mismanaged his financial affairs or had the *bon ton* simply tired of his shows? – James Graham took to the road, advertising extravagantly in the provincial press. Graham found provincial practice more difficult, since magistrates there were less tolerant of his sexual lectures and occasionally banned his performances.

Christine Hillam has similarly shown that numerous able and well-patronized provincial dentists maintained itinerant practices for decades – in some cases, son following father – during the eighteenth and nineteenth centuries, giving the lie to the superficial assumption that itinerancy was the invariable badge of roguery. Dentists would follow predictable circuits, moving on from town to town either at set months or as demand required; the public would learn of their anticipated arrival through the newspapers.

Historians have assumed that the itinerant quack was a species dying out like the dodo. It would be wrong, however, to kill them off prematurely. The young Francis Place enjoyed seeing Dr Bossy performing in full mountebank regalia in Covent Garden around the turn of the nineteenth century. John Galt thought that in Scotland at that time 'we have more mountebanks and Merry Andrews now, and richer cargoes of groceries and packman's stands'.[2] Not least, the advent of the railway gave mountebanks a new lease of life. If the traditional itinerant wended his way leisurely from town to town or, operating from a home base, plied his trade within a narrow radius, the locomotive massively improved his mobility. Records of early Victorian north-country quacks show that artists, once confined to a narrow radius, could, by boning up on the railway timetables, perform as far afield as Sheffield, Manchester, Preston, etc., more or less on successive days, thus vastly increasing their catchment area. Perhaps the most flamboyant quack ever to traverse England, 'Sequah', surrounded by tribes of 'Indian braves', flourished in the age of Pasteur.

The reason why historians have assumed that quacks were on the wane is because eye-witness accounts of them typically treat them with condescension and contempt. Thus Thomas Turner, the Sussex grocer, noted coolly on Wednesday 9 July 1760, that his wife 'walked to Whitesmith to see a mountebank perform wonders, who has a stage built there and comes once a week to cozen a parcel of poor deluded creatures out of their money, he selling packets which are to cure people of more distempers than they ever had in their lives for one shilling each, by which means he takes sometimes £8 or £9 of a day'.[3] Clearly, Turner thought it utterly beneath himself to participate in this charade. The significant fact is that his wife had also visited a mountebank in Whitesmith five years earlier – one imagines the same one – when she had purchased a packet of powders costing 12d.[4] It seems that this tradesman was well established – indeed, were he truly raking in the daily turnover that the envious Turner suggested, it would indicate a thriving traffic, especially for a sleepy rural area.

Over half a century later, the Northamptonshire peasant poet, John Clare, penned some lines, 'On the Death of a Quack', which once again sound like an epitaph, not just for the individual but for the breed itself:

> Here lyes Lifes Cobler who untimly fell
> By name of Doctor Drug'em known to all
> His frequent visits mad him known full well
> For where he'd business he ne'er faild to call
> Fools praised his power as great in saving Life
> And for that purpose many a journey made
> To village Lout and Tradesman's Wimsy Wife
> But some there must be to incourage trade
> For want of them full many a trade would stop
> And what wou'd doctors do if't wa'n't for fools?

Did this doctor's drugs work? They certainly packed the power to 'empty Pockets well as scour the Guts', conduded Clare – 'at this our Drug 'em was Expert enough'. The poet exposed the trade as a sham, fooling only the hayseeds. Eventually, he got his comeuppance; assailed by death, his pills did not avail:

> But Death feard naught – yet when the Physic flew
> The stick so nausious – made him turn about
> And forced him to retreat awhile to spew
> But frequent Sallies wore the Doctor out
> A Time to prove his Art was fairly bid
> Patients Expected – (Fools have little wit)

> That he would play his part (– well so did did)
> But then it failed and then the fools were bit
> They prove too wel! his Art of Getting Pelf
> But tother Art was either lost or past
> If he sav'd them he cou'd not save him self
> So here Poor Drug'em lies a Quack at last.

This quack, claimed Clare, 'made a boast of his ignorance by stating what he thought a better plea, in making his patients believe he was born a doctor by being the seventh son of a parent who was himself a seventh son and the seventh son of a seventh son is recknd among the lower orders of people as a prodigy in medicine who is born to perform miracles so he readily got into fame'. Yet if Clare despised this trickster, he did not disguise his brisk trade:

> The Art he practis'd knew it wondorous well
> While money lasted he ne'er faild of Stuff
> And Fools would by 'em – he knew how to sell
> And faith of Custom from his noted skill
> He never faild – his fame the Village spread.[5]

The carping comments of Turner and Clare do not show the quack as an endangered species, but they do indicate how such quacks experienced problems of securing credibility – having recourse on occasion to strange devices (boasting 'ignorance') to overcome such traumas. The problem of gaining credit was not one that uniquely faced quacks, however, but was common to all those operating as unknown factors in a milieu in which economic and personal transactions were traditionally conducted among familiars. What grounds did the public have for trusting an operator? What was to confer upon him his title to practice?

Regular practitioners acquired authority from attaching themselves to the norm, from following the standards of medical practice. Or, to take another example, the emergent scientific profession bid for authority through assuming lofty disinterest – theirs was a vocation dedicated to collective, co-operative search after truth. The problem of establishing a bona fide was more acute for the quack, however, since, lacking corporate identity, he had to behave rather in the manner of a Holy Roman Emperor and crown himself, and then, like a snail, carry his authority around with him upon his back.

Of course, this need for a pinch at least of charisma made him different, and that could in itself be a claim to fame. Indeed, many quacks (as we shall see in the following chapter) made effective play of their foreignness. Yet the native quack was no more a shaman than he was an exemplar of Weberian bureaucratic rationality. His true nature was to be a *bricoleur*, patching together some intellectual credibility from whatever shreds and tatters he could. In a highly precarious world, and with no routine institutional protection, quacks needed opportunistically to seize whatever props of power they could. Occasionally, they drew upon relatively intangible authority – for example, the mysticism of being a seventh son. Likewise, they would look to authorization from the wider world

Valentine Greatrakes, the Irish stroker. Oil painting.

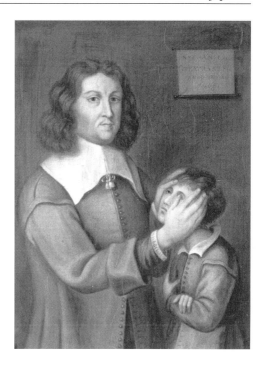

of the people, of the great, and of royalty. They were not alone in these tactics. For, as suggested in chapter 2, before that vast accrual of professional standing conferred by nineteenth-century reform and rationalization, medical power itself was a motley army. Certain strands of medicine possessed the sanctions of time and custom; some were backed by the popular voice; from the eighteenth century, the exchange values of the capitalist market-place became a further source of strength. Overall, the votes of the laity no less than the judgements of peers figured large in the legitimation of all manner of pre-modern medicine.

In respect of 'authorization', there was a lay power pyramid – with the king at the head – no less than a professional pecking order. Moreover, before the coming of the reformed modern state, it was by no means a foregone conclusion that central authority – monarch, court, and parliament – would see eye-to-eye with the medical profession. And, of course, the Crown represented the pinnacle of lay medical authority, through the personal exercise of thaumaturgical powers. Touching for the king's evil was resumed in England on a grand scale by Charles II, reaching an all-time peak under James II and continuing under Anne until the abandonment of the Divine Right doctrine by the Hanoverians terminated that theocratic healing rite. This ritual of the personal exercise of healing left the medical profession nonplussed, just as the medical top brass looked askance when Charles II's court seemed to countenance the reputedly miraculous faith cures wrought by the Irish stroker Valentine Greatrakes.

Lay patronage, at all levels from the monarch down to the masses, remained a powerful force in authorizing medicine at least through to the mid-nineteenth century (aristocratic and royal encouragement, for example, largely explains why smallpox inoculation gained a hold in England earlier than in France). Admittedly, from the early eighteenth century,

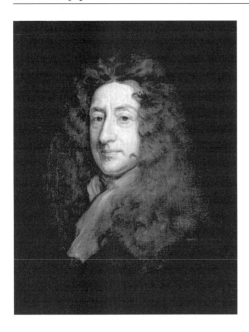

Sir Hans Sloane. Oil painting.

the importance of formal patronage to top artists, poets and architects may have been waning. Nevertheless, all the signs are that winning a post as physician or surgeon-in-ordinary to the king or to a lesser member of the royal family remained, for doctors such as Mead, Sloane, or Blackmore, a prize of inestimable professional and pecuniary benefit.

By parallel, anyone wishing to soar as an unorthodox healer had to look to prestigious lay patronage, above all from royalty. Such a task was made, paradoxically, easier by the fact that there always seemed an element of arbitrariness about the crown's choice of precisely whom to favour. Take the empiric Joshua Ward, to whom George II lent his patronage, apparently thanks to his being on hand at an opportune moment to rectify the king's dislocated thumb (the physicians had misdiagnosed gout). Duly impressed, the King granted Ward various privileges, including the much-trumpeted right to drive his coach-and-six through St James's Park and exemption from legislation empowering the College of Physicians to inspect medicines. Ward's nostrums became standard navy issue.

No less remarkable had been the rise of William Read. Originally a tailor, Read gained a reputation from the 1680s as an itinerant mountebank, specializing in eye diseases and in couching for cataract. Queen Anne suffered from poor eyesight; Read's services were called in. Finding favour, he was appointed oculist-in-ordinary to the Queen, and in 1705, partly because he ostentatiously gave his services gratis to treat the wounded in the war against France, the Queen conferred a knighthood upon him. Neither Ward nor Read managed to shrug off his notoriety as a mountebank but, as men of wealth of fame, charity and ebullience, they saw to it that they fraternized with the great and the literati. Both exploited court connections to the hilt in advertising their medicines, Read promoting his cures under the *Honi Soit Qui Mal y Pense* of the royal crest. The attempt to trade on a similar cachet shows in the scores of 'Sovereign Cordial Royal Antidotes', 'Imperial Pills', 'Royal Decachors', and suchlike also on the market. The famous Anodyne Necklaces, a charm to help infants' teething, carried a bill stating that 'The late Majesty Queen Caroline, sent monthly for these Necklaces for her Royal Children'.

As Read's case indicates, specialist fields such as eye diseases proved particularly happy hunting-grounds for irregulars possessed of a particular knack or technique and the confidence or temerity for handling difficult, delicate and dangerous conditions which the cautious surgeon might hesitate to tackle. Such men, not surprisingly, were much resented by the guardians of orthodoxy – specialization itself was long dismissed as quackery – as is evident in the fate of the Revd Dr Francis Willis, the Lincolnshire madhouse keeper called in to treat the delirious George III in 1788. Willis never escaped sneers and snubs from the king's regular physicians and was often called a quack. The antechambers to royal courts were open to empirics and irregulars, but their reign there was always uneasy. Possibly the most intriguing, and certainly the most ubiquitous, of all the mountebanks-cum-specialists haunting the courts of the *ancien régime* was John 'Chevalier' Taylor, whose three-volume reminiscences of a lifetime of adventures in treating eyes in all the courts of Europe bear casual comparison with the memoirs of Casanova.

An apothecary's son, Taylor was born in 1703 in Norwich, receiving a regular surgical education in London under Cheselden before starting up as an itinerant oculist. Until the early 1730s, he confined himself to England, but in 1733 he first travelled abroad, receiving MDs from Basle, Liège, and Cologne. After further travels in Holland and France, he returned to England in 1735, being appointed next year oculist to George II, a post he held to his death, when he was succeeded by his son, also called John.

But if Taylor made London his base, for the next thirty years he was almost permanently on his travels, operating upon eyes throughout the Continent and, above all, winning entrée into most courts of Europe. In 1736, he was in Paris; between 1737 and 1742, he toured Spain and Portugal; in the early 1740s, he was in France once more; around 1745, he travelled through Britain; and then in 1747, he passed over into Holland and Flanders. By 1750, he was practising in Germany. In 1751, he was called in to restore the sight of the Duke of Mecklenburg-Schwerin, *en route* visiting Hamburg and Denmark. Travels in Scandinavia followed, and then on to Breslau, Silesia, Warsaw, Mittau, Courtland Riga, St Petersburg and finally Moscow (where he claimed to watch cleansing rituals involving hundreds of woman prancing naked in the fields). On his return journey in 1755, he passed through Germany and Bohemia; he spent 1756 in Italy and then headed homewards via Vienna and Ghent, reaching London again in 1759. But that was not the end of his travels. Records show he was in Amiens and Rheims in 1765 and in Ghent in 1767; works of his were published in Hamburg and Leipzig in 1766, surely signalling his presence there.

Taylor was not a modest man. A puffing poem about him stated that he would 'make all Europe start', and in his autobiography he described himself as 'the most public man under the sun, being personally known not only in every Town in Europe, but in every part of the globe'. 'Introduced to the feet of the sovereigns' wherever he went, he listed among his acquaintance on the title-page of his memoirs 'The Kings of Poland, Denmark, Sweden, The Electors of the Holy Empire, The Princes of Saxegotha, Mecklenberg, Anspach, Brunswick, Parme, Modena, Zerbst, Loviere, Liege, Bareith, Georgia, &c.', dubbing himself there 'Ophthalmiator Pontifical Imperial and Royal'. He claimed that he had not only 'been personally known to every sovereign in all Europe, without exception', but that 'I have been also known personally to every man of distinguished character now living or has lived in Europe, in the present age, in every science, and in every part of useful knowledge'.

Taylor went on to apostrophize the high and mighty with extraordinary fulsomeness:

> Oh! thou mighty Oh! thou sovereign Pontiff Oh! thou great luminary of the church; given to mankind, in the sense of so many nations, as a star to the Christian world, The great excellence of whose diadem is faith Whose glory is the defence of virtue Who can believe, that you, most holy father, who art placed as the first inspector of the deeds of man, would proclaim to all the inhabitants of the earth, as you have done, your high approbation of my works, but by the voice of truth. Oh! ye Imperial – Oh! ye Royal – Oh! ye great masters of empire who have so far extended your benevolence, as to be witnesses of my labours Behold me at your feet – Oh! ye Empresses – Oh! ye Queens! Great partners of the governors of the people of the earth You, whose gentleness, whose goodness of heart, have so often engaged your awful presence on these occasions What satisfaction have you expressed at seeing the blind, by me, enabled to behold again the marvels of heaven! – And finding them prostrate at your feet, expressing their joy at what they first saw – Because, 'twas you they saw – The first object of their duty The highest in their wishes Have you not with your own gracious hands affirmed, that these things you have seen...[6]

What do we make of Taylor's claims to have rubbed shoulders with the good and the great? Given that he lived in the age when Baron Munchausen was published, that he was a contemporary of the impostor Formosan sage, George Psalmanazar, and overlapped with Count Cagliostro, we might be inclined to dismiss his assertions as a tissue of lies. And certainly we should not always take him at his word. His claims to have travelled as far as Persia seem, for instance, highly dubious, and his proud boast that he restored Bach's sight was at the least incorrect (he was possibly remotely responsible for the composer's death). But what is remarkable is not how many of Taylor's claims were a farrago of nonsense but how far they were true. He *did* operate in many courts, *did* receive diplomas and patents from many universities, courts, and learned societies (they are printed in one continuous footnote, running like subtitles, across sixty-eight successive pages of his autobiography) and he *did* come into contact with such eminences as Boerhaave, Linnaeus, Winslow, Haller, and Morgagni.

Historians want doctors to fit tidily into today's categories. Was a particular practitioner skilful, or a bungling quack? A pillar of the faculty or a coxcomb adventurer? A philanthropist or an opportunist? Taylor, however, resists being exclusively pigeonholed in such ways. In serving thus as a 'monster', he can illuminate the wider question of the authorization of the careers of quacks.

That Taylor possessed both science and skill in ophthalmology is beyond doubt. Through studying under Cheselden, he received the finest surgical education available.

His early book on the *Mechanism of the Eye* is an excellent compendium of contemporary science; it was criticized by Taylor's senior, Benedict Duddell, but criticized with respect. Taylor's extensive subsequent writings, in many languages, show that he kept up with the discoveries of the age. In certain fields, he probably made contributions of his own to the advancement of knowledge, as in his treatment of squint.

Furthermore, he was a skilled operator, though not always a judicious one. Of course, his standard itinerant oculist's practice of requiring several days of post-operative bandaging meant that by the time his failures came to light, he was already over the hills and far away. And there is evidence, particularly from late in his career, that he grew less cautious and less principled, operating (and taking fees) in cases he must have known to be hopeless – as in his treatment of George Frederick Handel. And it would be excessive to claim for him a major innovatory role in eye surgery. Initially by accident, and later by design, first Saint-Yves in 1722 and then the distinguished Jacques Daviel were to pioneer a new technique for treating cataract not by couching, or depression and displacement, as was traditional, but by extraction of the lens. It was to prove a profound development. But Taylor seems to have stuck to the old methods of couching in which he had been instructed. In print, he voiced his scepticism about the new method, and there is no firm evidence that he employed it till almost the close of his career. In so far as Taylor was an innovator, it was probably chiefly in treatments for squint.

But if Taylor was a traditionalist, there is no reason to impugn his hand. Dr William King, who met Taylor in 1748, reported: 'I was at Tunbridge in 1748, where I met with the Chevalier Taylor, the famous oculist. He seems to understand the anatomy of the eye perfectly well; he has a fine hand and good instruments, and performs all his operations with great dexterity.'[7] Many physicians on the Continent would have supported such a view. No less a figure than Albrecht von Haller called him 'a skilful man, but too liberal of promises'; Professor Mauchart of Tübingen testified to his candour, erudition, and operative dexterity, confirming that in Amsterdam he had failed to cure only fifteen out of 225 cases; and Dr Marteau of Amiens reported to the great eye surgeon Petit that he had watched Taylor practise for a month, being impressed by his techniques with gutta-serena and confirming that he operated '*d'une main aussi legère que sure*'. Not all contemporaries were so impressed, and Platner, among others, spoke of the contempt with which the learned world regarded Taylor's bombast, pretentiousness and temerity in treatment. Even so, the notion that he was just a bungling impostor clearly will not hold water.

Indeed, in a manner which we have seen already, Taylor was anxious to dismiss mere quacks and 'pretenders', to defend himself, with righteous indignation, against allegations of quackery, and to associate himself with pukka physic. In his first book, he warmly thanked the great Cheselden for the 'knowledge I have of this Branch of my Profession, such as it is'; seventeen years later, he dedicated one of his works to the President and Fellows of the Royal College of Physicians of Edinburgh. And Taylor's writings endlessly drop the names of the great, even if some of his references to them convey a certain studied aloofness, as when he records of a joint consultation with Boerhaave, 'The author had some difficulty, at first, to make this great physician comprehend the possibility of producing, by his new method, the effect desired but after being acquainted with his Theory, he highly approved of his method, and was himself witness of many instances of its success.'

What such examples show is that, typically of so many other eighteenth-century medical entrepreneurs, Taylor recognized he was better off throwing in his lot with the heroes of regular medicine than by exploiting his marginal status and cultivating an 'alternative physic'. Taylor's self-image was squarely as a regular physician; but, above all, it was as a specialist. He never tired of staking out a claim for ophthalmology as (to recall the phrase he blazoned on the title-page of his autobiography), 'distinct and independent of every other Branch of Physic'. Only specialists, he contended, could understand in sufficient depth the complexities of organs such as the eye (of which there were well over two hundred diseases, he claimed), and gain sufficient operative experience to protect the public ('What almost incredible exactment must be required in the movement of the hand to succeed in such a work as this!'). Such arguments resemble those used to legitimate other contemporary emergent specialities, for example, man-midwifery. Just as contemporary obstetricians, such as William Smellie, devised special models and apparatus for demonstrating their specialities to pupils, so Taylor had his own for the eye. In what was almost certainly a self-inserted plug in the *Grub Street Journal*, it was stated:

> We hear that Dr Taylor has brought with him from Italy, a specimen of a most exquisite piece of workmanship in enamel, intended to represent, in 385 figures, the several diseases of the globe of the eye, (made after his own designs) which he shews to the curious that honour him with a visit, at his house in Great Suffolk-street. 'Tis said, that this work (which is the only of its kind yet known) from its great use to his pupils, for instructing them in the principles of the science he professes, gave very great satisfaction to the academies of Paris. And this gentleman has now completely finish'd his apparatus for his curious operations of the eyes, and is so universally known to make no secret of any part of his profession, 'tis not doubted but curiosity will bring to him from the several parts of these kingdoms, as many spectators of distinction, and more particularly those who are related in the faculty, as he has been honoured with in foreign parts, it appearing that not a day pass'd but a multitude of persons, as well of superior quality as the first of those whose education led them to be judges, has been present on these occasions in every place he has pass'd through; and what has added greatly to their satisfaction, has been, that he has furnish'd their curiosity with seeing nearly 100 different operations on the eyes, amongst which there are upwards of 60 of his own invention; that he gives little or no pain in any of [his] operations; that they have never any painful attendants; and that, notwithstanding the delicacy of this sort of work, they are almost always attended with success; all which, 'tis hop'd, at this time can admit of no doubt, after his having been so often receiv'd for these his happy discoveries, not with respect only, but as a member of the body of physicians in several of the most celebrated universities abroad.[8]

If Taylor was thus a skilful operator, decrying quackish secrecy, then the arrant coxcomb in him grates upon us. Why such puffs, sycophancy, and egregious posturing? Of course, as argued at the beginning of this chapter, in the days before specialist hospitals, specialists had to be itinerant, and doubtless itinerants must advertise and cut a dash to drum up custom. Yet even so, Taylor chose to surround himself with an inordinate amount of ballyhoo. Standardly, on·moving to a new area, he would advertise his forthcoming 'audiences', both via handbills and in the press. Arriving in Northampton early in 1747, he advertised himself thus:

> To-morrow, being Sunday, the 20th (as usual on that day) the Gentlemen, the Ladies, the Clergy, and all of literature and Distinction, are hereby invited at Six in the Evening, at the Great ROOM, at the *Aed-Syon* to a *Phisico-Theological Declamation* in Praise of SIGHT, design'd both in Speaking and Action, agreeable to the Rules of ORATORY.
> – The SYLLABUS – will be given free to all present, and the Whole will be free.
> By JOHN TAYLOR, Esq., – Doctor of Physick, Oculist to the King of GREAT BRITAIN, Fellow of several Collegs of Physicians, etc. Being a Specimen of a Course many Years given in the several Universities, and the several Courts abroad *London, Edinburgh* and lately at Dublin. The Gentry are invited every morning to see his METHOD of *restoring* SIGHT, etc. At Six on Monday Evening next (the 21st Instant) he will certainly give the LECTURE on the Alterations of the EYE, etc. When the Eye will be dissected, and all its various Beauties displayed, in the Order of a Work lately published in Octavo, with Plates, at EDINBURGH. Notwithstanding the Many that usually attend on this Occasion, the ROOM will be so regulated that every Person present may see the several Parts of the EYE accurately examin'd.[9]

At the same time, Taylor would probably have distributed, presumably free of charge, other puffing works claiming to offer objective assessments of his merits, as, for example, a pamphlet entitled *A Parallel between the Late Celebrated Mr Pope and Dr Taylor, Oculist to the King of Great Britain, etc., by a Physician*, a work clearly written by Taylor himself or a hired hack. This established that the poet and the ophthalmiator shared one great quality – that of being calumniated by jealous enemies – and went on to laud Taylor's virtues (claiming that before Taylor, out of 243 diseases of the eye, only sixty were curable; now only sixty were not; and so forth). The pamphlet deploys blank verse to celebrate Taylor's talents:

> Hail, curious Oculist! to thee belongs
> To know what secret Springs of Vision move
> The Ball of Sight; what inward cause retards
> Their Native Force; what Operation clears
> A cloudy Speck, or bids the total Frame
> Resume the lustre of the lucid Ray…
> 'Tis thine to tell how veiled to gloomy Shade
> The darkling Eye retires, nor feels the Force
> Of solar Beam anon a darting Gleam
> Shoots thro' the Glass and gives the bright'ning Orb

To visit Light I see the Liquid stream
Flow, as the guiding Hand directs the Way
And bids it enter, where a total Gloom
Had drawn dark Cover o'er the Seat of Sight,
Whether in Choroied, or nervous Net
Fair Vision shines, thither the streaming Rays
Converge their Force; and in due Order Range
Their coloured Forms. Anon the Patient sees
A new Creation rising to the View In Living Light![10]

Taylor would then proceed to deliver his lectures in English, French, or Latin as appropriate. A good report survives from John Palmer, who heard Taylor in full cry in January 1747:

About ten days ago I crept over to Northampton, and luckily met there with the famous Dr Taylor, who operated every morning, and read lectures, as he call'd them, every evening to twelvepenny chaps, except on Sundays, when he gave gratis a Declamation (as you'll see by this advertisement enclosed, which was delivered to every house in town) . This gratis, I own, took me in for an auditor; and I'll tell you how it was carried on. The Doctor appeared dress'd in black, with a long, light flowing ty'd wig; ascended a scaffold behind a large table raised about two feet from the ground, and covered by an old piece of tapestry, on which was laid a dark-coloured cafoy chariot-seat, with four black bunches (used upon hearses) tyed to the corners for tassels, four large candles on each side the cushion, and a quart decanter of drinking water, with a half-pint glass, to moisten his mouth. He bowed, snuff'd the candles, descended and delivered out to the company his hat-full of Syllabuses, divided into Sections No. 1, 2, 3, etc. (such stuff, and so printed, as to be entirely incoherent and unintelligible). Then mounting his scaffold, he bowed very low; then putting himself into a proper attitude, began, in a solemn, tragical voice and tone: 'At Number 1 thus written you will find' and repeating this with some vehemence, he read No. 1 of his Syllabus, speaking for two hours in the same manner, and with the same air, gesture, and tone, and making a sort of blank verse of it, and always ending with a verb, for that, he says, is the true Ciceronian, prodigiously difficult, and never attempted by any man in our language before. In some instances, he said 'He equal'd the finest periods Tully ever wrote or spoke'; which always began with the genitive case, were followed by the substantive, and concluded with the verb as thus 'Of Th' Eye, the Beauties I will now declare—'. This was often repeated as his masterpiece; and he exulted and admired himself vastly upon it. When he had finished he came smiling among his Auditors, appealed to them publicly if it was not charming fine, and if they had ever heard anything like it. I must own I never did, or saw his equal; and therefore send you this sketch of him as a great rarity.[11]

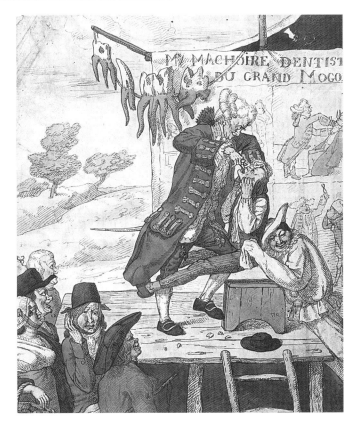

A foppish dentist extracting a tooth from a patient who is being restrained by a Pierrot clown. On the stage, a screen proclaims: 'M. Machoire dentiste du grand mogol'. Coloured etching by A. Auger, 1817.

One wonders about the precise psychology underlying such performances, as similarly with the rather comparable cleverly self-mocking and self-dramatizing shows put on a generation later by the sexologist James Graham. Certainly, like Graham after him, Taylor attracted both a barrage of unfavourable verdicts (Dr Johnson called him the 'most ignorant man I ever knew' – he probably meant ignorant of Latin – an 'instance of how far impudence will carry ignorance') and a stream of satire, such as the Edinburgh lampoon *A Faithful and Full Account of the Surprising Life and Adventures of the Celebrated Doctor Sartorius Sinegradibus*, which related, in Martin Scriblerus fashion, the portentous events surrounding the birth of the noble doctor, and *The English Impostor Detected, or the History of the Life and Fumigation of the renowned Mr J———— T————- , Oculist.* A ballad opera called *The Operator* featured Taylor in the persona of Dr Hurry, an oculist, and included the following scene in the doctor's house:

> The assembled patients have heard that he does not take money, but it is rumoured that there is a secretary who 'holds out the palm'. The doctor, they are informed, has thirteen lords and dukes with him that morning. Presently he enters; there is a general distribution of snuff, which, he assures them, is a panacea for all diseases. When the people remind him of his advertisements of free treatment he replies that the fees which he exacts are to supply remedies for the poor. To one woman who says she has nothing,

he answers that it makes no difference at all, but he happens to be exceedingly busy that morning. He tells some medical men who visit him, that he can cure gutta serena 'with one drop of my collyrium', and confesses that he 'purchased a diploma for gold at Padua'. Asked his opinion of Sir William Read [another famous quack, oculist to Queen Anne], he calls him a 'mere nurse, a mere washer-woman, in respect of what I do'. He quotes, with approval, the father's advice: 'Get money honestly, son, if you can: however, get money'. He admits that when he began to practise he blinded 300 people. A supposed blind man is brought in, and Dr Hurry is adjured to tell the truth for once; he promises to do so: there is no hope. It turns out that the man sees perfectly. In the last scene the doctor treats all his duns and creditors at a tavern, and then decamps, leaving them to pay the bill, whereupon the pawnbroker consoles the others with the following couplet:

> 'But let us be gay, and our losses despise,
> And rejoice that we've safely escap'd with our eyes'.[12]

Being thus satirized – not least, of course, in Hogarth's 'The Company of Undertakers' – may have flattered Taylor's vanity, and he probably operated on the maxim that all publicity is good publicity. Certainly, despite sneers from commentators such as Horace Walpole, who warned a friend against Taylor's practices thus: 'I need not desire you not to believe that stories of such a mountebank as Taylor; I only wonder that he should think the names of our family a recommendation at Rome; we are not conscious of any such merit; nor have any of our eyes ever wanted to be put out', there is no sign that his fame was a flash in the pan, readily discredited, or that his customers increasingly came only from the riffraff or the really desperate. The fact that he treated Edward Gibbon in his childhood and George Frederick Handel nearly twenty years later may suggest that in England, where, presumably, he was best known, the darts of satire could have been indices of his success rather than an obstacle to it.

Taylor was probably prepared to take his chances in these ways, risking his reputation with the public at large, because it could be traded off against his remarkable success in gaining entrée at court, and thereby in winning favour and patients in the highest circles. Indeed, the fact that he was persona grata at court clearly secured him privileged access as well to the nobility and their households, and not least (if we accept Taylor's own autobiographical account) to establishments such as convents – he claimed to have been inside 'almost every female nunnery' in Europe, and seen their 'beauties'. Success bred success. Decked out in style, he travelled at what he called 'the crisis of his grandeur' with 'no less than two coaches and six, above ten servants in livery, besides gentlemen, my companions, in my own pay', in a coach emblazoned all over with eyes, bearing the motto *Qui dat videre, dat vivere*. Mimicking the parade of nobility (after all, he styled himself 'Chevalier'), he proceeded armed with testimonials and patents from half the rulers, cities, and learned societies of Europe.

There is no sign that fashionable and courtly custom ever dried up. There must always have been patients at court whom local physicians had failed to cure or had pronounced incurable. At Saxe-Gotha, he recalled, 'the first lady of the palace passed thro' my hands

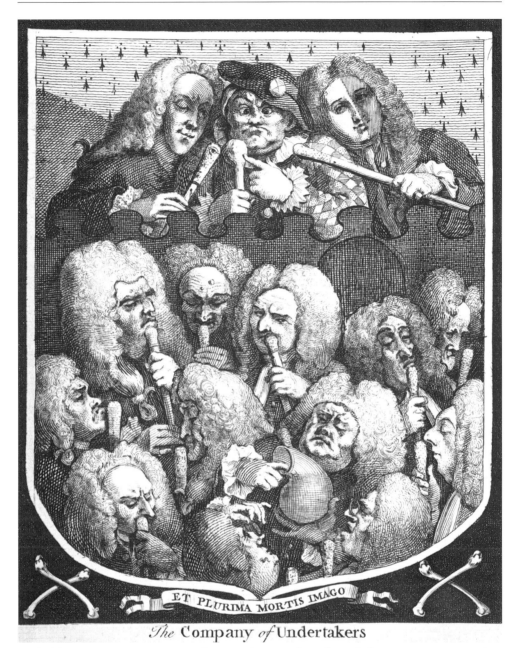

ET PLURIMA MORTIS IMAGO

The Company *of* Undertakers

A shield containing a group portrait of various doctors and quacks, including Mrs Mapp, Dr Joshua Ward and John Taylor. Etching by W. Hogarth, 1736, after himself.

for a defect of sight'. In any case, it seems as if notables were glad to offer Taylor a welcome because they enjoyed the vicarious frisson of watching their own servants, or even total strangers, being operated on by this consummate showman. And, furthermore, Taylor probably made it his forte to perform semi-cosmetic surgery of his own devising upon the eyes and faces of beauties at court, as this account of an ectropion operation indicates:

> Being in one of the principal courts abroad, I saw a lady in the drawing-room of a great court, who had the lower lid of her left eye fallen down, by an accident from fire, which left part of her eye uncovered, this defect destroyed the beauty of one of the finest faces I ever saw. I approached her excellency… and spoke to this effect; 'permit me lady to tell you that one half of that face of yours is exquisitely pretty. Well, Sir, she said, and what do you say to the other? Why, the other, Madam, said I, is so much the reverse that it strikes me with horror; how, Sir, said the lady with great quickness; What insolence is this?'

Taylor reassured her he would not have made that seemingly rude remark, did he not possess the extraordinary power of making both sides of the face equally handsome…

> Having sent for my instruments, therefore, and having retired with the lady to a private apartment, I immediately passed a needle through the skin of the temple, near the lesser angle of the eye, and with my lancet dissected, to about half an inch diameter, the skin of that part from the muscles. Whilst thus employed, her excellency often called out to me, "you hurt me! you hurt me!" And I as often answered "remember lady, beauty! beauty!" and with this charming word beauty I softened her pain in such a manner that she kept her courage to the end of the operation, which was to draw the edges of the wound together and fix them so by passing the needle threaded through them as to tie them together. Thus I brought that upper eyelid into its place without touching it, and after putting on the wound now closed, a small plaster, which seemed rather an ornament than a blemish, I conducted the lady back to the courtiers in the palace. Seeing her thus changed, they all appeared astonished, and looked as if this business had been done by some miracle.

Peddlers of rare expertise such as Taylor would make a beeline for court patronage. The courts of Europe were still quite easy of access to exotic and entertaining artists and performers, successors to the jesters, alchemists, astrologers, and magicians who had filled the renaissance courts of rulers such as Rudolf II. Moreover, if we may take Taylor at his own word, in the erotically titillating atmosphere of the rococo court, a physician could readily be both a welcome diversion and a useful practical client for bored ladies.

We know from the affair of the court physician-cum-statesman Struensee with Queen Caroline Matilda at the Danish Court at a slightly later date how service as a physician could open doors to intimacy. Certainly, Taylor's narrative of his adventures gives many examples of how the special opportunities of the eye-doctor – not least the abundance of eye-to-eye contact, the darkened rooms, the bandages – were exploited by 'the fair' at court, and even by nuns, as occasions for playful love-making. Taylor had a contemporary reputation for his looks and for being a ladies' man.

Her certainly made it his business to ingratiate himself at court. For one thing, he advanced a series of anecdotes and maxims on the art of pleasing ('so necessary to the happiness of man') resembling the almost contemporary letters of Lord Chesterfield to his son. Dedicating a volume to David Garrick ('who, Sir, like you can please?'), Taylor contended that instructing in these arts of pleasing was integral to his vocation:

> Before I proceed on this admirable subject, I believe it will be expected of me, as a courtier, that I should give my thoughts on the art of pleasing, as being so essential to the happiness of man, though so little known, and much less practised, but amongst the great, and persons of high life, by discovering in myself some judgment in this useful knowledge; I cannot fail of throwing such a lustre on many of my adventures, as to engage at least the noblest part of my readers.

Explaining that the topic was almost inexhaustible – 'I could talk whole days on this most interesting and delightful subject, and I believe all who know me, will agree, that such have been my opportunities to acquire knowledge this way, and such is my acquaintance with men and things, that on this topic I could furnish a perpetual variety; but it becomes me here to put a period.' – he confined himself to the central elements: the art of compliment, the capacity to elevate the self-esteem of others without descending to gross and transparent flattery. An element of plain speaking, he argued, befitted the physician, and particularly the Englishman, in encounters with princes and other nobles. By contrast, the proper performance with 'the fair' consisted in the supreme ability, as Taylor put it, to 'play with words'.

Taylor's discussion of the delicate balance between the physician and the courtier throws great light on contemporary quackery. It reveals that Taylor was profoundly aware of the precariousness of his position. He was always in danger of being abruptly and unceremoniously booted out of court – Frederick the Great's way with him. Taylor attributed that action not to the policy of that enlightened ruler (who probably thought Taylor a spy) but to the schemings of rival courtiers. And he could be put on the spot (according to his memoirs) by imperious ladies who summoned him to their bedchambers and impugned his honour (and doubtless his manhood) if he declined. In the cold intrigues of court or the heady glitter of the masquerade, one false step would have been fatal to the fortunes of the English doctor in the company of the great (if he masqueraded as a grandee and disarmed the defences of a duchess, what would happen when he was unmasked and reality was revealed?). But (he reassured his readers) he had always carried off the act with supreme *savoir-faire* and aplomb.

Taylor recognized his career hinged on more than his skill as an operator upon eyes. He had to operate on minds and hearts as well. In response, he unfolded a philosophy, a mystery, a romance of the eye, 'that beauteous, that inestimable, that divine little Globe', which when restored by the oculist, 'again its native Power reclaims, again becomes a Lucid Orb'. Making a mystique out of sight and light was not difficult. The age of the Enlightenment was, naturally enough, preoccupied with seeing and with the victory of light over darkness, in the light of such scientific works as Newton's *Opticks* (especially bearing in mind Pope's 'God said Let Newton Be, and all was light'), philosophical books such as George Berkeley's *Treatise on Vision*, and psychological speculations stemming from William Molyneux and carried on in Diderot's *Lettre sur les Aveugles*, on the relations of seeing as sensation and seeing as understanding, perception and conception, sight and insight – on how the physiological fact of blindness could threaten the qualities of humanity. Taylor exploited such speculations. Above all, he aimed to turn the eye-doctor into a privileged moral agent. His prime skill was, Christ-like, to give sight to the blind. But in addition, he saw his vocation as being to confer moral vision as well, to remove moral blinkers from patients' eyes. Of such higher services he related many examples:

> At Prague, a young libertine of distinction, who, having an aged father blind, was intrusted with the management of a large fortune, which he disposed of with great imprudence. On my passage I was requested to draw the curtain from before his father's eyes, that he might behold his worthy child before he left the world. Finding but little delicacy in the son's conversation, and no great inclination that I should succeed in such an attempt, I judged that he wanted respect both to his father and myself, and being determined to shew him his error, I took the veil from before his father's eyes, and soon enabled him to be that way a witness of the vices of his son.

Such episodes find an intriguing echo in a mid-eighteenth-century play possibly stimulated by Taylor's career, *The Oculist*, written by the Revd Phanuel Bacon, vicar of Reading, which weaves a moral allegory around the figure of a quack oculist, who, besieged by the greedy and the grasping, the vain and the vituperative, opens their moral eyes, gives them insight, and turns his patients into reformed characters who have seen the light.

Alongside that therapeutic, didactic mission, Taylor offered his services, informally and tacitly at least, as a character reader, blessed with second sight. Stressing that the eye is 'index of the mind', he assumed the tradition of physiognomy which had operated so powerfully throughout the early-modern period, backed by the occult arts and aesthetics:

> I shall here only say, with regard to the changes of the eye from the affections of the mind, on which I have given, in different languages, and in various nations, so many discourses; that though it is difficult for us to conceive how that which is not matter affects that which is, or, in the sense I am speaking of, how the parts of the eye are changed from the affections of the mind; it is agreed by all, that the eye is the index of the heart, and that there are painted the passions of the soul. But to bring this knowledge into rule, so as to determine by the eye, the then present business of the mind, is a study that requires much knowledge of human life, and what I have taken more pains to bring to a certainty, than perhaps any who lived before me.

In a way prefiguring Lavater's doctrine of the physiognomist's 'additional eye', Taylor argued that skilful reading of people's eyes is the perfect litmus test of sincerity and the heart's intentions: 'I mean that of judging by the eye, the will of the heart. There is scarce a crowned head or sovereign prince in all Europe, but before whom I have occasionally, in their own palaces, held discourses on this subject.'

Thus the apothecary's son from Norwich amply seized the opportunities the open world of the *ancien régime* offered to a man with the talent, showmanship, and, one might add, gall to transcend an apothecary's career. But he was able to go so far because he perfectly understood that he needed to mobilize all the modes of authority and credit available, above all, public popularity, academic respectability and court privilege. A supreme illusionist, he was like a man whose financial resources were overstretched and his credit shaky, yet who, by transferring funds from one bank account to another at great speed, was able to sustain the appearance of wealth. Before his popular audiences, he paraded his scientific contacts and court testimonials. 'In anatomy', he declared, dropping names like petals, he knew,

> Albinus, Morgagni, in whose presence I was created doctor in chirurgery in the university of Padua: Winslow, Hainalt, to both whom I was well known: Hunter, Nicols, Monro, Brathwaite, with who I sometimes studied anatomy. In surgery, Morand, Petit, Carengeot, &c. and all those of eminence in our own country. In botany, I was well acquainted with the celebrated Linnaeus, in Upsal, Sweden. In my own way, and from whom I received the first rudiments in the science I profess, Woolhouse, St. Ives, Annel, Petit the physician, once my great protector… [and so forth].

Before the faculty and the university ('Oh! ye learned Great in the knowledge of physic Excellent in virtue'), he would authenticate himself by parading his thousands upon thousands of cures amongst the people. And when cutting a figure at court, he would pointedly give what he called 'academic lectures', emphasizing his bona fide as a scientist and surgeon. No wonder then (and here the Taylor balloon rose into the air, buoyed up on its own puffery), given his success at court, the public in turn should trust him:

> From the sovereign I was naturally introduced to the knowledge and protection of the nobility. Their confidence in me was such, as to submit themselves under my care, as appears by the number of princes, and other great personages, who, in various nations, have happily passed through my hands; greatly exceeding what any physician now living can say but myself; and as the people could not fail to follow the example of their superiors, it is no wonder that I left every country with so much satisfaction to the public, and honour to myself.

Thus Taylor explained his success. He avoided reliance upon the *vox populi*. Instead, success at court guaranteed secure enjoyment of all the sources of medical authority: 'Thus instead of beginning with the people, which was the case of all those contemptible

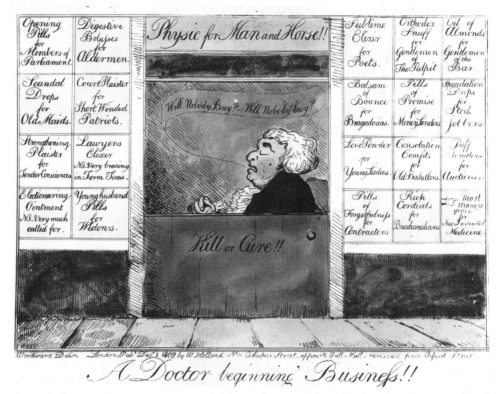

Opening Pills for Members of Parliament.	Digestive Boluses for Aldermen.				Sublime Elixir for Poets.	Orthodox Snuff for Gentlemen of The Pulpit	Oil of Almonds for Gentlemen of the Bar
Scandal Drops for Old Maids.	Court Plaister for Short Winded Patriots.				Balsam of Bounce for Bragadocios.	Pills of Promise for Money Lenders	Speculation Drops for Stock Jobbers
Strengthening Plaister for Tender Consciences	Lawyers Elixir NB Very bracing in Term Time.				Love Powder for Young Ladies	Consolation Comfits for Old Batchelors	Puff Powders for Auctioneers
Electioneering Ointment NB. Very much called for.	Young husband Pills for Widows.				Pills of Forgetfulness for Contractors	Rich Cordials for Bacchanalians	Most Money given for New Invented Medicine

Physic for Man and Horse!!

Will Nobody Buy? — Will Nobody buy?

Kill or Cure!!

Woodward Delin. London Pub. Dec.r 1. 1802 by W. Holland. N.11 Cockspur Street opposite Pall Mall – removed from Oxford Street.

A Doctor beginning Business!!

A quack doctor in his premises, surrounded by medicines. Coloured etching by G.M. Woodward, 1802.

dabblers, whom I have met from time to time in my travels, and who were ever neglected by the great, and by the learned; I, on the contrary, was ever by the great protected, by the learned esteemed, and by the people respected.'

Taylor thus shrewdly grasped the fact that, so long as he kept all his balls in the air at once, reinforcing authority upon authority in one great barrage of noise and bluster, and not least, so long as he kept on the move, he could succeed, keep the money rolling in and satisfy that great *ancien régime* ambition: to see the inside of a court. A quack might stare at a queen.

'Chevalier' Taylor made a career out of being an itinerant, more or less dying in the saddle. Medicine on the move was a way of life, a way of authentication, mirroring the picaresque mode that so fascinated contemporary novelists. It provided Taylor with career success. His son, John, followed him into the eye business, but it is significant that Taylor junior ceased to operate as an itinerant, settling down in London.

Performing on the road was, I have argued, a necessity for many quacks (and, as the 'Chevalier' Taylor's career shows, it could clearly have positive advantages). Yet its drawbacks are equally obvious: it meant a life of uncertainty, and of endless wear and tear. Many commercial doctors preferred, if possible, to establish fixed premises. But this posed equal problems. Could they count on sufficient casual trade seeking out their special skills and distinctive medicines? It was one thing to keep shop as a regular druggist or apothecary, for customers would call to buy all manner of medicaments and preparations; it was a very different enterprise to be a sedentary quack, whose public reputation depended upon claims to the special efficacy of one or two particular nostrums. To achieve sufficient sales, would a purely local trade be sufficient? Jonathan Barry has argued how, in any locality, the dice were loaded in favour of the regulars, contending that the quacks' recourse to saturation advertising may be a sign of desperation, not success.[13]

It was not an easy business decision. For the aim of generating sales outwards from a fixed centre of practice was fraught with dangers – of over-extension, fraud, and, not least, of other dealers pirating one's products. For this reason, certain quacks felt obliged to emphasize, perhaps making a virtue of necessity, that they and they alone sold the real McCoy. Aiming thus to exclude imitators, Comelius à Tilbourg boasted, apropos of his 'Orvietan' poison antidote, 'you must have it from my own hands, or not at all'. 'I have deputed no Person to sell it for me', he averred, 'so that all Pretenders in that Nature, are Cheats'.[14] John Pechey likewise warned readers that only one retail outlet existed – himself – for his medicaments, so as to prevent counterfeiting. How was the reader to know he was getting the genuine article? By identifying the practitioner in person: 'I ride in a Calash with one horse' – important information, he asserted, so that potential patients may be 'better able to know me as I pass by'.[15] But choosing to sell one's product from a single source must have been a rather risky enterprise.

That is surely why other quacks were keen to transcend face-to-face and over-the-counter selling, and instead to develop more sophisticated distribution networks. From Restoration times onwards, some made considerable play of the virtues of postal sales, which had the obvious advantage of promising anonymity. The proprietor of 'The True Spirit of Scurvy-Grass' was proud to announce that:

> By the new ingenious Way of the Penny-Post, any Person may send for it, from any part of the City or Suburbs, writing plain directions where to send it to them: if for half a dozen Glasses, they will be brought as safe, as if fetch't by themselves, and as cheap as one. But who sends this way, must put a Penny in the Letter (besides Six Pence for each Glass) to pay the carriage back; for no body can think the profit great: therefore a Penny must be sent for every Parcel. From one Glass to six, makes a Parcel. None need fear their Money, in sending by the Penny-Post, for things of considerable value, are daily sent with safety by it, security being given for the Messengers. There are Houses appointed in all parts of the Town, to take in the Penny-Post Letters.[16]

Did this procedure work, however? Or did it prove too cumbersome? Certainly, most proprietary medicine vendors preferred to get their wares to the people not through the post but through intermediary dealers, by developing chains of outlets – at the time, a rather novel form of salesmanship. Some promised discounts to wholesalers and retailers willing to serve as stockists. 'Merchants and shopkeepers', announced the proprietor of Radcliffe's Royal Tincture, 'may be supplied with these drops with good allowance to sell again, at Lloyd's Coffee House, Lombard Street, London, Price 1/- a bottle'.[17] In the same vein, the vendor of the Elixir Magnum Stomachicum advised 'if any Captain or Seaman want any Quantities or any keeping a Publick House to dispose of, or sell again, they may be furnished at any time by Letter, or otherwise, from Mr Colbatch's, Stationer'.[18]

It was presumably through clinching such arrangements that many late seventeenth-century vendors were proud to announce dozens of sales outlets for their products. There were about thirty retailers – called somewhat optimistically the vendor's 'trusty friends' – for Jones' Friendly Pill, including stationers, shoemakers, a cane shop, a chandler, a slop shop, a potter's shop, a worsted shop and a toy shop. Already, by the turn of the eighteenth century, a few products were advertised as available nationwide: thus one could buy Stoughton's Grand Cordial Elixir at some fifty shops the length and breadth of the country, including ones in Nottingham, York, Barnstaple, Banbury, and Evesham; and Salmon's Pills were similarly available in London, Worcester, Newbury, Braintree, Ruthin, Lichfield, Stafford, Dorchester, Devizes, and Gloucester, even being sold by a certain Martha Fripp at Cowes on the Isle of Wight. Even these numbers cannot compare with the hundreds of retailers for the Balm of Gilead listed by Samuel Solomon a century later. Not least, like manufacturing chemists, quacks began to look to export markets. Salvator Winter told readers he hoped merchants and mariners would come forward to help sell his medicines 'to France, Germany, Italy, Virginia, New England, Barbadoes, Jamaica and many other places'.[19] Thanks to such developments, the traditional person-to-person quack was perhaps becoming less prominent than the operator acting as the faceless name behind the product.

With such developments, new opportunities, but also new problems, presented themselves. On the one hand, the sedentary quack, the spider at the centre of a distribution web – these were often located in the eighteenth century in Covent Garden – had a much larger potential turnover than the itinerant or the stall-holder. On the other, he was more vulnerable to loss from inept or dishonest subordinates, thus explaining why quacks were so paranoid about counterfeiting (to avoid mistake, Dr John Turner advised readers that his lozenges were sold only in papers, and 'every Paper hath the Impression of the same Coat of Arms with which they are Sealed stamped on the Backside of them').[20] Above all, as the doctor became the 'invisible man' behind the product, still further credibility problems emerged: upon what criteria was this reified healing to be sold?

We have seen the labour which 'Chevalier' Taylor put into investing his own person with authority. What then was the right strategy for an invisible quack? Was he to promote himself, or his product? Whence was his credit to derive? The next chapter will explore the development of advertising tactics as an attempt to grapple with this dilemma, and will show the further problems that such media images created.

Female quacks

I have just been examining the techniques by which irregular practitioners claimed career credibility in the Babel of the medical marketplace. All those discussed were men. But, in fact, quacks were far from exclusively male.

Though the orthodox medical profession was primarily men-only, healing was, of course, an office commonly exercised by women in early modern England – nurses, midwives, Ladies Bountiful, clergymen's wives, and so forth, not to mention 'witches', all operated as healers, some for love and some for money. Possibly, as feminists have argued, the status and practice of such female healers were coming under threat during the long eighteenth century, as the male-dominated medical profession flexed its muscles and expanded into certain traditional women-only domains, such as midwifery. Though research in depth is awaited, there is abundant evidence of the continuing activities of amateur or occasional women, and of their acceptance amongst sufferers, male and female alike, at this time.

Soaring above such 'village Nightingales', a handful of women made names for themselves in the Georgian medical arena. Mrs Joanna Stephens owned a lithontriptic nostrum which she sold to Parliament for £5000 in what was surely the best deal ever clinched by a quack in English history; Sally Mapp, the Epsom bone-setter, was probably the most hailed manipulator of the day; and Bridget Bostock, the Cheshire healer who cured by spittle, won quite a following in the 1740s.

And there were scores of active, if lesser known, female quacks besides, commonly the wives, widows, sisters, or daughters of male quacks. Late in the seventeenth century, 'Agnodice: The Woman Physician, dwelling at the Hand and Urinal' boasted of her Italian Washes and Spanish Rolls good for the 'Scotch Disease, or the Itch'.[21] Or there was a 'gentlewoman on the corner of Coventry Court in the Hay Market' who sold an 'excellent paste for the shaking and trembling of the hands after hard drinking'.[22]

One might suppose that female healers plying a trade for gain were by definition quacks, since they were excluded from the regular medical *cursus honorum* until the late nineteenth century. This is, however, to overstate the case, since it was possible for women to obtain seals of official approval to practise medicine, and when they did so they made as much of them as a Brodum or a Solomon made of his MD. Mrs Mary Green of Chancery Lane boasted in 1693 that she possessed the Archbishop of Canterbury's licence and was expert at curing the 'stoppage of the stomach, Coughing, Shortness of Breath', to say nothing of her ability to discharge 'windy Vapours'; everybody she had treated she had 'perfectly cured', even 'those who have been given over by their Doctors and Chirurgeons'. To prove her skills, she appended testimonials from those a 'long time under the Hands of many Eminent Doctors and Chirurgeons, and found no Relief, and who were in a short time perfectly cured by her'.[23]

It would be foolish, however, to get bogged down in the purely semantic issue of deciding whether all female operators were necessarily quacks, merely by virtue of their gender – the line certainly adopted by contemporary misogynists. Male quacks were despised as the 'bastard brethren' of a male profession; female quacks were sneered at for practising medicine at all. What is beyond dispute, however, is that women healers were no less adroit in exploiting market potential than were the men, putting out bills, advertising in newspapers, and vending distinctive products. Indeed, in one respect, female quacks were in clover. For they had virtually no female regulars against whom to compete. This practically guaranteed them two attractive sections of the market.

On the one hand, they could seize the opportunities for vending products and pills associated with their own sex, not least, beauty preparations. Thus there dwelt a 'Gentlewoman' at Blackfriars, next door to the Sugarloaf, who had 'very rare complexion waters' for the face, and 'makes age look youthful, and takes away freckles, morphew, or sunburn, or any redness or pimples in the face' . She would cure all sorts of women's conditions, including green-sickness, 'with many other things in women not fit to be mentioned'.[24] Various other female quacks also specialized in nostrums for female conditions, for instance, Sarah Cornelius de Heusde, widow of Dr Sasbout, who excelled at curing the 'suffocation or rising of the mother' and 'descending or hanging out of the mother', as well as rendering 'fruitful' 'women or maidens who cannot get their natural Flux'.[25]

At the same time, female quacks could capitalize upon that body of women sufferers unwilling to consult with, or to be examined by, a male doctor. By no means all women had such scruples (as the rise of man-midwifery demonstrates) But some undoubtedly did; for example, Isabella Duke, who wrote to John Locke asking him for his medical advice, stating that failing that, she would go to 'some Quack Doctress', 'for I will never apply myself to any of your sex, if you do not help me'.[26]

Very commonly male and female quacks operated in partnership. A quack bill, signed by a male, would frequently invite female patients so disposed to consult with his wife or sister instead. Abraham Souburg, for example, told readers that if women did not want to consult with him personally, they could see his 'sister', who had been 'brought up all her Life in the knowledge of Physick'. Likewise, Cornelius à Tilbourg appealed to any woman with a condition (such as a 'Rupture or any foul Venereal Distemper or is subject to Obstructions'), which she 'is ashamed to discover… to me', by informing her that she can 'speak to my Wife', who will 'relieve them very secretly'.[27] Along the same lines the proprietor of the 'Herculeon Antidote against the Pox' told women too bashful to consult him that they were welcome to see his wife.[28] Regular doctors can hardly have had this measure available to them, thus giving quack practice one notable advantage over orthodox, and rendering it more 'user-friendly'.

It is noteworthy that the medical colleges and magistrates appear to have taken so little action against female quacks – their practice might well have seemed an abomination in itself, even without the clear hints at procuring abortions contained in certain bills. Female quackery exemplifies how irregular medicine could genuinely be to the fore in providing types of medicines (or, one might say, exploiting patient susceptibilities) which the more rigid structures of orthodox medicine could not match.

4 Quack culture

We have now examined the careers of quacks in their socio-economic milieu: a century of economic growth, rising personal expectations, the extension of commercialization, and consumer spending. Marketing, the service sector, retailing, and the distribution trades were all blossoming. From pills to porcelain, brand-name products became conspicuous items of sale, beneficiaries of advertising, emulative spending, and consumer psychology. The nostrum trade represents the medical aspect of these developments – indeed, the commercialization of healing to become a sector of capitalist innovation.

In this age when people were said to be 'sick by way of amusement' and fashion supposedly dictated people's choice of illnesses, doctors, and medicines, it is not surprising that a sophisticated medical service sector emerged, equipped with manufacturing depots, warehouses, nationwide wholesale and retail marketing facilities, and mass advertising, to cater for, or cash in on these needs. But to grasp the dynamics of consumerism, we must understand the key role played in it by the semiotics of salesmanship, with its seductive soft-sell collusion between manufacturer and customer; no small innovatory part in that was played by medical nostrums, dealing in healing. There is a marked contrast with France.

Quack medicine boomed in England during the long eighteenth century because it went hand in glove with socio-economic dynamics. Quackery was that branch of medicine which boldly promoted itself through the spoken and printed word, to gain the ear and eye, and so captivate the mind of the public. This chapter will dissect quack publicity, exploring the performances, the theatre of the quacks, examining their messages and mythologies, overt and covert, and the resonances they played upon.

With quacks it was publicize or perish: unless they could woo with words and entice with images, their marginal position left all the dice loaded against them. Yet there was nothing so unusual or particularly disreputable *per se* about self-promotion. After Gutenberg, all literate people were in the business of proving – both to their fellow literati and also to *hoi polloi* – that the tongue was a rapier and the pen mightier than the sword. The post-renaissance era was, after all, as Jean-Pierre Agnew emphasizes, the great age of the stage, the courtier, humanistic rhetoric, pulpit oratory, and the euphuistic prose of compliment and dedications. Rhetoric was pivotal to the trivium, itself the foundation-stone of a classical education. Neither was eloquence restricted to words alone. Peter Burke has demonstrated how in the public, pre-bureaucratic, urban cultures developing from the Renaissance, the attention-seeking, strutting, presentation of the self – expressed through posture and gesture, dress and address, carriage and carriages – constituted a magniloquent idiom of its own.

Regular doctors were no dumb-dogs, innocent of, or indifferent to silver-tongued display. As befitted aspirant gentlemen, they set great store by their own mien and demeanour. Even lowly barber-surgeons made themselves conspicuous with their striped poles; and in their shop-windows, apothecaries traditionally displayed medicine-filled

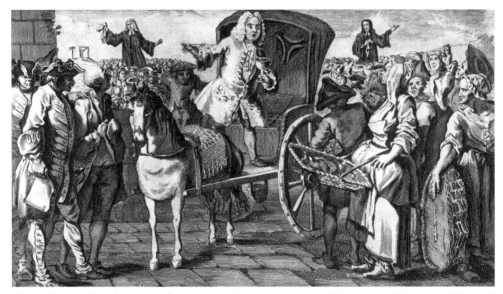

Doctor Rock selling his wares from a horse-drawn carriage on Kennington Common. John and Charles Wesley are preaching in the background. Engraving, 1743.

carboys, stuffed alligators, and pestles and mortars to impress passers-by. Physicians, for their part, sported unmistakable wigs and canes. In Georgian England, it became the mark of the successful physician to lord it in a coach.

Not least, given that so few of their 'cures' worked, it was especially important for the medical profession to present themselves civilly and genteelly. Polite society wanted its physicians to be gentlemanly – explaining why a Classical Oxbridge education remained a passport to success for the fashionable doctor, despite the patent inferiority of the medical training given there to that provided by Leiden or Edinburgh. And a good bedside manner – comforting and consoling where medicine couldn't cure – was, quite properly, as medical ethics manuals pointed out, the *sine qua non* of the humane as well as the unctuous clinician. The princes of the profession in the latter part of the eighteenth century – such men as William Hunter, William Heberden, and Matthew Baillie – were all admired for their culture and breeding.

Not least, doctors spoke their own lingo. Consider the scene in *Tom Jones* in which Fielding shows the surgeon, summoned to treat the hero after his fight with Northerton, being questioned by the lieutenant:

> 'I hope, sir,' said the lieutenant, 'the skull is not fractured.' 'Hum,' cries the surgeon, 'fractures are not always the most dangerous symptoms. Contusions and lacerations are often attended with worse phaenomena…'. 'I hope,' says the lieutenant, 'there are no such symptoms here.' 'Symptoms,' answered the surgeon, 'are not always regular nor constant… I was once, I remember, called to a patient who had received a violent contusion in his tibia by which the exterior cutis was lacerated, so that there was profuse sanguinary discharge;

and the interior membranes were so divellicated, that the os or bone very plainly appeared through the aperture of the vulnus or wound. Some febril symptoms intervening at the same time (for the pulse was exuberant and indicated some phlebotomy), I apprehended an immediate mortification… But perhaps I do not make myself perfectly well understood?' 'No, really,' answered the lieutenant, 'I cannot say I understood a syllable.'[1]

Fielding may or may not have had an honest ear for faculty jargon. But he knew how to show that doctors, deliberately or not, would mystify with words, thereby creating their own mystique (or presumably, if that failed, exposing themselves as pompous, prating asses).

Here we encounter a fundamental ambiguity about the uses of language. On the one hand, the logos was truth ('in the beginning was the Word'), and speech possessed a healing power long before Freud, or rather 'Anna O', spoke of the 'talking cure'. Yet the verbal, or rather, the merely verbal, was suspect. Not least, seventeenth-century philosophy and the 'New Science' espoused a philosophical nominalism that preached radical distrust of language, preferring *res* to *verba*. Philosophical empiricism denounced as a pernicious confusion that forced marriage of words and things, names and power, traditionally endorsed by Scholasticism, by magic, and not least by Christianity itself. To stop such contamination, indeed to prevent diabolism, reality and its verbal signs had to be systematically disengaged (so argued Bacon, Hobbes, and Locke). Otherwise, truth and humanity would be alike enslaved to the idols of the marketplace, tribe, cave, and theatre. 'Words are wise men's counters', pronounced Hobbes, 'they do but reckon by them; but they are the money of fools.' '*Nullius in verba*' echoed the motto of the Royal Society. Words could thus embody the gospel but all too easily, after Babel, they could be cant and casuistry. In view of all this, publicity was fraught with paradox: it could mean bringing information before the public, but it might be lies. Advertising doubtless served honest purposes. 'Blessings on the man… who first invented the loud trumpet of Advertisements', sang Edward Gibbon, after a newspaper insertion succeeded in letting a property of his; but almost contemporaneously, Samuel Johnson was more guarded about their 'promise, large promise'.

In championing the spoken and written word, the quack was thus seizing opportunity, but he was also on the horns of a dilemma and could readily fall into a snare. For in endeavouring to charm his auditors, he had to disarm the suspicions his very presence excited, primed as they were to suspect words as engines of fraud.

How then are we to read quacks' own performances, their bid for the public ear and eye through street-theatre, oratory, handbills, broadsides, verse and, increasingly, pamphlets and newspaper publicity? For one thing, we must note that quacks' use of speech involved important divergences from the verbal exchanges of regular medicine.

The pre-modern regular physician needed, as we have seen, to cultivate an open-ended dialogue with his patient, because only through attending to the patient's history, as narrated to him, was he likely to reach a diagnosis – or, at least, one negotiable with the patient. Some regulars, such as Erasmus Darwin, were noted for their reliance upon more indirect techniques of interrogation – picking up important clues in roundabout ways – but such methods were somewhat controversial. In turn, what the doctor told the patient

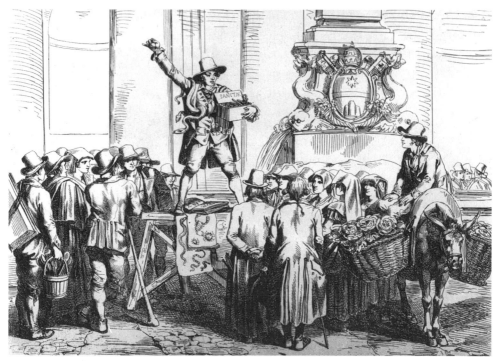

An Italian medicine vendor adorned with a snake sells his wares from a mobile stage. Etching by B. Pinelli, 1821, after himself.

likewise weighed heavily, since the astute clinician's words were held therapeutic in their own right. The good doctor, judged Giorgio Baglivi, needed a 'well-hung tongue'.

The quack was bound to use word-power in rather different ways. Gaining custom in the first place required strong or smooth sales-talk or advertising copy. And then effective psychological persuasion might well be essential to the 'cure' itself (whether or not the sickness was acknowledged to be psychosomatic). Living off his wits, the quack would be wielding words to sell himself and his products.

Thus quackery is a one-way speech system. Unlike the dialogue of regular medicine, the quack's patter is more like monologue or soliloquy, instilling confidence, exercising persuasion, disarming resistance, even – dare one say it? – out-arguing illness. Quackery supposes an impersonal audience (or readership), a crowd of strangers, without a formal speaking part within the 'script'. Though not 'captive', it is expected to be receptive (when did the sick not crave to be well?). The quack's clientele may be compared to a demagogue's auditors, a preacher's congregation, or to theatregoers, without forgetting that the playgoers of the past often answered back.

The words quacks spoke were stage-managed as part of a larger ritual. The traditional quack in renaissance Europe, modelling himself on the Italian *ciarlatani*, prefaced his act by defining a public space, a theatre where his word was king. The mountebank performed from a mobile stage or improvised rostrum to give himself the advantage of height – or, like a general, declaimed from horseback, with the additional advantage of a ready getaway.

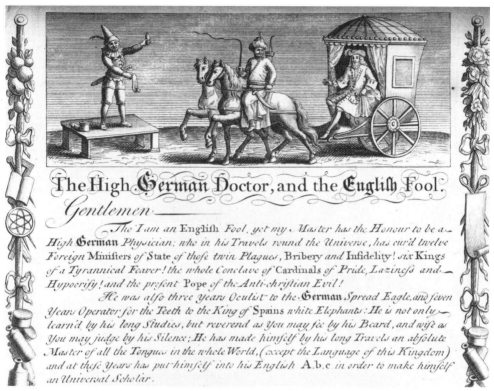

The High German Doctor, and the English Fool.

Gentlemen

Tho' I am an English Fool, yet my Master has the Honour to be a High German Physician; who in his Travels round the Universe, has cur'd twelve Foreign Ministers of State of those twin Plagues, Bribery and Infidelity! six Kings of a Tyrannical Feaver! the whole Conclave of Cardinals of Pride, Laziness and Hypocrisy! and the present Pope of the Anti-christian Evil!

He was also three Years Oculist to the German Spread Eagle, and seven Years Operator for the Teeth to the King of Spains white Elephants: He is not only learn'd by his long Studies, but reverend as you may see by his Beard, and wise as you may judge by his Silence; He has made himself by his long Travels an absolute Master of all the Tongues in the whole World, (except the Language of this Kingdom) and at these Years has put himself into his English A.b.c in order to make himself an Universal Scholar.

An English fool acting as spokesman for a Dutch quack doctor. An ornate border composed of the paraphernalia of quackery surrounds his proclamation. Engraving by G. Bickham.

He appeared in eye-catching garb, something exotic or hinting at an official uniform. He was generally accompanied by a stooge – a harlequin, clown, or zany – whose job it was to draw a crowd and soften up bystanders with fooling, dumb-show, doggerel, conjuring and tumbling, and often to serve as an emotional surrogate for the audience. The act would be backed up by props such as cats, snakes, monkeys, skulls, stuffed alligators, alchemical apparatus and surgical instruments. Banners and bunting would create an atmosphere, music would drum up excitement (and drown the cries of patients having teeth extracted, boils lanced, etc.). Testimonials supposedly penned by satisfied customers and 'patents, certificates, medals and great seals, by which the several princes of Europe have testified their particular respect and esteem for the doctor', festooned the scene.

Some quacks did all the patter themselves. Others – especially foreigners whose English was broken – left the big-talk to their barker, and basked in the mystique of the silent sage. Like all the best circus or vaudeville acts, quack routines blended the familiar and time-honoured with the original, the funny, the thrilling, and the bizarre. The audience was to be won over through a stylized performance that may have had its own placebo effect: a bit of fun and distraction made the sick feel better already.

The tricks of the quack doctors' tirade are familiar. They decried quackery, abhorring it from their very bowels. Yet the regulars were no better – jealous, monopolistic wolves, preying on the people. Mountebanks laid claim to infallible nostrums and pledged to heal the incurable. Many had some special gimmick; 'The Famous High German Operator', John Schultim, was one of many who boasted 'no cure, no money' – detractors retorted that that didn't mean that you escaped fees if you did not get well but that if you had no money, you'd not get treated at all! Some specialized in bargain packs, free pamphlets with every purchase, silver measuring spoons, sugar-coated pills, violin-shaped bottles, treatment gratis for unfortunates or soldiers back from the wars (Sir William Read's special offer), and so forth. Others performed dazzling stunts – their side-kicks would swallow 'poison', and then make miraculous recoveries thanks to wonder antidotes. Most offered reassurance, promising confidentiality for those suffering from unmentionable disorders.

Above all, quacks stirred the emotions. They exploited the psychology of persuasion, mingling hard and soft sells, excitement and amusement, bathos, pathos, surprise, titillation. In playing upon the susceptibilities of the sick, they did not miss a trick – witness, for example, this broadside publicizing James Graham's lectures and healing acts, which conveys some sense of the fever-pitch electricity of his performances:

> NOW OR NEVER. You must come forward to hear and to see, and to receive what never more can be heard or seen in London, or in any other place, so long as the world endures. GRATIS – LECTURES, and a Display of the Celestial Brilliancy of the Temple of Health, before its final close and dissolution, Dr. GRAHAM'S FINAL WILL, LAST BLESSING, and most PATHETIC EXHORTATIONS to the inhabitants of London and Westminster. As the Sale of Dr. GRAHAM'S Furniture and Apparatus is to be next week, he desires respectfully to inform the Public, that THIS, and EVERY EVENING till the Sale, he will have the honour of delivering Gratis, a LECTURE on certain means (without medicines) of preserving life, till at least an hundred and fifty years of age. In the course of the Lecture, he will show mankind, how grossly they have been blinded and imposed upon, and robbed of their health property, and lives, by the Physicians and Apothecaries.
>
> The rooms are now crowded, and over flow every night more and more, as all London, especially the Ladies, seem determined to see this celebrated place – this enchanting elysium in full glory, before its final dissolution – as it now exceeds in splendour, elegance, brilliancy and magnificence, every Royal Palace in the world.
>
> Singing by a Young LADY. + + + Ladies are requested to come very early. The Lecture begins at Half past Seven o'clock.
>
> Free admission to the whole, to every Lady and Gentleman who purchases, price only one Shilling, The Guardian of Health, Long Life, and Happiness.
>
> N.B. As the Temple has overflowed by several hundred persons, each of the three last nights, those Ladies and Gentlemen who wish earnestly to be admitted, must come, indeed, very early.[2]

How are we to assess showmanship such as this? Graham excelled in over-the-top, blatant hyperbole, promising the impossible – and more besides. Did he expect it to be believed? Did, indeed, audiences believe it? Were they so credulous? Or are we witnessing theatricality, astutely carried to the point of self-parody, the cultivation of pure make-believe, accepted as such on both sides? Perhaps it was of the essence of the quack's act that his blarney was known to be baloney. Was, then, getting people to listen, and entertaining them with tall stories, the name of the game? Did some quacks even want to rouse disbelief at the preposterousness of it all, provoking chaffing, catcalls, and heckling?

Let us address more systematically the rhetorical language of the quack, from reports of their live shows, handbills, and publicity. Quack doctors perfected the ringmaster's patter, what John Wilmot, Earl of Rochester, jokingly called their 'damn'd unintelligible gybberish'. Their cadences aimed at the heart, the pocket, the eye, and their skilful blend of the technical, absurd, and humorous was perfectly caught in Ned Ward's satiric vignette of the charlatan in full cry before the 'Listening Herd', demonstrating 'a Pacquet of Universal Hodg-Podg':

> Gentlemen, you that have a Mind to be Mindful of preserving a Sound Mind in a Sound Body, that is, as the Learned Physician, Doctor *Honorificicabilitudinitatibusque* has it, Manus Sanaque in Cobile Sanaquorum, may here at the expense of sixpence, furnish himself with a parcel, which tho' it is but small, yet containeth mighty things, of great Use and Wonderful Operation in the Bodies of Mankind, against all Distempers, whether Homogeneal or Complicated; whether deriv'd, from your Parents, got by Infection, or proceeding from an ill Habit of your own Body.
>
> In the first place, Gentlemen, I here present you with a little inconsiderable Pill to look at, you see not much bigger than a Corn of Pepper, yet in 'this Diminutive Phanpharmica so powerful in effect, and of such excellent Vertues, that if you have Twenty Distempers lurking in the Mass of Blood, it shall give you just Twenty Stools, and every time it operates, it carries off a Distemper; but if your Blood's Wholesome, and your Body Sound it will work you no more than the same quantity of Ginger bread. I therefore call it, from the admirable Qualities, *Pillula Tondobula*, which signifies in the Greek, *The Touch Stone of Nature*; For by taking of this Pill you will truly discover what state of Health or Infirmity your constitution is then under… [and so forth].[3]

The quack's spiel manipulated a rhetoric combining assurance, hyperbole, and bombast. Addressing the public, not his peers, he first softened up his auditors with flattery. 'Beloved Women', cried Stephen Draper, 'who are the Admirablest Creatures that ever God created under the Canopy of Heaven, to whom therefore, I have devoted my studies to the preserving of your Beauty, Health, Vigour, Strength and Long Life',[4] unfolding to them his skills as a man-midwife and his techniques for making the barren conceive. The operator then needed to establish his own credentials, by stating his pre-eminence and boasting a roll-call of celebrated cures. For example, though modestly denying being 'an infallible worker of miracles', James Graham offered himself not just as 'a graduate Physician of a British College'

– not, strictly speaking, accurate – and as 'an experienced and loving Minister of NATURE', but also as 'a student of that university of truth… whose omnipotent Founder and eternal Chancellor is the infinitely glorious Creator and Preserver of the Universe'. With an eye to the *ton*, John Taylor, self-styled 'Chevalier', liked to fanfare himself as 'The Chevalier John Taylor, Ophthalmiator, Pontifical, Imperial, and Royal, who treated Pope Benedict XIV, Augustus III, King of Poland, Frederick V, King of Denmark and Norway and Frederick Adolphus, King of Sweden'[5] – with a list of further notable patients as long as your arm.

Before the nineteenth century, however, quacks did not commonly 'graduate themselves' – regale themselves with phoney professional qualifications, invented degrees, or diplomas from bogus institutions. Quacks' colleges were a nineteenth-century vanity. It was much more common – and was believed to be far more impressive – to assume rank, connections, and charisma; hence quacks often portrayed themselves as hyper-experienced 'artists' and 'masters' of arcana, having acquired the most profound wisdom through tireless travels and by squatting at the feet of sages. For example, the 'High German Doctor, who by his great Study, and constant Practice in several Parts of the World, as well in Princes' Courts, as in Hospitals, and War-like Expeditions hath obtained such a Physical Method, as to Cure all external and internal Distempers (if curable)'. This operator made much of his 'Testimonials, not only from Kings, Dukes, and Electoral Princes', but also, nearer home, 'from the right honourable the Lord Mayor of London'.[6]

Next, they bragged of the extraordinary virtue of their nostrums. One favourite claim was that they would cure all, as with Bromfield's 'Pillulae in Omnes Morbos, or Pills against all Diseases', which would particularly eradicate all the 'chief Signs of the Scurvey', including 'Giddiness in the Head, sudden Flushings, Heat, and Redness in the Face, and Body, Putrification and Stinking of the Gums, Tooth-ach, Stinking-breath, Blackness and Looseness of the Teeth, want of Digestion, much Wind and unsavory Belchings, and by thick Vapours arising from the HYPOCHONDRIA to the Midriff'. Bromfield was playing a devious double game, because he also disclaimed hyperbole – unlike those vermin, the quacks – trusting that the 'Reader will not judge the worse of me or my Pills, because I have not herein commended them with high-strained praises and boastings, which way of setting off any thing, I am very sure, the wise man likes not.' Disclaimers aside, he was, nevertheless, too public-spirited to hide his light under a bushel, for the 'Pillulae in Omnes Morbos' were, beyond doubt, the 'most excellent medicine [that] was ever in like manner disposed of'.[7]

There were other panaceas. John Case termed one of his seven preparations the 'Universal Medicine', the 'Mundus Sanitatus, or his World of Health' (it had the added virtue of keeping 'for forty years').[8] Case had an eye for the bold, even brazen, headline. One of his bills was headed in great gothic letters: 'A Most Infallible, and Sure, Cheap, Secret, Safe and Speedy Cure for a Clap', continuing with the sub-heading: 'Of him the Sick may have Advice for Nothing', followed beneath by, 'And good Medicines cheap'.[9]

Likewise, John Newman's pills were 'never-failing', and William Patence ('dentist and physician to several of the Royal family') similarly presented his 'Universal Medicine or Supreme Pills' as a 'catholicon', or panacea, with the usual rigmarole of knockdown prices and 'money-back-if-not-satisfied' guarantees. 'I shall offer no apology for my medicine', apologized Patence,

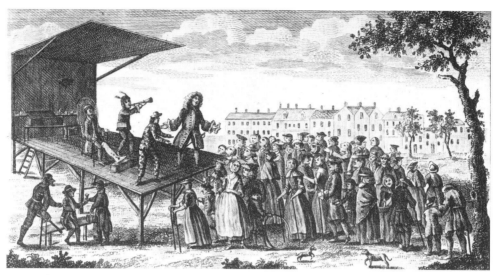

A 'High German Doctor' promoting his wares before an audience of townspeople. Etching by T. Kitchin.

which is well-known to give ease and satisfaction in palsies, gout, rheumatism, piles, fistulas, cancers of any sort, King's Evil, hereditary infections, jaundice, green sickness, St. Anthony's Fire, convulsions, consumptions, scorbutic diseases, pains in the head, brain, temple, arteries, face, nose, mouth, and limbs, for which nothing upon the earth is surer, softer or better. The Universal Medicine also restores lost hearing and sight, renews the vital and animal vitalities, gives complexion to the face, liveliness to the whole structure, and many times has given unexperienced relief on the verge of eternity… if they do not answer the end proposed, I will return the Money. The real worth of a box is Ten Guineas, but for the benefit of all, with proper directions, it is sold for three shillings; with personal advice, ten and sixpence.[10]

If Patence healed all known diseases, the 'High German Doctor' went one better, curing 'many other Distempers which no Physician can give name to'. His boast that 'he hath cured such when given over by others as incurable' was irresistible. Many quacks spelt out great lists of diseases their powders would pulverize. Thus the bill of an anonymous 'Physician in High Holbom' claimed his medicines were excellent for venereal disease, not to mention,

Consumptions
All sorts of Fevers
Pain in the Head and Stomack
Such as cannot hold their Water
Stone in the Bladder or Kidneys
Convulsions Rickets

Ptisick or shortnesse of breath
Red hair may be changed
Gouts several sorts
Wind Cholick
Sore leggs or old Ulcers
Dropsies, as Timpany, &
Barrennesse
Abortiveness
Old Surfeits Agues
Sinewes sprained
Pain in the Back of Limbs
Stoppage in the Urine
Kings Evil Falling sicknesse
Worms Ruptures
Rheumatick Defluctions
Yellow Jaundice
Cankers Sciatica
Loosenesse
Sore Eyes Freckles
Piles and Emrods
Obstructions of Women
Immoderate Fluxes…

'with many others', he concluded his tabulation, adding darkly, 'some not convenient, others too tedious to be here inserted'.[11]

The miracle cure was the Himalaya of hyperbole. 'He Cured a Child (next Door to the Black Horse in Market Lane near St. James's Market)' – ran the bill of another 'High German Doctor' – 'that was Born Blind, in 13 days time. John Humel of the Parish of S. Thomas in the City of Bristol, aged 72, and Alice Diddel of the Parish of Temple in the said City aged Fourscore Years, and that they had been Blind 9 Years, he restored their sight immediately, and perfectly cured both them and others in 14 days.'[12] Hyperbole was of the essence of the quack bill. Sometimes it came in full-frontal form, as with the bill which presented 'Three Infallible Cures', felling scurvy, the pox, and gonorrhoea, 'without hazzard either of BODY, PURSE, or REPUTATION'. The proprietor of the 'Pulvis Benedictus' begged to announce that his preparation was 'more like a Miracle than a Medicine, especially as a worm cure, for 'raro corpus nostrum sine vermibus'. The pious quack heading his bill, 'Nothing Without God', disclosed that the Lord had been so good that 'he hath given to me many large Talents', thanks to which he possessed 'a perfect Cure for Consumptions, Coughs', etc., – all these, 'with many other Diseases, are by the Blessing of God by me Cured.'[13] Almost out-hyperboling hyperbole was the 'Incomparable Extractum Humoreale called also Panaseton, from that Universal Operation it hath upon all Humoral Diseases', prepared by that public benefactor, Edward Ewel, who signed himself 'doctor of physick'.[14]

On occasion, hyperbole came with a jolly swagger, as in the 'Panoplia Medica or a Medicinal Armour for the Whole Body, Proof against the Invasion of Sickness, being

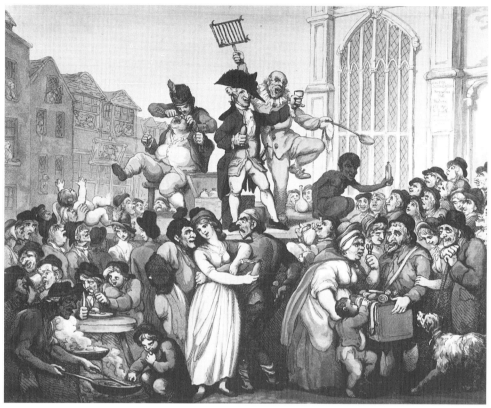

'Doctor Botherum', perhaps based on Doctor Bossy, sells his wares to a raucous crowd with the aid of assistants. Coloured engraving by T. Rowlandson, 1800.

Composed of the greatest Arcana' – a fistful of different medicines prepared by Edward Andrews, MD, which included the 'Great Stomach Pill', for the support of that 'noble Part', a 'Grand Antiscorbutick' called 'Anima Cochleariae', the 'Alexiterial Balsamick Lozenge' for the Lungs, and the 'Tincture of Mars' for Melancholy – four medicines which between them would cure all ills.[15]

What's in a name? When it came to nostrums, the answer was anything. The brand-labels of the preparations were naturally carefully chosen to evoke their promise. Certain tags traded on the fame of their begetter – Dr James's Powders, or Daffy's Elixir, the latter immortalizing a Stuart clergyman and still on sale this century. Many incorporated superlatives, sailing under such flags as the 'Infallible Powder', 'The Only True Plague Water', 'The HERCULEON ANTIDOTE', or the 'Sovereign Cordial'. Or there was 'Rose's Balsamick Elixir', 'The Most Noble Medicine that Art can produce... a signal Restorative for Consumptive persons and there is not such another preparation in the whole world... It cures the English Frenchify'd beyond all the other medicines upon the face of the Earth. It removes all pains in 3 or 4 doses and makes any man, tho' rotten as a Pear, to be sound as a suckling lamb.'[16] Quack-bill headlines evoked total cure, health, and happiness. As a contemporary indictment, Daniel Turner's *The Modern Quacks*, snarled, 'at the end of each of these Remedies (being part of the Bait), I find some very inviting Term, such as Angelic, Royal, Incomparable, Odoriferous... Specifick, (which is now become the universal Epithet, if it were but for a Remedy for broken-winded or founder'd Horses; so that in a little time we shall doubtless have Specificks to kill Rats and Mice (about which their Time and Medicines would be better employ'd) as there are already for Lice and Fleas) and most of them Admirable, Infallible, or Never-failing."[17]

Alongside such verbal extravaganzas went the exploitation of 'hard names' – authentic or bogus jargon calling to mind scientific discoveries, the occult, or craft mysteries. This orotund cant, making free with neologisms, doubtless traded on the spellbinding associations of conjuring, the lure of the obscure, the sublimity of the arcane, with a bravura topping of virtuoso pyrotechnics. 'I am a High-German Doctor', announced a German quack of the seventeenth century (there were many around):

> who, by the blessing of Aesculapius on his great Pains, Travels and Nocturnal Lucubrations, has attained to a greater share of knowledge than any person before him was ever known to do. IMPROMIS. Gentlemen, I present you with my 'Universal Solutive', which corrects all the Cacochymick and Cachexical Disease of the Intestines, Hydrocephalous, Epileptick Fits, Flowing of the Gall and many other distempers not hitherto distinguished by name. Secondly, My 'Friendly Pills' call'd the Never Failing Heliogenes, which by dilating and expanding the Gelastick Muscles, first of all discovered by myself. They clear the Officina Intelligentiae, correct the Exorbitancy of the Spleen, mundify the Hypogastrium, comfort the Sphincter and are an excellent remedy against Prosopo Chlorosis or Green sickness. They operate seven several ways viz. Hypnotically, Hydrotically, Cathartically, Proppysinatically, Hydragogically, Pulmatically, and lastly Synecdochically, by corroborating the whole Oeconomia Animalis.[18]

Within this rhetorical phantasmagoria, quacks were deft at manipulating quite specific allusions carrying 'pull' and prestige. Many annexed the buzz-words of natural philosophy, aiming to blind with science. Some boasted their powers of natural philosophy, as, for example, Gustavus Katterfelto with his expertise in the 'Philosophical, Mathematical, Optical, Magnetical, Electrical, Physical, Chemical, Pneumatic, Hydraulic, Hydrostatic, Proetic, Stenographic, Blaenical and Caprimatic Arts'. Product names often drew on the authority of seats of learning, such as the 'Oxon Pills' for scurvy (*nomen est omen*), or on the fame of top doctors and scientists: 'Dr Boerhaave's Aurea Medicina' (whose vendor modestly confessed 'I cannot venture to say of them, as Quacks do of their Trash, that they will infallibly cure everything'), or 'Dr Radcliffe's Famous Purging Elixir', 'or the General Rectifier of the Nerves, Head and Stomach [which] corrects all irregularities of the Head and Stomach by hard drinking or otherwise.... It is the best purl in the world: in beer, ale or wine, or purl royal in sack.'[19]

Similarly, the 'Chevalier' Taylor endlessly name-dropped the geniuses he had met on his travels – Boerhaave, Haller, Morgagni, Winslow, Monro, Linnaeus, and the Hunters –

dedicating his monograph, *An Exact Account of Two Hundred and Forty-Three Diseases to which the Eye and its Coverings are Exposed* (1749), to the Royal College of Physicians of Edinburgh: 'grateful for the Remembrance I have, of the Attention which some of your Body judged me worthy of, by so frequently favouring me with their Presence at my Lectures, and Method of Practice, and by their giving me such undeniable Proofs of the good Opinion they have of me, from the many they have recommended to my Care.'

Many nostrum-mongers thus quested cachet by latching on to the lights of science and physic. The 'Pilula Salutiferens' was claimed by its proprietor to have been first prepared by the 'famous Dr. Sydenham for his own use, who afterwards prescribed it with incredible success throughout the vast extent of his laborious practice'. Salvator Winter boasted his 'Elixir Vitae' was recommended by Sir Kenelm Digby. Another vendor traded on the prestige of none other than Robert Boyle as 'the inventor of an Effectual pill': 'That the world may no longer be deceived by the false and ignorant pretenders to Physick, of which this City has more than enough; I present to all the ingenious, the most Effectual Pills of which the ever-honoured Esquire Boyle was the Author.'[20]

Dr Paul Chamberlain, marketer of a teething necklace for children, staked his claims to the secrets of dental health on 'a treatise dedicated to the Royal Society', and Daffy's Elixir similarly bore a label attesting the blessing of 'Dr. King, physician to Charles II and the late learned Dr. Radcliffe'. When, early in his career, he made great play of the vogue science of electricity (calling one of his medicines the 'Electrical Aether'), James Graham was glad to trace his own pedigree back to Cullen, Whytt, Priestley, and Franklin (he later dissociated himself from such yesterday's men).

Passing off remedies as the brainchildren of modern masters was a plausible ploy because, as we have seen, regular physicians themselves lent their names to market-brands. And so the practice multiplied, Dr Adair being outraged to find that 'the names of FOTHERGILL, HUNTER and SOLANDER have been prostituted to those knavish purposes'.[21] It exemplifies how the 'advertising professors' strategically appropriated the prestige of scientific discovery and progress. Leading Stuart and Georgian quacks were not repudiating the physic of the great and the good, but hoping to hitch their own waggons to its star. Yet if the 'new science' held great appeal for the quacks, as eclectics they did not neglect the selling power of traditional cosmologies and the arts of magic, alchemy, and astrology. Thomas Saffold and John Case, in particular, cast horoscopes as well as dealing in nostrums.

Take, for example, the manipulation by quacks of the 'natural symbols' of the cosmos. Quacks needed to suggest they were masters of universal power, adepts at tapping the arcana of nature, and distilling them into the compass of a pill. Now hinting at the new science, now harking back to the old occultism, nostrum-mongers made great play with the associations of the elements and the precious metals. Mercury, a specific against syphilis, united the secrets of alchemy and astrology with the vaunted efficacy of the new heavy-metal medicines. Gold-remained another potent icon of natural power, appearing, for example, in the form of potable gold ('aurum potabile') and in the best-selling 'Cordial Balm of Gold', manufactured by the late eighteenth-century Liverpudlian Dr Samuel Solomon, who, in his *Guide to Health* – dedicated to Lord Mansfield, no less – described it as 'extracted from the seed of gold, which our alchemists and philosophers have so long sought after in vain'.[22]

No less symbolically charged were the heavens. 'Solar' medicines enjoyed a great vogue, perhaps focusing the Enlightenment's fascination with light. There were James Graham's pills, 'a pure extract drawn by the sunbeams', Lionel Lockyer's 'Pilulae Radiis Solis Extractae', which Lockyer astutely stipulated were to be swallowed before one fell sick, 'England's Solar Pill against the Scurvy', Fletcher's 'Panacea', a 'medicine of a Solar (or Gold like) nature', and, not least, the Hatton Garden quack, Dr George Jones's 'Famous Friendly Pill', 'being the Tincture of the Sun, having dominion from the same light, giving Relief and Comfort to all mankind… a wonder among other wonderful medicines'. Dr Ebenezer Sibly, empiric and mason, patented a 'Reanimating Solar Tincture or Pabulum of Life', but probably made more money from his 'Lunar Tincture', which, with its hints at menstruation, was aimed at female complaints.

The appeal to science was thus often complemented by the more traditional aura of the occult and of alchemy. Yet the 'advertising professors' clearly believed the kudos of science invaluable, for no proprietary drugs boasted of exploding the newfangled heresies of modern science and physic. True, various remedies were still marketed whose allure was essentially homely, for example, 'Mother Bedlicot's Drink for the Dropsy', or such folksy drugs (mocked in *The Modern Quacks*) as a 'Coal-heaver's Decoction, and Old-Woman's Plaister and Oyntment, [and] a Tarpaulin's East India Oyl'. What is noteworthy, however, especially in contrast to Victorian popular medicines, is the absence of a call to radical alternatives. Eighteenth-century proprietary medicines did not carry primitivist 'back to the earth', 'back to nature', purity crusades; quite the reverse, for Georgian empirics and their nostrums basked in the reflected glory of the Enlightenment.

Eager for legitimation, quack medicines also latched on to religion, or, in a critic's very palpable hit, 'you will say you committed yourself to Providence as well as Prunes'. A handful of healers claimed a personal thaumaturgical mission, as perhaps James Graham, who in his born-again years, styled himself 'Servant of the Lord O.W.L. [O Wondrous Love]', or the theatrical designer, Philip de Loutherbourg, who practised mesmeric healing and claimed to have 'received a most glorious power from the Lord Jehovah viz; the gift of healing all manner of diseases incident to the human body, such as blindness, deafness, lameness, cancers, loss of speech and palsies.'

Others appealed to Christian healing through charity, for instance, Henry Hippen, whose regular cures cost forty shillings, but 'FOR THOSE THAT HAVE NO MONEY AND DESIRE IT FOR GOD's SAKE, HE WILL CURE GRATIS';[23] or the 'faithful physician lately arrived in this Kingdom' whose claim was 'The poor I cure gratis'.[24] But most common in nostrum publicity were verbal hints of supernatural qualities: sometimes miracle cures were alluded to ('miraculous anodyne necklaces'), sometimes divine physic authenticated by the Bible, as in the many 'Balm of Gilead' preparations on sale.

Often the religious overtone was ecumenical, and not even specifically Christian. Thus James Graham evoked pagan mythological healing with his 'Temple of Health and Hymen', equipped with its 'Apollo Room' and a priestess styled 'Hebe Vestina', the 'Goddess of Youth and Health'; significantly, Graham occupied the Adelphi Building off the Strand, designed by the Adam brothers, at the height of the neo-classical vogue. Even 'Mecca Pills' were, perhaps surprisingly, on offer, marketed by the Jewish Dr Solomon;

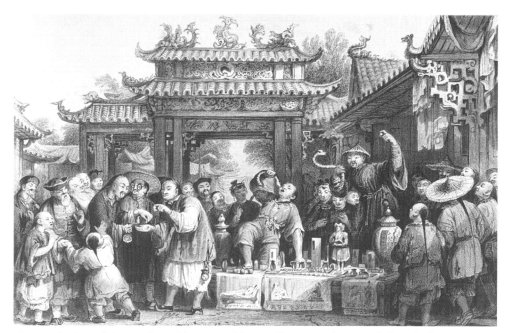

An entusiastic medicine vendor in Tien-sing, China, sells to an audience with the aid of assistants and snakes. Engraving by P. Lightfoot after T. Allom.

here it was presumably the oriental rather than the specifically Islamic references that were meant to catch the eye.

In the nostrum trade's annexation of holiness what is most intriguing is the range of overt references to Roman Catholicism. Saints and Catholic worthies were commonly invoked, as in the 'Pulvis Benedictus' ('rather a miracle than a medicine'), the 'anodyne necklaces' made from the bones of St Hugh, and 'Fuller's Benedictine Pills'; but there was also 'Friar's Balsam', the 'Catholique Medicine' (catholic having the connotation of universal), and, most explicitly of all, Dr Trigg's 'Golden Vatican Pill', at two shillings a box. Of course, healing and holiness are etymologically of a piece, and 'patter' comes from the Pater Noster, but the prominence of Catholic thaumaturgy is intriguing in a land of belligerent 'No Popery'.

Its presence was, indeed, a source of great anxiety. The author of *The Modern Quacks*, Daniel Turner, demanded that all such 'Popish Trumpery' be cast into the fire, lamenting over the anodyne necklaces, 'Ah England! England! that it ever should be said of thee, that even the meanest Masters of thy Families (since Popery and Superstition have been banish'd hence) should permit, or the Mistresses thereof desire, such Childish Trinkets (fit only to amuse Ideots or Fools) to be brought in, or hung about their Children's Necks, in Expectation of Advantage by the same?'[25] Turner feared that medicine-chests would prove Trojan horses: unable to convert Britain by open proselytizing, the Vatican was clandestinely infiltrating the nation through its ailments. A few eighteenth-century operators, such as Joshua Ward, did, indeed, have Jacobite sympathies; many had spent time travelling in Catholic Europe; and, of course, plenty of the quacks operating in

England were natives of France, Italy, and Poland, where it was routine to capitalize on the healing powers of hallowed waters, rosary-style beads, and the laying-on of hands. Salvator Winter, the preternaturally long-lived Italian who vended restoratives, thus opened his spiel, 'Seeing the great wonderful Success it hath pleased Almighty God to bless this my Elixir with…'

As Ramsey, Devlin, and others have shown, holy healing continued in France within overtly ecclesiastical protocols. But, saddled with a confession that regarded the mystical and sacramental apparatus of healing as superstitious, vulgar, and fetishistic, Protestant Englishmen had to slake their thirst for holy healing outside their own Church – either in the residual folklore of witchcraft and magic or through the mystique of patent medicines. Such an interpretation, endorsed by Keith Thomas,[26] echoes the contemporary judgement of Lady Mary Wortley Montagu that the relics of popish superstition, expelled through the door, simply flooded back in again through the window, transmogrified into quackery. 'The English', she contended,

> are easyer than any other Nation infatuated by the prospect of universal medicines, nor is there any country in the World where the doctors raise such immense Fortunes. I attribute it to the Fund of Credulity which is in all Mankind. We have no longer faith in Miracles and Reliques, and therefore with the same Fury run after Receipts and Physicians. The same Money which 300 years ago was given for the Health of the Soul is now given for the Health of the Body, and by the same sort of People: Women and half-witted Men. In the countries where they have shrines and Images, Quacks are despis'd and Monks and Confessors find their account in managing the Fear and Hope which rule the actions of the Multitude.[27]

In addition to science and religion, medical entrepreneurs showed an eye to the main chance in exploiting the suggestive power of language in other ways. Scores of seventeenth- and eighteenth-century nostrums and health advice pamphlets were marketed with brand-names, letter-press, and tags in foreign tongues. Of course, mirroring the kudos of orthodox physic, Latin was the favourite language, though a few, such as John Badger's 'Olbion' cordial, also squeezed in the occasional Greek maxim from Hippocrates. Nostrums whose very names were Latinized include the 'Elixir Vitae' of Salvator Winter, the 'Elixir Magnum Stomachicum' of Richard Stoughton, Dr Pordage's 'Pilulae Anti-Scorbuticae', Bromfield's 'Pilulae in Omnes Morbos', Edward Ewel's 'Panaseton, or Extractum Humoreale', Edward Andrews' 'Gremelli Pulmonates', and Lionel Lockyer's 'Pilulae Radiis Solis Extractae'. There were numerous 'Aurum Potabile' and 'Aqua Coelestis' products, and one could also buy the 'Arcanum Magnum', the 'Solamen Miseris', the 'Elixir Proprietatis', the 'Pilula Salutiferens', the 'Panchimagogum Febrifugum', and dozens besides. Numerous quacks plumed themselves on their classical erudition, 'Chevalier' Taylor, in particular, claiming to lecture in 'the true Ciceronian, prodigiously difficult and never attempted in our language before'. These pretensions were constantly ridiculed, for example in an anonymous pamphlet of 1676, which accused the quack of engaging some 'friend that's Book-learn'd to correct the false English and sprucify the sence, and interlard it with Proverbial Latin and Cramp words, as a gammon of bacon is stuft with green herbs and cloaves'. Throughout the century, in the endless pamphlet skirmishes involving quacks, many took great delight in nitpicking rivals' French accents, Latin syntax, and terminations.

In parading their classical technical terms and proverbs, quacks recognized that the medium was the message, and clearly hoped to have their cake and eat it. Conspicuous skills in learned languages would help to assimilate them to 'high medicine', while also leaving the ignorant awestruck. If Classical words were all Greek to them, *hoi polloi* would at least have to acknowledge that quack doctors belonged to the same genteel world of erudition as liberal professionals such as parsons and lawyers. In any case, it would be patronizing to presume that none of the purchasers of proprietary medicines had any familiarity with Latin. And if, as suggested, a fair segment of quacks' clientele actually came from the more affluent and educated ranks – and some must have, for nostrums sold at prices up to half a guinea – Latin offered a cosy rapport between practitioner and customer, an earnest of ability.

Classical tongues conjured up the mystique of venerable tradition. But hardly less common in quack medicines was an appeal to faraway places with strange-sounding names, peddled by practitioners claiming to hail from, or to be steeped in the wisdom of distant parts. Pepys deplored 'the absurd nature of Englishmen, that cannot forebear laughing and jeering at anything that looks strange'. Yet, in medicine at least, the foreign carried kudos, surely because so many of the leaders of the fine and performing arts in early modern England came from the Continent. The public looked abroad for the spring of medical innovation – for instance, a certain foreign 'Unborn DOCTOR' claimed to cure the pox without fluxing, by a 'Method never in England till now'.[28]

There were certain brews that traded on native loyalties, such as the 'Pilulae Londinenses', the 'British Pills', the 'British Oil', and the 'Scots Pills' ('excellent after hard drinking'); but exoticism was seductive, and rich pickings beckoned the foreign-born quack doctor from 'beyond the Seas' to the English circuit. Up to the end of the seventeenth century, the Italian mountebank was perhaps most common, both in the flesh and as caricatured in drama and satire. Generally licensed by the Crown, Italians such as Salvator Winter – later succeeded by his son – promoted elixirs of life, and, above all, poison antidotes, especially the 'Incomparable Orvietan', the link with poisons being hardly surprising as Italy was synonymous in the public mind with Borgian skullduggery. French quacks were also much in evidence, offering themselves as nonpareil in treating the morbus Gallicus (or French pox), with remedies such as the 'Paris Pill';' but by the close of the seventeenth century, quacks were pouring in from all parts, High and Low Germans, and Germanic Jews, such as Drs Bossy and Brodum, becoming common in the eighteenth century. A sprinkling of outlandish cures even came from as far afield as Poland and Turkey, before the nineteenth century brought its massive influx of alternative medical systems from the New World (though a 'Paraguay tooth-powder' was on sale in the eighteenth century).

Exotic tags for nostrums were clearly a favoured selling feature. In 1698, Frederick van Neurenburg – like so many others long billed as 'just arrived' – was offering a one-man Cook's tour round the pharmacopoeia, vending the 'Persian Balsam and Powder, which cures all Fluxes and sharp corrosive Humours in the Blood. The Asian Balm, the American Balsam and Essence, by the use of which the Americans are generally strangers to the Gout. The Japan Powder which expels all manner of worms. The Chinese Antidote for rheumatism. The Empirical Pill for the Ague. The Grecian and Turkish Antidote which prevents fainting. The Arabian Antidote that prevents and cures the Ptysick and Consumption. The Balsam of Gilead for internal pains…'[29]

Trading on the mysteries of names, many quacks hinted that exotic wisdom had brushed off on to them on their serpentine travels, as for example: 'a most famous, German, Turkish and Imperial Physitian can shew his testimonials from Three Emperors, Nine Kings, as also from Seven Dukes, and Electoral Princes, as the Romish, Turkish, and Japanese Emperors; he can shew his testimonials in 36 languages, which no other doctor can shew. He hath cured the brother of the Turkish Emperor, which was blind thirteen years and hath obtained his natural sight again. This German Physitian has travelled through three parts of the world.'[30] 'I believe', Joseph Addison slyly remarked in the Tatler, 'I have seen twenty mountebanks that have given physic to the Czar of Muscovy'[31]

It was, after all, the seventeenth and eighteenth centuries that saw European receptivity to the wisdom of the East reach high-water mark. Before the nineteenth-century Evangelical and Utilitarian new brooms, Europe was still respectful towards Semitic wisdom and the allure of the Levant and the Orient – an awe magnified in the branding of proprietary medicines. Cagliostro touted 'Egyptian Pills', powdered 'mummy' was a favourite long-life preparation, and inoculation was brought to England from Asia Minor, not long after those other health aids, coffee and the hummums. Some came from farther afield, such as the 'Indian Gattee' for scurvy. Significantly, Bishop Berkeley chose to unfold the secrets of his tar-water cure-all in a work entitled *Siris*, the old Ethiopian name for the Nile (tar-water itself was supposed to be concentrated, etherealized sunshine).

All the hullabaloo about 'Eastern promise' offered sitting targets for satirists and detractors. 'We have Salves and Waters without Number', mocked Daniel Turner: 'some of them as far fetch'd as Jerusalem, tho' they never travelled perhaps a Mile from the Exchange; …for the Toothache, Tinctures, etc. and to whiten them Dentifrices, or Powders from Morocco, China, and Japan; for the Mouth, Gargles and Washes, many; for the whole Face and Hands, Chymical Washballs, besides Pearls, Cream Balls, White-Pots, and Custards, some from Rome and Italy, others from Venice.'[32] Yet this orchestration of symbols also shows medical entrepreneurs trying to cash in on a smart Enlightenment cosmopolitanism. Commercial medicine was not yet selling the line that healing, like charity, began at home (a view revived in the Victorian folksy piety that God had blessed each nation with cures for its own diseases).

One further source of prestige tapped time and again in quack medicine publicity and puffery was social cachet. The labels of proprietary medicines read like a bottled *Burke's Peerage*, echoing the titles of the high and mighty. Alongside 'Sintelaer's Royal Decachor', you could try James Graham's 'Imperial Pills' or Samuel Major's 'Imperial Snuff'; then there was the 'Duke of Portland's Powder' for that aristocratic disease, the gout; 'Lady Moor's Drops' and the 'Countess of Kent's Powder' for plague, tapping the tradition of

George Berkeley. Line engraving.

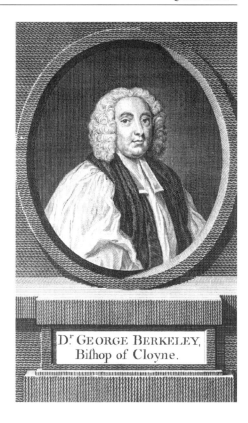

Dʳ GEORGE BERKELEY,
Biſhop of Cloyne.

Lady Bountiful as dispenser of household medicine; and, not least, the 'Princesses Powder', precisely as used by 'four great beautiful European princesses'. Any many quack doctors cried up their (real or Mittyish) connections with royalty.

Quacks endlessly dropped names. A 'High German Doctor' headed his bills 'By the KING and QUEENS Authority'; Cornelius à Tilbourg, a Netherlandish quack, claimed to have been 'Sworn Chirurgeon to the late King Charles the Second', and was saving lives with his 'never failing Remedies' under William and Mary by 'their Majesties Special License and Authority'. Major Choke proudly announced his elixir had cured the Duke of Buckingham of an ague 'when all physicians had left him' Similarly, the vendor of an 'excellent Cephalick Water, or Liquid Snuff', which 'cures Swimmings in the Head, Giddiness, Dizziness, or Vapours, proceeding from intemperate Drinking', boasted he had prepared it 'for our late most Gracious Queen' (Anne) and traded under a royal crest. Possessing a licence or patent could be turned to commercial advantage, for the seal seemed to imply royal use or endorsement. So in 1695, Madam Gordan of Goodman's Fields headed her medical bill 'By His Majesty's Authority' (a common headline) and rounded it off 'VIVAT REX'

This lightning tour of quack publicity has highlighted its hidden agenda of mythologies. Commercial medicine cashed in on the prestige symbols of the times, aiming to make medicine smart, intriguing, and even fun. Some further distinctions are, however, called for. The passage from the Restoration through to the Georgian heyday saw certain modifications in medium and message. This chapter will conclude by examining such changes.

Late-Stuart London was awash with quack handbills. You could not enter a coffee-house, Ned Ward remarked, without being blasted by advertisements for: 'May Dew, Golden Elixirs, Popular Pills, Liquid Snuff, Beautifying Waters, Dentifrices, Drops, Lozenges, all as infallible as the Pope. 'Where', as the famous Saffold has it, 'everyone above the rest, Deservedly has gained the name of best'; good in all cases, curing all distempers; every medicine pretends to nothing less than universality.' 'Indeed', bantered Ward, 'had not my friend told me 'twas a coffee-house I should have took it for the parlour of some eminent mountebank.'[33]

In the mid-eighteenth century, Oliver Goldsmith similarly had his fictional Chinaman in London take note of the modus operandi of the public doctors and the preoccupation with health that sustained them, saying that: 'every wall is covered with their names, their abilities, their amazing cures, and places of abode. Few patients can escape falling into their hands, unless blasted by lightning or struck dead with some sudden disorder… before I was a week in town, I was perfectly acquainted with the names and the medicines of every great man, or great woman of them all.'[34] The very real Prussian traveller, Von Archenholz, was no less amazed, a few years later, by the high-pressure salesmanship of English advertisers, who seemed medical almost to a man: 'One person informs you that his MAD-HOUSE is at your service; a second keeps a boarding-house for idiots; a good natured man midwife pays the utmost attention to ladies in certain situations, and promises to use the most scrupulous secrecy. Physicians offer to cure you of all manner of disorders, for a mere trifle.'[35] Why this novel phenomenon? Such intensive, frenetic levels of publicity were explained as the logical outcome of metropolitan life. 'In a great and populous City like this', mused *Mist's Journal*, 'where the Inhabitants of one End of the Town are Strangers to the Trade and Way of Living of those of the other, many Things which prove of singular Use and Benefit could never be known to the World by any other Means but this of advertising.'[36]

The street-side quack advertising of Charles II's reign was vastly different from the billboard hoarding of today. The reasons for this lie, in part, in technological considerations (we have at our fingertips photography, colour, and indefinite size), but they are also cultural, a function of the kinds of messages quack publicity needed to convey, and of contemporary philosophies of persuasion.

The seventeenth-century bill was primarily a document, designed to be read. The maximum possible number of words was crammed on to the sheet. Some contained an illustration of sorts – occasionally a royal coat of arms, sometimes a woodcut of the doctor himself (James à Tilbourg appears clutching a pair of forceps with a bladder-stone between the blades), or perhaps an apothecary's shop; stereotyped small heraldic devices also appear. But the paucity of eye-catching illustrative material is noteworthy.

The same holds for layout. The bill sporting a bold or offbeat headline, in huge capitals or Gothic script, or garnished with intriguing and arresting sub-headings, by-lines, catchy phrases, jingles, jokes, lines of verse, or other verbal devices to attract the eye, is the exception, not the rule. Such features are, of course, not absent. The 'Unborn Doctor, Seventh Son of the Seventh Son' thus offered some doggerel rising to this climax:

> So to conclude, and make an end,
> I to you this Paper send,

> That you may see God's Gift is great to me
> By which I cause the Lame to go, and the Blind to see.[37]

Verse was said to be effective. Joseph Addison remarked that the couplet, 'Within this place, / Lives Dr Case', made that clap-cure peddler more money than Dryden ever earned with all his verse. Case was more enterprising than most. One of his bills elegantly tabulates his sundry medicines in the left-hand column, with the disease against which they were specifics in the right: the punter could see at a glance which to buy.

Yet these are exceptions. In general, prose predominates, produced in continuous blocks of text, often down a couple of congested, cramped columns. Some attempt at stylistic animation is conveyed by capitals, italicization, and the like; but the print is generally small, and up to two thousand words are often squeezed on to a bill measuring about ten inches by eight; sometimes the text slips into a still smaller font near the foot: evidently, the advertiser believed every word counted.

To some degree, the welter of information wedged into these bills was unavoidable, for purely practical reasons. For example, vendors naturally wished to list all retail outlets for their goods – usually confined to London, though sometimes they stretched across the nation. In the days before networks of specialist chemists' shops existed, the public would not be sure precisely where individual pharmaceutical products could be purchased, for vendors sold perforce through an oilman here, a cheesemonger there, this stationer, that coffee-house, or simply Mr So-and-So at the Duck and Drake. Itemizing some thirty or forty addresses ate up space.

But the sea of words followed from more than mere practical necessity. Naively or not, the philosophy underlying such layout banked on the assumption that weight of words would prevail. The more the symptoms listed, the greater the roster of diseases vanquished by the medicine, the more global the itinerary of the empiric's travels, experiences, and so forth, the more comprehensively plagiarists and rivals were ground into the dust, and, not least, the longer the tail of testimonials and affidavits from thrilled customers, with full documentation of their names and addresses, the more – advertisers seem to have believed – the reader would be convinced.

The quack evidently felt the need to blitz the public, to overcome the ambivalent anonymity of his mode of trading: presumably, most purchasers of the pills promoted in the bills never actually saw Stoughton or Saffold, Jones or Anderson, face to face, unlike the familiar local apothecary. So every possible scrap of information had to be jammed into the bill to compensate. But the credibility gap mentioned earlier also had to be resolved by the 'advertising physician'. If rhetoric roused suspicion, and words were the stuff of lies, wherein lay the solution for the word-juggler? Quack advertisers evidently concluded that they needed to counter-establish a fabric of reality through saturating the reader with the maximum quantity of just that kind of documentary prose, brimful of hard facts, which Defoe was perfecting to impart an equivalent air of conviction to his fictions, his novels. A discreet brass plaque on the door, or a neighbourhood reputation, would have achieved credibility at minimal effort for the regular. The quack, by contrast, has to trumpet his own fame, yet through means that would not corrode his credit; he had to

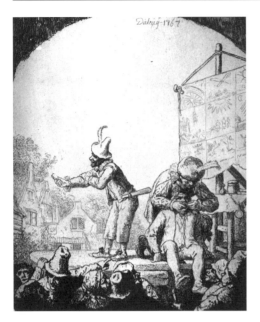

An itinerant medicine vendor crying up his wares while his assistant draws a man's tooth. Etching by Diebiey, 1767.

create his renown without thereby wrecking his reputation. It was fortunate that quacks were used to performing miracles.

In placing their faith in black and white, quacks traded upon a certain trust that the culture held in the permanence of print. Contemporaries often remarked upon the quasi-magical status easily assumed by the printed word in a partially literate culture in which, for many readers, access to reading matter was still quite limited. Print still had a certain magic aura. People were perhaps not so blasé about hand-outs as today. Many citizens, finding a quack bill thrust into their hand as they bustled along the street, treated it doubtless, as today, as throw-away literature – indeed, literally as bumf. Doctor Trigg, vendor of the 'Golden Vatican Pill, Famous for the Cure of Most Diseases in either Sex', appealed: 'Reader, Be not so injurious to thy Self as presently [that is, instantly] to commit this Paper to the Worst of Offices; it designs thy Good. Therefore first Read; three Minutes performs the Task.' A realist, Trigg concluded, 'after which, use thy discretion'.[38] But many readers surely did not actually own much reading matter or have anything new to read. Under such circumstances, cramming all those words on to a bill may have been a shrewd stroke: perhaps every last word was actually read by people without a daily newspaper or television; maybe it was even read out loud to wider circles.

The itinerant mountebank, haranguing the crowd, had to excel in bravura showmanship. The same man, doubling as the advertiser of salves and services through handbills, had to couch his hyperbole in a more sober format, so as to cash in upon the equation of the printed, the authentic and the real. Or is this to read too much sophistication into the post-Restoration quack handbills? Certainly by the early eighteenth century, Joseph Addison was remarking upon the inventive verve of the advertisements then appearing, with their bold experiments in layout and typographical devices. Products such as the anodyne necklace, as Francis Doherty has elegantly demonstrated, were to create their own fantasy world through the running stories attached to them, designed to divert and entertain potential buyers. By the mid-eighteenth century, Samuel Johnson could go one step further, and proclaim 'The trade of Advertising is now so near to perfection, that it is not easy to propose any improvement'.

By contrast to such refinement, however, the bills of almost a century earlier look rather unsubtle. One wonders whether 'Glad Tidings to all Unfortunate Venereal Patients' was really the best way to greet sufferers, though that quack at least showed some enterprise in actually addressing the reader. For although some bills tried out the vocative ('Beloved Reader'), most did not establish any direct rapport between the doctor and his readers – beyond, perhaps, variations on the stiffly pompous 'This is to give Notice, That here is lately arrived…', etc.

Perhaps the Restoration handbill should be read as a utility text, a workmanlike attempt to communicate a body of information to a disparate and indeterminate public. The Restoration advertiser's grasp of graphics was perhaps rudimentary. It is noteworthy how little these early quacks rang the changes in their promotions. Their copy seems stereotyped and standardized: relatively little differentiates the bills of many different doctors. When John Case took over Thomas Saffold's pills and practice, he also assumed his publicity, almost verbatim. That may have been sensible strategy; it may, however, betray a poverty of propaganda imagination.

Advertising in newspapers

Advertising was the soul of the Georgian newspaper, particularly the provincial press. Without advertising revenue, it could hardly have been financially viable. In any case, as Jeremy Black has recently argued, newspapers were probably bought largely for their advertisements and notices of markets and auctions, of property for sale, concerts and assemblies – all of which helped animate the local economy. Looney has shown that real estate and tradesmen's advertisements formed the largest categories of inserts; but among commodities offered for sale, proprietary medicines easily commanded pride of place.

Medical matters made up no small part of the contents of Georgian newspapers. Regulars advertised in them, usually in a discreet way (for example, bringing readers' notice to a change of address or the addition of a new partner), though sometimes more boldly (as when touting for trade as surgeon-inoculators). Poems or facetious medical items were common, for example, a set of verses telling the shocking story of a 'Newcastle Apothecary' who (as one might predict) killed off his patients, but, in the public interest, took up midwifery:

> This balanced things – for if he hurl'd
> A few more mortals from the world
> He made amends by bringing others into't.[39]

Yet among medical items, it was quack medicines and operators that occupied by far the most column inches. One powerful reason for this lay in the fact that drug wholesalers and newspaper owners were often partners or business cronies. Printers acted as distributors of medicines, typically selling them from their offices or bookshops (where they also sold the medical books advertised in their papers), and even delivering them, through their agents and newsboys, with the newspapers themselves. Through such means, nostrum advertising directly supplemented the editor's revenue. Thus the *Reading Mercury* in 1746 was regularly carrying advertisements inserted by the printer announcing that he personally had for sale:

> Dr Hooper's Female Pills, Anderson's Scotch Pills, Aurea Medicina, or Boerhaave's Scots Pills Improv'd, the True British Oil, Friar's Balsam, Daffey's Elixir, and Squire's Grand Elixir, Greenough's Two Tinctures, the one for preserving the Teeth, the other for curing the Tooth-ache, A Tincture, to cure the Itch by smelling, Golden and Plain Spirit of Scurvey Grass, Godfrey's Cordial, Hypo Drops, Golden Cephalick Drops, Lady Moor's, Bateman's Stoughton's and Chymical Drops, Pile Ointment, The Liquid Shell for the Stone and Gravel, The best Sort of Issue Plaisters, Hungary and Lavender Water.[40]

Newspaper proprietors standardly listed the nostrums they stocked. Thus the printers of the *Bath Journal* in the 1780s catalogued in most issues the 'following Genuine Medicines':

Ague and Fever Drops, a certain cure, 5s and 2s 6d
Anderson's True Scots Pills Bennet's Antiarthritic, for the Gout, 5s 5d
Becket's Sovereign Restorative Drops for Barrenness, weakness 10s 6d
His much-esteemed Drops, for venereal complaints 3s
Bateman's Pectoral Drops ls
Cinnamon Drops for Disorders of the stomach, colds, chills, 3s 6d
Famous Corn Salve, for hard or soft Corns, and gives immediate ease ls 6d
The Cordial Cephalic Snuff, for the head and eyes, 6d
Debraw's Asiatick Toothpowder for preserving and beautifying the teeth 2s 6d
Tooth brushes from Indian hair and pattern ls
Daffy's Genuine Elixir ls 3d
Maredant's Drops, for the Scurvy, Leprosy, and all breaking out, 5s 3d
Oriental Vegetable Cordial for disorders in the stomach and bowels, 5s
Famous Patent Ointment for the Itch, a safe and effective remedy, ls 6d
Pectoral Lozenges of Tolu, for coughs or colds ls
Radcliffe's purging Elixir ls
Restorative Electuary, a sovereign remedy for Venereal Complaints 6s
Admirable Essence of Life, for preventing the Venereal Disease taking place, 6s
Squire's grand elixir, for consumptions, ls 3d
Spilsbury's Surprisingly efficacious Drops for the scurvy, leprosy 4s and 7s
Dalby's Carminative for colicky disorders, ls 6d
Essential Salt of Lemons, for taking Stains or Spots out of Linen, ls

Hickman's Pills for the stone and gravel, 3s

Hamilton's Tincture for the tooth ach, scurvy, & 2s 6d

Hooper's Female Pills, ls

James's Fever Powder, 2s 6d

His Analeptic Pills, of great efficacy in fevers, rheumatic complaints 4s 6d

Jackson's celebrated Tincture for the gravel ls

Jackson's British Powder for the teeth and gums ls

Leake's Genuine Pills much used for effectually curing the Venereal Disease in a
short time

Norris's Drops for Fevers Rheumatisms & 2s 6d

Godfrey's Cordial 6d

Steers' Opoldelduc, for chilblains, or chaps in the hands, or feet, bruises, sprains,
2s

Turlington's Balsam of Life, for the gravel ls 9d

Vandour's Nervous Pills as so universally esteemed for their good effect in
lowness of spirits, melancholy, and all Nervous Disorders, 2s 6d

Vegetable Syrup, for venereal complaints, scurvy, & an amazing purifier of the
blood and juices 8s 6d Walker's Jesuit Drops, for the Venereal Disease, 2s 6d

WARD'S MEDICINES Celebrated Anti-Scorbutic White Drop 2s 6d

Essence for Head-ach ls 6d

Red Pills for Rheumatism ls

Emetic Sick Drop 6d[41]

Without the newspaper, how would customers have even known these preparations were available? Would any shop have bothered to stock them? Would manufacturing them have been profitable?

There was thus good reason to believe that the advent of newspaper advertising constituted an epoch in quack medicine promotion by vastly multiplying the number of potential buyers accessible to a vendor. By the close of the eighteenth century, names such as James's Powders or Solomon's Balm of Gilead were featuring literally in millions of copies of newspapers per year. As early as 1719, a reader of *Mist's Journal* had pinpointed the transformation, complaining that the quack advertisements being printed in that paper 'spread death and desolation to every part of the nation', whereas 'were they to keep to their stage, and only harangue the gaping crowd, from an eminence of eight or ten foot high, their voice would not be heard very far and some parts of the Kingdom would escape their infection.' The advent of the press had changed all that. In Christopher Anstey's *New Bath Guide* (1766), a tale of a family visiting Bath, two of Sir John Hill's empiric preparations are taken by Tabby Runt, the maid, who then ails and has to be treated by the doctor:

> He gives little Tabby a great many Doses
> For he says the poor creature has got the chlorosis,
> Or a ravenous pica, so brought on the vapours
> By swallowing Stuff she has read in the papers.[42]

Of course, people exaggerated. The writer who asserted in the *Publick Register* in 1741 that 'one fourth part at least of all the papers that are now extant, is filled with quack advertisements', himself engaged in quackish hyperbole.[43] Nevertheless, medical advertising made quite a splash. As P. S. Brown has emphasized, there were perhaps a couple of dozen products whose names one could reliably expect to find cropping up in paper after paper – familiar products such as Dr Mead's Vegetable Balsam, Dr Smyth's Restorative Medicine, Dr James's Analeptic Pills (for rheumatism), Sir John Hill's Pectoral Balsam of Honey, Essence of Pearl and Pearl Dentifrice, Leake's Pilula Salutaria, and Spilsbury's Drops for the Scurvy – all of these figured, for instance, on a single page of the Bath Chronicle on 8 October 1778, many trailing elaborate testimonials, including one for an 'Attenuating Tincture' attested by the intriguingly named 'Mark True'.

Some inserts for individual preparations were extraordinarily long: publicity for Dr James's Fever Powders occasionally stretched to more than a column (it was probably put in by the newspaper owner as a 'filler'). The *Bath Journal* for 18 June 1744 contained an advertisement for Greenough's various tooth-powders that covered no less than a column and a half – the public was informed that powders could be obtained at the printing office, along with half a dozen other preparations. Continuous runs of mid-Georgian newspapers commonly reveal that every single copy carried advertisements for such products as Dalby's Carminative Mixture (recommended for all sorts of stomach disorders, especially for infants), Walker's Patent Genuine Jesuit Drops (openly stated to be a cure for venereal disease), Doctor Bennet's Specific for the Sciatica, Dr Anderson's Scots Pills, and so forth, to say nothing of the ominously named Rooke's Matchless Balsam.

Does comparison of the quack handbills of the post-Restoration age with the newspaper advertisements of a century later reveal any significant transformation in pitch and public? I suggest it does, and that the shift classically exemplifies MacLuhan's dictum that the medium is the message. For the newer advertising medium, the newspaper, presupposed a rather more literate and sophisticated readership than the street-crowd traditional mountebanks or handbill-distributors were attempting to influence. Moreover, the typical newspaper insert – an inch or two long – could not possibly match the large handbill in opportunities for prolixity: hence the newspaper advertiser was under pressure to stake his claims for his product briefly and evocatively. (He could, however, rely upon the undoubted advantage of ready repetition: the reader was more likely to experience multiple exposure – with its subliminal possibilities – to a much-used newspaper advertisement than to a handbill.)

Not surprisingly, therefore, the nostrums advertised in mid- or late-eighteenth-century newspapers carry rather different profiles from those prominent in the Restoration posters. For one thing, as befits their undoubtedly middle-class audience, they are rather more expensive. As the list reproduced above from the *Bath Journal* shows, many of the nostrums advertised in the 1780s were selling at three or five shillings per item – contrast the shilling or two much more normal earlier (inflation would have been a marginal factor).

For another, the prominent late-Georgian nostrums were far less likely to be claiming to be panaceas. It probably made sense for an itinerant mountebank, or the author of a one-off bill to claim to cure everything. A pageful of panaceas vying for attention in a newspaper would, by contrast, have been self-defeating. Hence a division of labour insensibly sprang up, whereby individual preparations staked out special patches for themselves: some (as can be seen) were for scurvy, some for the head, some for colic, some for chills or chilblains. Moreover – and the link is obvious – whereas almost all the nostrums advertised in Restoration handbills claimed to cure serious, usually fatal conditions, a century later, no small proportion of preparations were being targeted at lesser disorders – corns, blemished complexions, coughs, and colds. Their vendors apparently felt confident that they did not have to promise everything in order to clinch a sale – or, to put the same point another way, it would appear (as intimated in chapter 2) that by the late-Georgian age, consumers were used to buying a multiplicity of commercial medicines, one product for each type of malaise.

A further sign of growing market maturity is noteworthy. Seventeenth-century advertising was direct, assertive, and factual: a century later, such would have been seen as naive and uncouth by a culture pleased to flatter itself upon its superior sensibility. The Enlightenment mind took enormous delight in seductive suggestion, in the self-conscious play of art and artifice, in forms of speech light, easy, allusive – indeed, *Spectatorial*. The Georgians turned publicity into style – a perception never better encapsulated than in the character, 'Puff', in Sheridan's *Critic*, whose vocation was to charm with words in such a way that the deception, far from grating, became a pleasure in itself. Rather than selling by direct blasts at the public, Puff excels in the art of gentle persuasion, of the subtle seductive use of diction, to ingratiate himself with the public. His forte is high-flown idealization:

> from me [people] learned to inlay their phraseology with variegated chips of exotic metaphor; by me too their inventive faculties were called forth: – yes, sir, by me they were instructed to clothe ideal walls with gratuitous fruits – to insinuate obsequious rivulets into visionary groves – to teach courteous shrubs to nod their approvation of the grateful soil; or on emergencies to raise upstart oaks, where there never had been an acorn; to create a delightful vicinate without the assistance of a neighbour; or to fix the temple of Hygeia in the fens of Lincolnshire.[44]

Some strokes of this civilized sales-talk may be seen in the promotion of quack medicines in late-Georgian newspapers. Language tends to be softened in the direction of decorous euphemism. The widely promoted New Canada Balsam, for instance, was recommended as excellent for 'Weaknesses in either Sex, Whether Occasioned by Excesses, Ill-Habits or Diseases'. The precise nature of these weaknesses was left to the reader's imagination, though its author planted a broad hint for educated readers by suggesting that the most exhausting of all diseases was the 'single passion of DIOGENES', from which 'dreadful ills' followed, including decaying memory and mind, poor eyesight, and back pain.

William Brodum was another late-Georgian expert in insinuating understatement, almost too delicate to mention a disease by name in front of the sufferers. Brodum – who, in time-honoured fashion, stressed that he was a 'regular physician', 'not a nostrum vendor', and that his 'motive for publishing' advertisements was to 'secure the health of the public' – presented his Botanical Syrup as a 'Cure for the Indiscretions of Youth', and wrote at large about the incomparable importance of 'Cleanliness', as so wisely advocated by Lord Chesterfield.

Another who advertised widely in a similarly allusive, but perniciously anxiety-making style was Samuel Solomon (who presented himself in the *Bath Herald* as MD, FRHS). Solomon developed a delicately devastating sales pitch. In his newspaper publicity, he chiefly restricted himself to the respectable endeavour of drawing attention to his book on proper living, the *Guide to Health*, a 'valuable and interesting Work founded on many years experiences of the calamitous consequences of youthful indiscretions'. The work, he explained, was not even primarily to be bought by sufferers, but, for the sake of prevention, by 'parents, guardians, superintendents of large seminaries', and so forth, in the hope that the 'wholesome and salutary advice contained therein will guard against an accumulation of misfortunes, both temporal and spiritual'. Of course, sickness was involved as well, but its existence could fortunately be implied without stooping to specifics: 'There is likewise a system laid down for the radically curing a certain fatal disorder in all its stages, and infallibly removing all Scrophulous and Scorbutic Diseases, and every Impurity of the Blood, concluding with Advice to School Boys, against a most destructive solitary Passion.' Only finally did Solomon get round to puffing his own products, though still hardly mentioning a disease by name. Solomon's Cordial Balm of Gilead, he claimed, was: 'a certain and effectual Remedy for nervous disorders, juvenile indiscretions, head-aches, debility, seminal weakness, lowness of spirits, female complaints, loss of appetite, relaxation, indigestion, coughs and colds, consumptions, weaknesses, impurity of blood, an ill-cured lues, gleets...'[45]

This sophistication of mature quack advertising lies in trading upon the conventions of civility. Disease takes a back seat, and quack medicines are praised for treating those vague malaises forming the penumbra to the 'English malady'. Thus Vandour's Nervous Pills were ideal in 'Nervous disorders, lowness of spirits, headaches, tremblings, vain fears and wanderings of the mind, frightful dreams, catching, startings,... specks before the eyes... relaxed fibres'. And certain medicines catered quite explicitly for up-market hypochondriasis: 'To those of either sex who are troubled with Lowness of spirits, Horrors of Mind, Anxieties, Confused Thoughts, Troublesome Sleep, groundless Fears and the Like', ran one much-printed newspaper advertisement, the 'so-much famed Hypo-drops' were the answer, bringing relief to minds 'where nothing but Horror reigns'. The author cannily added that the true terror of hypochondria was the 'prodigious variety of its symptoms', which he helpfully proceeded to list, including 'sour belchings' and 'depraved appetite'. Others suffering non-specific disturbances of the head were recommended 'Royal Patent Medicinal Snuff, Just Cured'.[46]

These themes – especially the insinuation of quackery into the market for sexual disorders – will be further explored in the next two chapters. It should be clear by now, however, that the economy of quack medicine (and, by analogy, of regular medicine too) inscribed doctor and patient, disease and treatment, within a particular loom of language. The development of publicity machines afforded heightened opportunities during the long eighteenth century for manipulating consciousness about health and sickness.

5 Health, disease and cure

Was quack medicine 'alternative medicine'?

Nowadays, the medical establishment is challenged by a multiplicity of medical movements whose contention is that the basic conceptions of health and disease, of the economy of the body, and of the strategies of treatment enshrined in official, allopathic, scientific medicine are radically misguided. In turn, they offer something fundamentally different – including homeopathy (like cures like) in place of allopathy (cure by opposites), the wisdom of alien cultures (for example, Chinese acupuncture), or the power of mind over matter (faith cures). As John Harley Warner and others have stressed, the appeal of the medical sects luxuriating during the last century lay precisely in presenting themselves as the medical equivalent of 'radical dissent', the antithesis of an orthodoxy that could be accused of being no less therapeutically foolish than ethically and professionally corrupt.

In the pre-modern era too, alternative medical philosophies clearly existed. Belief was widespread that sickness and its cure might lie beyond the realms of nature, science, and pharmacy, being explicable rather in terms of cosmic struggles between the Deity and the Devil; thus some people looked to prayer, holy water, the invocation of saints, etc., for relief. In Catholic nations, such strategies received a certain ecclesiastical blessing in the form of shrines and pilgrimages (they still do); in Protestant, anti-superstitious England, they persisted chiefly as vestigial rural survivals, as did folk medicine itself, with its armoury of charms, spells, amulets, and the practice of sympathetic magic.

But was quackery – that is medicine as practised in the market-place by commercial operators – an alternative medicine? Obviously, it was in a purely banal sense, in that it boasted a wisdom and powers lacked by regulars, culled from adepts steeped in Oriental wisdom and similar sources. But did seventeenth- and eighteenth-century quackery mutiny, radically repudiating regular medicine and developing an alternative epistemology and ontology of its own? Above all, was it perceived by the public as offering a different – more scientific, popular, grassroots, ethical or more experientially plausible – scenario for understanding falling sick and getting better?

Certain facets of quackery suggest that this might have been so, and are thus worth examining. For example, various prominent post-Restoration quacks, such as Thomas Saffold and his successor, John Case, advertised astrological as well as medical skills (the two were of a piece). Yet casting horoscopes did not mark a man out in those days as particularly heterodox. As Patrick Curry has emphasized, astrological convictions and practice formed part of the world-view of perfectly mainstream Stuart practitioners from Richard Napier to William Lilly. If Georgian quacks had publicized astrological healing as a symbolically privileged facet of their trade, that would have appeared as a bid to present the public with something heterodox (for regular physic, in line with Enlightenment science, by then had, indeed, abandoned astrology). But that did not happen. Even movements such as mesmerism (with its vision of human health depending upon ethereal cosmic fluids, a view which might have been expected to draw upon the quasi-mystical associations of astrology), signally did not choose to encumber themselves with what was seen by then as an obsolete cosmology (though hostile critics and cartoonists drew the link).

Uroscopy affords a certain parallel. Various Restoration quacks boasted their skills at urine-gazing (that is, making diagnoses and prognoses from inspecting a patient's urine, even in the absence of the patient himself). The 'Famous High German, Turkish and Imperial Physician', for instance, proclaimed that he 'doth cast all sorts of Humane Urine'.[1] Obviously, the 'pisse prophet' expected to win celebrity from this prodigious feat. But uroscopy had its pragmatic side, too. It allowed the sick person to be treated without actually having to rise from his bed to see the healer – possibly a dangerous, or a socially embarrassing act: a urine-flask could be fetched by a servant. Diagnosis at a distance had many attractions.

By the close of the seventeenth century, urine-gazing as a self-sufficient medical art (rather than as part of a battery of diagnostic procedures) was becoming stigmatized as a special trade-mark of quackery. Various unorthodox healers kept up the art in country areas through the eighteenth century. The Hon. John Byng dubbed them 'country Myersbachs', alluding to the notorious Theodore Myersbach, whose career will be discussed in chapter 7. Yet there was nothing inherently alternative about recourse to urine as a diagnostic tool: far from it – it had been one of the stocks-in-trade of the medieval and renaissance regular, fully sanctioned by Galenic and classical medicine. Urine-casting never became a party badge of the quacks, remaining rather the idiosyncrasy of a few.

The pointers become unambiguous if we look at other fields in which quacks might be expected to have staked out theories and practices radically differentiated from orthodoxy. Did they, for instance, go in for explicitly thaumaturgical forms of cure, including faith healing? Despite parroting of such pious platitudes as *nihil nisi dominus*, the answer is no. There seem no connections between the group faith-healing exercises of the early Quakers, or, later, of certain Methodists, and the operations of the quacks (who were conspicuously without specific denominational affiliation). Or, did they claim to heal by spiritual power, by white magic, charms, or preternatural powers? As witchcraft became discredited, did quacks assume their mantle in a more sanitized mode? Their rhetoric indeed hints at occultism, but their practice belies it.

Eighteenth-century France boasted many *maiges* whose forte was a rigmarole of healing by faith and unique personal thaumaturgical powers; but it is noteworthy that after Valentine Greatrakes at the Restoration, not a single eminent English quack specialized in faith cures. Nor were there even many charms on sale. The rather ominously named Major Choke sold necklaces ('no heavier than a nutmeg') which eased 'children breeding teeth' (one had sped the recovery of a child of the Countess of Northumberland). These seem to have worked like magic. But they were unusual amongst quack products.

Alternatively, one might suppose that quack medicine would have tried to carve out a distinctive identity for itself through championing novelty, and, in an age of science and technology, patenting a wave of gadgets to bamboozle the public. Certain instances come to mind: James Graham set up his 'Celestial Bed', hooked up to electrical currents and magnetic fields, and pledged to ensure fertility. Similarly, the mesmerists had their magnets

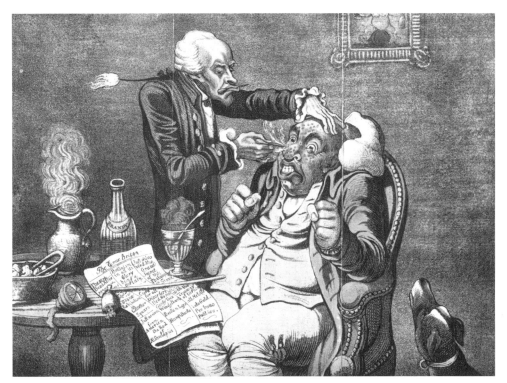

Benjamin Perkins, an American quack doctor, operating on the carbuncled nose of an obese patient. Coloured aquatint after J. Gillray, 1801.

and baquets, storing animal magnetism; the Perkinses, *père et fils*, introduced their metallic tractors for drawing out disease, and various operators unleashed electrical currents upon nervous diseases. Yet it is not the superabundance of machines and gadgets, but their relative paucity which is striking. The grotesque proliferation of junk technology – ozone boxes, masturbation-suppressors, electrical belts, thermal socks, hydraulic pimple squeezers, and the like – is a product of late-Victorian quackery (a reflex response, one suspects, to the introduction of laws regulating quack pharmacy). Georgian quacks probably drew upon the medical potential of electricity no more than their regular colleagues.

Did the quacks colonize domains of disease relatively neglected by the regulars? The answer seems, by-and-large, no. Take, for instance, the question of suffering. People clearly suffered appalling pain in the early modern period. Regular medicine had few effective analgesics and did not trouble itself unduly about pain-control (for example, opium was used relatively rarely to reduce pain in surgical operations, and the profession dragged its feet about the introduction of anaesthetics). So, did quacks cash in on this, fanfaring their own capacity to quell pain? After all, pain-relief is, perhaps, the prime selling point in the slogans of proprietary medicine today. Yet that is not what we find. Either pre-modern patients were such Stoics that pain-control really was not a high priority to them; or, once again, we find quack medicine not so much playing a pioneering role but rather treading in the footsteps of orthodoxy.

117

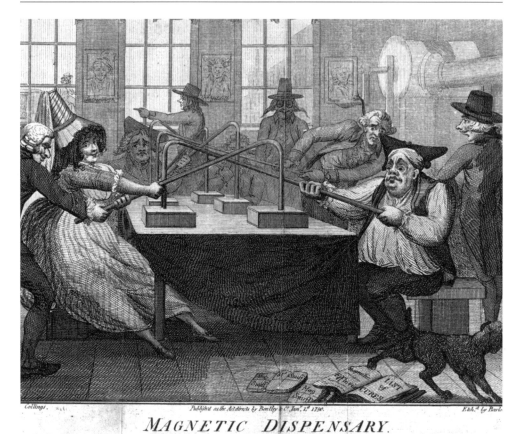

MAGNETIC DISPENSARY.

A group of patients undergoing magnetic treatment at the hands of a quack doctor. Etching by J. Barlow, 1790, after J Collings.

We must not confuse quack rhetoric and quack reality. To some degree, their public relations obviously made them sound different: they were, after all, touting for trade. In reality, as we shall now explore, their notions of health and disease, and therapeutic orientation were remarkably convergent.

And this is borne out by the fact that the sick during the long eighteenth century mixed regular with quack medicine. There is considerable evidence that many Victorian patients repudiated regular medicine – became total abstainers, as it were – and abandoned themselves exclusively to some alternative system of their choice. But there is little sign that Georgians took rigid ideological stands for or against regular medicine. As Jonathan Barry has shown in his admirable study of the Bristolian William Dyer, people drew now on regular, now on irregular medicine, as it suited them, often using both at the same time.[2] In his *Medical Ethics*, Thomas Percival was reconciled, albeit grudgingly, to the idea that the patients of regular doctors would also be taking quack nostrums.[3]

Jewson's view of the 'patient-centredness' of the Georgian medical milieu, discussed in chapter 2, offers a plausible explanation for this. If, as Jewson contends, patients were calling the shots (more so, at least, than today), medicine – all medicine, regular and quack

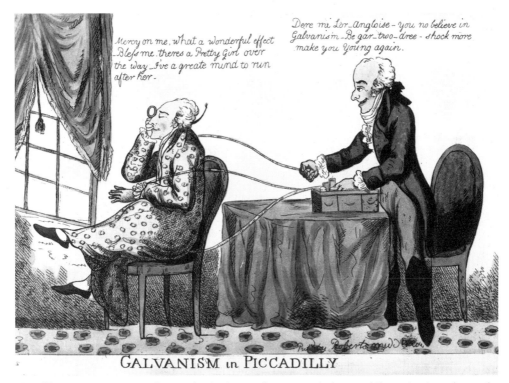

GALVANISM in PICCADILLY

An affluent man receiving galvanic electric therapy from a quack doctor while staring intently out the window. Coloured etching by Roberts.

– would necessarily be relatively 'user friendly' (otherwise it would hardly be used). It had to offer visions of health, sickness, and recovery, which made sense from the sick person's point of view – verbalizations and visualizations of the body's workings, telling plausible stories, accounting for pains and perturbations, and permitting some degree of co-operation on the part of the sick person in working towards recovery.

The hospital milieu and scientific medicine that gained effectiveness in the nineteenth century arguably put paid to this anthropocentrism (Jewson speaks of the 'disappearance of the sick man from medical cosmology'). The ensuing vacuum, left by the demise of patient-centred medicine, came to be filled by fringe sects that continued to make some sense of sickness. But before the Victorian era the need for such alternatives was perhaps small. Georgian quacks had to beat the regulars at their own game.

Health

Health-consciousness ran high in pre-modern England. People rarely ignored their physical well-being till they fell sick: life was too precarious, and medicine too feeble, to permit that luxury. The spectre of the hypochondriac shows how readily health anxieties got out of hand. The goal of positive health, and the duty of nurturing it, were widely acknowledged in quack writings. 'As there is hardly anything of this World more deservingly welcome to Mankinde, than Health and Long Life', announces one of Bromfield's bills, 'so whatever contributes most thereunto, ought to have a fair reception and high value in the thoughts of all men.'[4] Another contemporary bill-monger bade readers 'Try the Preserving of Health' (adding piously 'Nihil Absque Deo'), and made particular play of his capacity to overcome 'chronick and stubborn distempers'.[5]

Quacks, like the lay public and regulars too, thus concerned themselves not just with disease but with positive health (the cynic would say it was their way of enlarging their domain). Many claimed to have medicines to fortify the body against the onslaught of sickness. Thus Charles Peter's Famous Head Pill was a 'great Preservative to Nature', which 'prevents Convulsions and Apoplectick Fits'. Its prophylactic powers were remarkable: 'one dose, taken once in Twenty Days, preserves the Body in Health; for it resists all putrefaction, and will continue good Seven years or more'. Thus these Head Pills were especially valuable for the likes of sailors embarking on voyages, without regular access to medical help on tap. Not least, Peter's remedy, like many others, appealed to those too busy to take to their beds, needing what we might call 'convenience therapies': 'those that take them, may safely go abroad about their Business, and need not observe any Diet'.[6]

Other quack remedies played upon the entrenched belief that the key to health lay in a sound constitution. Even a healthy system would, if neglected, decay in time. Hence the appeal of the quack who presented himself as 'The Great Restorer of Decay'd Nature', pitching his advertisement at 'all those who desire to make their lives Happy and Long'. He had in his possession a medicine designed to 'retard that Natural Decay, which old age brings upon Humane Bodies', being, above all, a specific against 'Impotency in Love Affairs', for it would render 'Old Men, and Women, of three or four scores, as Youthful, in this point, as those of twenty or thirty years of age', thanks to augmenting the 'supply of vital spirits'.[7]

There was clearly a brisk market in restoratives for countering fatigue, ageing, and function loss. Concern with longevity was underlined in Salvator Winter junior's Elixir Vitae, which passed itself off as 'an excellent Life-Preserving Remedy, be the Distemper never so Chronical', for it was 'So speedy a Reviver of the Spirits, and Restorer of decayed Nature'. The proprietor claimed that his father had lived to the ripe old age of ninety-nine by 'having always a Bottle of it in his pocket, and drinking a spoonful therefore 4 or 5 times a day and snuffing it up very strongly into his Nostrils, and bathing his Temples'. Mirabile dictu, his elixir has even 'revived great Numbers of people supposed to be dead'.[8]

Pandering to basic worries about health and the desire to fortify failing systems, many quack preparations – as, of course, many orthodox medications – offered themselves as general cordials or tonics, designed to ensure the vitality of the system. The virtue of Rose's Balsamick Elixir, for instance, was that it 'quickens all the Senses, and gives Life and Vigour even to Old Age. It is so great a Restorative, that for Consumptive Persons, there is not such another Preparation in the Whole World which gives a healthful countenance and a lively Humour, keeping the Spirits in the true Temper.' Overall, Rose's preparation 'gives or restores to Nature what's wanting, and takes away what's hurtful': what could be simpler? Unusually, it was a preparation also said to ward off specific diseases in the first place: in particular it 'prevents the Small Pox'.[9]

The Grand Balsamic Or the Health Procuring and Preserving Pill possessed comparable virtues. 'Adapted to all Ages and Constitutions', this medicine would 'sweeten and purifie the whole Mass of the Blood, and maintain its Circulation'. Not least, it would 'reform the Digestion of the Chylus, the bad Concoction of which is the Original of most Diseases' – the consensus of contemporary medicine was that the stomach was the seat of most disorders – and furthermore 'sweeten the Blood, promote Circulation, and correct the Imperfections of Concoction', overall aiding the 'animal spirits' to perform 'their proper Functions' . As with Peter's Head Pills and many similar preparations, it was specially urged upon seafarers, but women suffering from 'barrenness and green sickness' would also particularly benefit.[10]

Disease

The greatest operating dilemma facing the 'advertising professor' lay in handling those sick of some particular disorder. The beauty of the modus operandi of regular medicine lay in the fact that the physician would carefully take the patient's history and, on the basis of vast experience, form a considered diagnosis. Thence a course of therapeutics would be initiated, which could be tucked and trimmed as necessary, as a result of almost daily visits. Thus – for those who could afford such cosseting – everyone's treatment was bespoke, perfectly tailored to his condition.

The quack's practice precluded such niceties of clinical diagnosis. His consultations – where they existed at all – were likely to be perfunctory and not repeated, and he would not even see the consumer of his nostrums if the patient heard about them through advertisements and bought them through retailers. Hence the quack, by the very logic of his trade, had to press the astonishing claim that his medicines, made up in advance wholesale to a standard formula, would conquer all diseases in all people. In those circumstances, quack advertising had to serve as a substitute for the diagnostic process.

Fortunately for quacks, they could trade upon the assumption commonly held amongst the sick that they knew in advance what was wrong with them (merely drawing upon the physician for confirmation and treatment). Thus the strategy of the typical quack bill lay not in a general appeal (as made later by the dispensaries) to the sick, to come and submit themselves to the practitioner's powers, but in tabulating a comprehensive list of the ailments from which readers or auditors would already believe themselves to be suffering and which his skills or pills would conquer. In this, the scope for exploiting the sick person's suggestivity was obviously quite boundless.

The ailments listed in the typical seventeenth-century quack harangues or bills include, of course, conditions from which people died (as a glance at the Bills of Mortality will show). But they were not primarily the most lethal, acute diseases. Quack bills did not set themselves up, above all, as ready and infallible conquerors of, say, plague smallpox, typhus, pneumonia, or the other virulent epidemic infections. The reasons are obvious. For one thing, the typical by-stander or reader would not actually be suffering from (or even think he was suffering from) these diseases: if he were, he would be too sick to be sitting in the coffee-house or shoving and pushing round the stage. For another, only a foolish quack would blatantly pretend to specialize in curing conditions from which his customers were very likely to die in a day or two (not least, there would be no repeat prescriptions).

Rather, quacks presented themselves as godsends to those suffering principally from serious, painful, and unpleasant, but not immediately fatal diseases – ones which largely left them on their feet, still trying to earn a living or going about their business. The typical patient might well have tried, but found scant relief from kitchen physic or from an apothecary. Thus the bill for the Pilula Homogenea explained that it was a medicine – nay more, a 'miraculous pill' – tailor-made for 'Curing those Chronick Distempers reigning in this Age, viz the Scurvy, Dropsy, Gout, and Agues of all sorts, with many more Maladies incident to Mankind all which ariseth from an ill habit of the Body'.[11]

Those diseases – dropsy, gout, agues (that is, malaria or similar fevers), scurvy-crop up again and again, alongside asthma, consumption (meaning general wasting conditions), worms, rheumatism, arthritis, the king's evil (scrofula), jaundice, colic, wind, and all manner of other complaints of the gastro-intestinal system. These were the sorts of conditions the 'advertising physicians' felt confident they could handle. Thus Jones's Friendly Pill was sure to get rid of worms in children, because it 'works seven several ways', and had the further advantage that it 'purges so gentle'.[12] Equally wonderful for worms was the Pulvis Benedictus, which 'carries off all manner of Corruption and Putrefaction, expels Wind and Water, Sweetens, purifies, and enriches the whole Mass of Blood' in the process.[13]

Likewise prominent amongst the disorders quacks could conquer were long-term surgical conditions such as fistula, stone, ruptures, wens, and carbuncles. Deformities and 'crookedness' were also commonly mentioned. There were many eye specialists and benefactors of the deaf (though they usually specified they could help only if the deafness were caused by external obstruction). All such conditions were claimed to lie within the compass of the quacks. The 'High German Doctor', for example, 'helps all Bursten or Broken Bellies', claiming that he could effect rupture cures, unlike most, without recourse to a truss.[14] Likewise, there was a Dutchman who promised help to 'all such whose Members of their Bodies are out of Shape or order, that is to say, such as are inclin'd to be Crooked'.[15]

Appearance was of vital importance in the face-to-face encounters of early modern society, as Margaret Pelling has insisted, not least because so many people were born somewhat deformed, or had become unsightly through smallpox, skin disease, eye complaints, accidents, and suchlike. Not surprisingly, therefore, cosmetic medicine loomed large in the promotions of the quacks and the minds of their customers. Radical cures were, naturally, part of the rhetoric; but many quack bills also laid great stress upon their capacity to patch people up effectively, removing growths, sores, scabs, and ulcers. Thus the 'Unborn DOCTOR' was a dab hand at healing all 'Wounds, Swellings, Tumors, Cancers, Ulcers, old Running Sores, King's-Evil, Ring-worms, Redness in the Face', to say nothing of making good 'all sorts of Ruptures in Men, Women and Children'; he could also 'set the Head upright', and work the 'cure of crooked children'.[16]

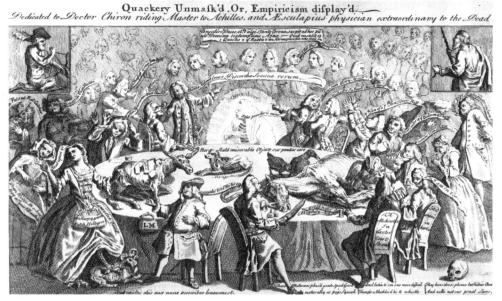

A large table in a lecture hall with many medical practitioners of dubious fame seated around it. In the background are tiers of spectators. Engraving, 1748.

But if quack remedies made great play with external, visible disorders, they equally promised relief for various non-specific internal complaints, offering respite from that general sense of unwellness so pervasive in the past. Many patented preparations were targeted at the sufferer experiencing a general sense of constitutional debility: his blood in poor condition, his stomach out of temper, his bowels sluggish. To counter such sensations, 'The Most Excellent Spirit of Ground Ivy' thus assured the public that it 'infallibly cools and sweetens the Blood, and helps mightily to keep the Stomach in order'.

The term serving in the latter part of the seventeenth century as an umbrella for a constellation of possibly interconnected malfunctionings and distempers was 'scurvy' – a name that clearly included the classic mariners' disease, but which was popularly used far more expansively (compare today's colloquial usage of terms such as gastric 'flu or glandular fever). 'Scurvy' had become 'a Disease spread all over this Nation', claimed the bill forEwel's Extractum Panaseton; the vendor of the Herculeon Antidote deemed it a 'popular disease', while, according to the poster for the Catholick or Universal Pill, 'amidst all Diseases that afflict Mans body, there is none so Epidemical and Raging at this time as the Scurvy'.[17]

Scorbutic conditions, as popularly understood and as mirrored and magnified in regular and quack accounts alike, were thought to manifest themselves in skin disorders, including ulcerations and scrofulous swellings, swollen gums, loosened teeth, bad breath, bleeding, weakness, lack of appetite, and the like, all of which were thought to be the products of bad blood, poor digestion, and peccant humours within (especially a surfeit of melancholy, which darkened and thickened the blood). Indeed, its symptoms were

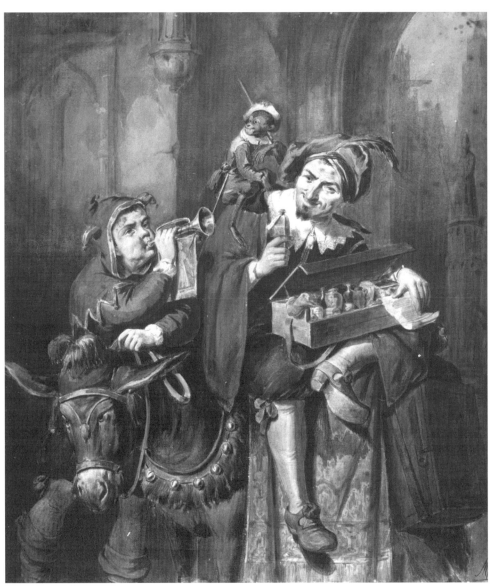

An itinerant medicine vendor sitting on his donkey with his boxes of medicines. A monkey sits on his shoulder and a fool blows a trumpet at them. Watercolour by M. Calisch.

protean and numberless, claimed George Jones, maker of the Friendly Pill, but they especially included

> pains in the Head, Face, Nose, Shoulders, Arms, Back, Breast, Belly, Thighs, Knees, Legs, Shins, Feet and Joints, with swellings or Tumours in the Hands; Arms, Thighs and other Parts, with loss of appetite, and a general weakness of the whole body. The Scurvy causeth sore Throat, Gums, and Looseness of Teeth, with red Knobs in the Face and Body, briny sharp Humours behind the Ears, and in other parts; it bring the Dropsie, Consumption, Feavers, Agues, Gout, and many other Diseases...[18]

'all which' – luckily for the sufferer – 'are cured with this Pill'. Many other quack bills offered similarly all-embracing lists of symptoms. Were you suffering from 'Swimming and Dizziness in the Head'; was your 'Body dull and Heavy', or your complexion 'swarthy'; did you have 'Flushing in the Face, Worms, black, loose and aking teeth, sore and bloody Gums, strong and stinking breath, streightnesse of Breath, Difficulty in breathing, ready to die, Sour Belchings, Wateriness at Stomach, Weariness of the Limbs, Faint Sweats towards Morning', not to mention 'Spots red, blewish or purple in the legs'? If so, you had scurvy, a 'popular disease' (identical phrases crop up again and again in the quack bills), which you should instantly counter with Nendick's Popular Pill, which had the bonus effect of also being an 'excellent Head Purge, good for over-drinking'. In other words, scurvy was the 'cause' of no end of 'tedious and difficult Diseases'.[19]

If, as widely accepted, scurvy produced this melange of symptoms, precisely what was it? According to Nendick, it was: 'bred from corrupt humours which strangely taint and foul the blood, and fill the vessels with Obstructions, raising Vapours.'

Another bill expanded upon these same themes:

> The Scurvy is a certain evil habit of the whole Body, turning all the Aliment we receive into evil Humours, taking its Original from Crude and Melancholy Humours, the Cause whereof is for want of good Digestion in the Stomack, caused either by great Obstructions of the Spleen, Liver, or Mesentery, and sometime from Obstructions of the Sweetbreds, as also from a raw and undigested Blood in the whole Body, but chiefly in the Hypochondries or Sides, which offends by a certain specifick Putrefaction arising from our Diet.[20]

All in all, the author concluded, after this tour de force, which further referred the reader to the works of the great Thomas Willis, scurvy was 'proteus like'.

Medicines against scurvy thus had to combat the great evil of the age. The Herculeon Antidote – which proclaimed that there are 'few Diseases, but have a spice of the scurvey, which corrupts the Blood' – promised to effect a 'cure by cleansing of the Blood, Purging by Urine, and gently by Stool': act fast, urged the author, before the disease radicated itself into the system and thus turned dangerously constitutional.

It was of the essence of quack medicines that their contents were kept secret from the public. Rarely did a quack bill reveal what a nostrum contained – though often the proprietor boasted of the cesspit of harmful ingredients, such as mercury, from.which his particular compound was free. Things were slightly different in the case of scurvy, since a freely-growing plant, scurvy-grass (cochlaea), was readily available, which had a good reputation as a folk remedy. Quacks dealing in antiscorbutics thus needed to develop a response to scurvy-grass. Typically, they claimed that recourse to the grass in its crude, rough, unpurified form would inevitably produce deleterious side-effects. Far better was the use of the herb properly distilled, for instance in the form of The Essential Spirit of Scurvey Grass Compound, the 'Invention and Preparation of the Sieur de Vernantes, a German born', who had 'Graduated in Physick in those famous Universities, Montpellier, and Padua in Italy'.[21] His compound was free of all the rough effects of the grass itself, had good keeping properties, and was further excellent for dropsy, strengthening the stomach, and stimulating the appetite.

Numerous other preparations similarly claimed to present cochlaea in more palatable or beneficial forms. Bateman's Spirits of Scurvy-Grass – far superior to the crude scurvy-grass – came in two different forms ('plain' and 'golden'), and was especially indispensable for those sick as a result of 'large suppers or over-drinking', and racked with 'sower Blenchings'. Robert Bateman was pleased to reveal that the famous Dr Dyke, who practised near Taunton, allowed his name to be used in support of his preparation.[22]

Or you could try Blagrave's Spirits of Scurvey-Grass – according to Bateman, a pirated form of his own medicine. As well as overcoming scurvy, this was also good for cholic, scabs, spots, wind, and for bringing away 'gravel in the kidneys' -indeed, for much more besides, such as: 'Dropsie, Stone, Wind Collick, Gravel in the Kidneys, Opens Obstructions, Cures and Green Sickness, and causeth a fresh ruddy Complexion; Evacuates Cold Phlegmatick Humours from the Stomach, Liver, and Spleen, wasting the swelling and hardness thereof… and recovers a lost Appetite.'[23]

How did such scurvy-cures work? Like so many other medicines made by quack and orthodox alike, they operated by purging – by opening up the passages and vessels within, and by expelling noxious substances. Thus John Case's Cordial Elixir overcame scurvy by 'opening Obstructions of the Spleen and purging Melancholy Humours from the Blood in every vein'. In so doing, not only did it remove scurvy, but would also 'purge Choler and Flegm too'.

Purging was the vital operation performed by all such medicines, which promised to rectify general malaises of the blood, digestion, and internal organs. Thus Ewel's Panaseton did not merely cure scurvy but also eradicated 'Obstructions, Flushings, windy Belchings, Fumes, Heachachs, Surfeits, Gripings in the Guts, Vomitings, Loosness, Fainting, Loss of appetite,... and leaves the Stomach mightily strengthened' – overall it 'purges away those salt, briny, melancholy, sharp humours, which so universally indispose the Body'.[24] Yet another antiscorbutic trading upon the universal faith in purging could be had 'over against the Golden Faulcken in French Alley': this was a 'Famous Cordial Spirit', which 'takes away the Scurvy out of the Body, Root and Branch, and the Dropsie to Admiration'.[25]

Scurvy was thus the archetypal disease of the late seventeenth century. It produced multifarious symptoms of malaise; it was rooted in the stomach and the blood, and it could be conquered by dosing oneself with the appropriate proprietary purges. Complementary medicines – such as Anderson's Scots Pills – were also advocated for cleansing the system of all manner of other ailments and disorders. The Grana Angelica ('universally known and approved by Physicians and others of all Ranks'), would, for instance, serve as a 'Sovereign Remedy against Diseases or Pains in the Head, Stomach, or Bellies of Men, Women and Children; but especially against Giddiness and thick Humours, Worms, Paleness, Green-sickness, Defluctions on the Lungs or Joyntes, Gravel, Stone, Scurvey, Dropsie Chollick or Gripes and all Obstructions'.[26]

And to augment the action of such medicines designed to rid the body of poisons, crudities, and foul humours, a pick-me-up was obviously required, or a tonic or cordial, such as the Elixir Magnum Stomachum, which was 'not purging but cordial only', 'the best purl in the world' – that is, a bitter meant to impart an appetite, bracing and strengthening the stomach lining, 'especially after a surfeit of hard drinking'.[27] (It was precisely such a habit of alternating drinking binges with medication which, Thomas Trotter deplored, ruined the stomach and was the slippery slope to alcoholism.)[28]

The allure of the typical late-Stuart quack medicine was thus that it would not merely vanquish disease, but by taking 'away all sordid humours' (as Cornelius à Tilbourg claimed) restore the metabolism to its pristine, natural efficiency. Therein lay the appeal of such 'cleansers' as the Universal Scorbutick Pills, which worked as a 'Radical Purifier of Nature': 'Operating by Purgation and Urine, with the greatest ease and success in various Diseases and Infirmities: gntly cleansing the whole Body (by those two principal evacuations) from all Scorbutick, Corrupt and depraved Humours; thereby casting out the Seeds of diseases.'[29]

Such claims to restore the entire system to health continued to orientate the rhetoric of quack medicine throughout the eighteenth century. But a certain change in terminology and in the accompanying image of disease can be seen. Mirroring shifts in regular medicine itself, Georgian quackery came to construe the roots of general indisposition as lying not so exclusively in a scorbutic constitution or in the explanatory framework of the humours, but rather in the nervous sensibility, determined by the nervous system. Thus it increasingly appeared that remedy lay less in the traditional hydraulics of purging and flushing, but instead in operations such as strengthening, vivifying, renewing tensility, and energizing. Medicines increasingly promised to recover the vital powers, indeed (with electricity in mind) to galvanize the system. Such developments will be explored in greater detail in the following chapter.

Quack medicines

What were quack medicines like? Official pharmacopoeias – for instance, that published by the Royal College of Physicians – remained a hodge-podge, and our knowledge of the prescribing habits of the average apothecary is scanty. Under such circumstances, and assuming the painful workings of the law of trial and error, it is unlikely that empiric preparations which commanded their share of the market for fifty or a hundred years – or more! – were decisively worse than those prescribed by regulars. Indeed, as was repeatedly

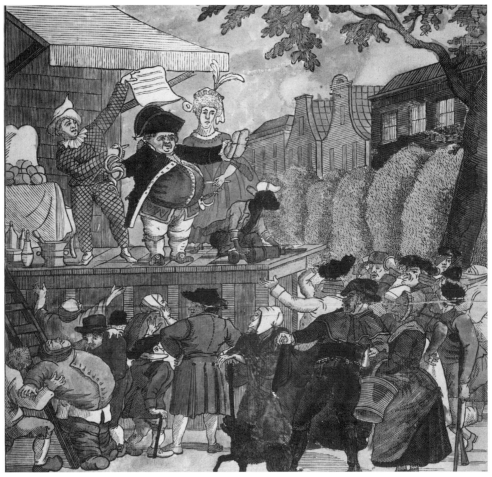

A nostrum-vendor performs his patter before an excitable crowd. Coloured wood engraving by J. Oortman.

pointed out, regular doctors themselves often prescribed patent and propietary medicines. Proper research is needed on early modern pharmacy, and it is beyond the scope of this section to analyse the ingredients contained in quack medicaments or to evaluate their efficacy. Rather, I wish to explore some of the arguments proposed by quacks themselves, demonstrating why their own drugs excelled those of the regulars, and to hazard some assessments of why the sick actually purchased them.

Quack doctors, as we saw in chapter 4, commonly asserted point-blank that their medicines were universally effective and therapeutically nonpareil. But while exploiting the appeal of the panacea, they also championed the 'specific', with its plausible rationale that one particular sort of drug was fatal to a particular disease (rather as artillery would destroy fortifications while cavalry would prevail on the battlefield). After all, it was becoming more widely accepted that certain specifics truly worked – for example, Jesuit's Bark (quinine) against ague or marsh fever – and the enhanced prestige of chemistry was

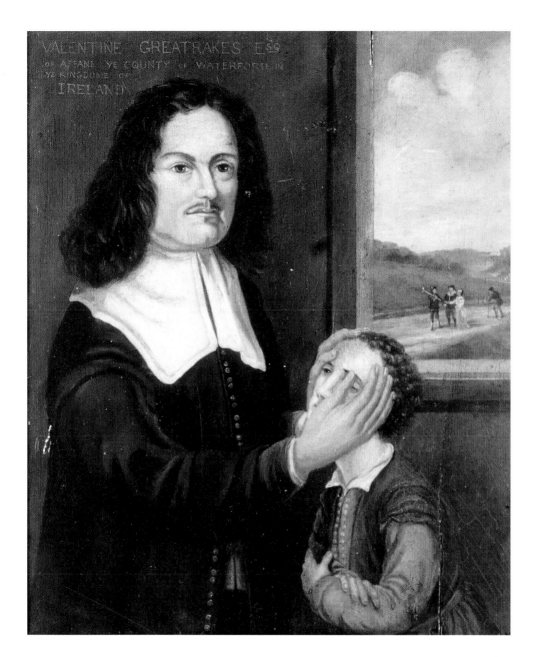

Valentine Greatrakes, the Irish stroker who was a favourite of Charles II. Oil painting.

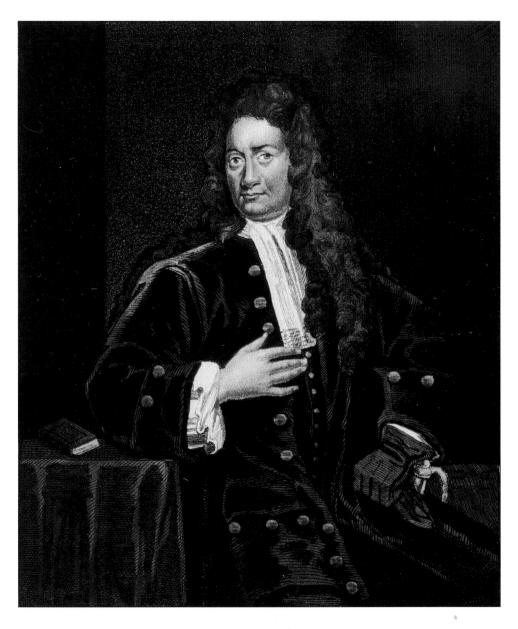

Dr Radcliffe, founder of the Radclivian library and creator of Radcliff's Purging Elixir. Coloured stipple engraving after M. Dahl after Sir G. Kneller, 1710.

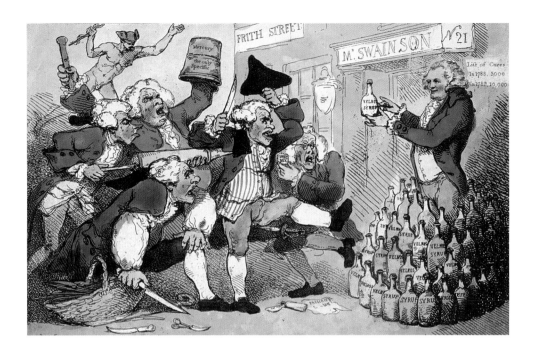

'MERCURY and his ADVOCATES DEFEATED, or VEGETABLE ENTRENCHMENT'
Isaac Swainson promoting his Velno's syrup in the face of rival practitioners advocating mercury.
Coloured etching by T. Rowlandson, 1789.

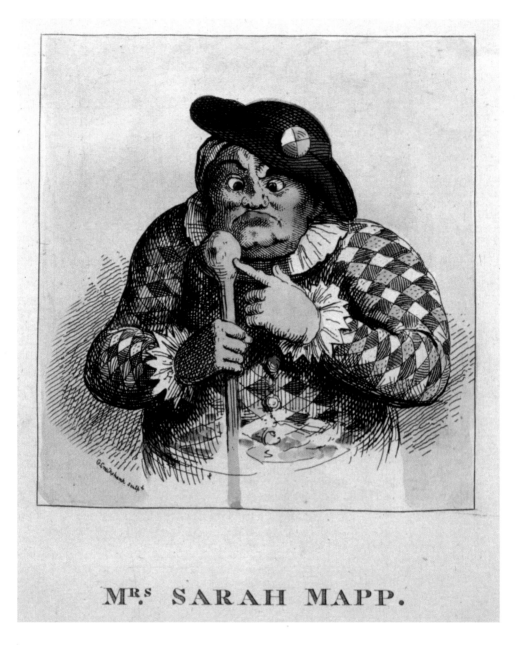

M^{RS} SARAH MAPP.

Sarah Mapp, the bone-setter of Epsom, as she appeared in Hogarth's 'The Company of Undertakers'.
Coloured etching by G. Cruikshank, 1819, after W. Hogarth.

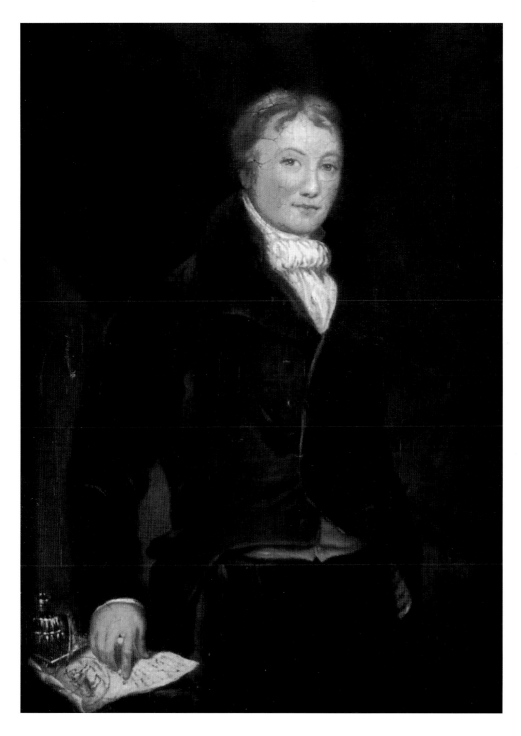

Edward Jenner, vaccination pioneer and creator of indigestion lozenges. Oil painting.

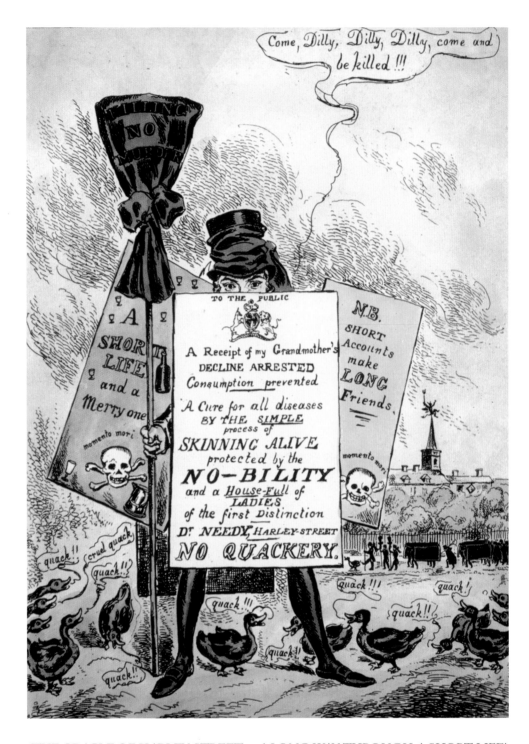

'THE ORACLE OF HARLEY STREET or A LONG WAY THROUGH A SHORT LIFE'
John St John Long, who specialized in consumption cures, is shown dressed as a funeral mourner and
carrying placards promoting his dubious practices. Coloured etching, 1830.

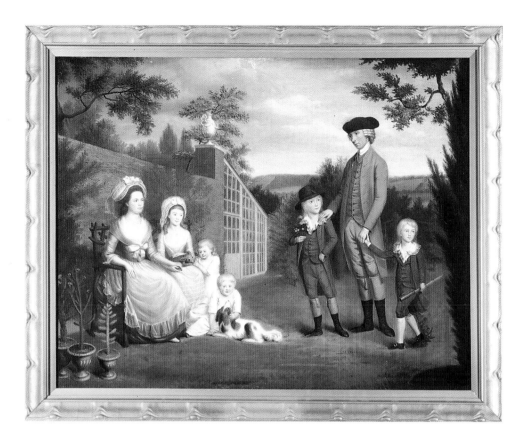

John Coakley Lettsom, an eminent London physician who campaigned against quackery, particularly the urine-gazing of Theodor Myersbach, in his garden at Camberwell. Oil painting.

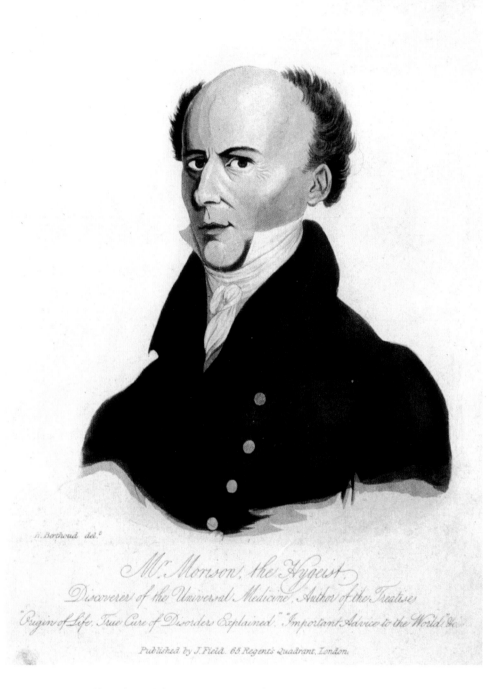

James Morison, self-proclaimed 'hygeist' and creator of Morison's Universal Pills. Coloured aquatint after H. Bertoud.

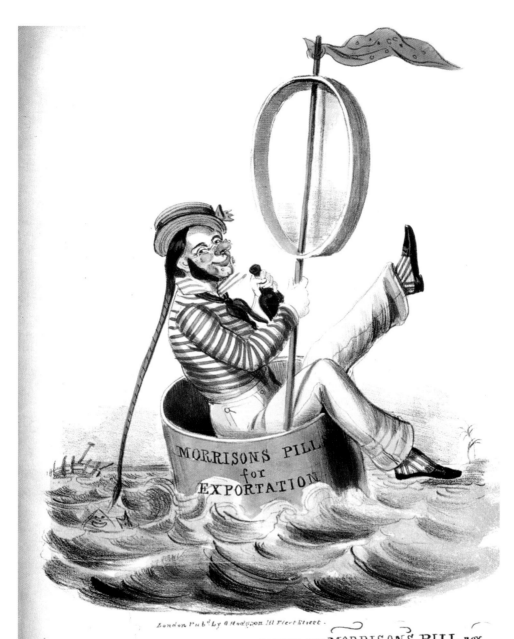

London Pubd by G Hodgson 111 Fleet Street

THE LIFE OF A BRITISH SAILOR SAVED BY MORRISON'S PILL BOX

Never go to sea without a large box of Morrisons Pills they will save your life said the doctor and sure his honour was right and no mistake when we were wreckd and all aboard perishd I swallowd the Pills jumpd into the BOX and here I am going with a fair wind safe ashore. —

A sailor owes his life to Morison's Pills after a shipwreck. Coloured lithograph.

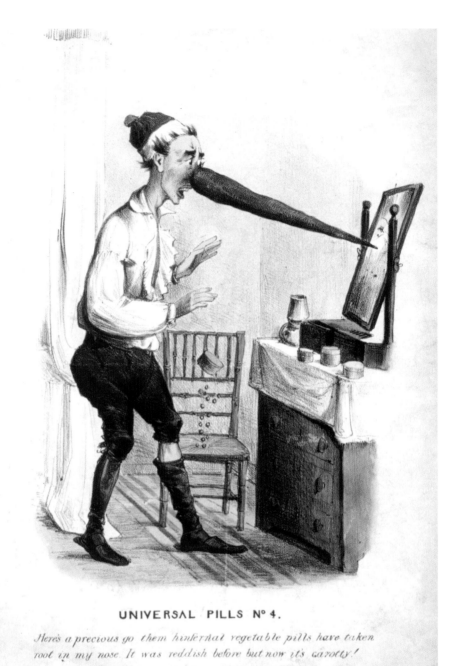

UNIVERSAL PILLS Nº 4.

*Here's a precious go them hinfernal vegetable pills have taken
root in my nose. It was reddish before but now it's carotty!*

W. Spooner, 377 Strand

A horrified man discovers the unexpected side-effects of Morison's vegetable pills. Coloured lithograph.

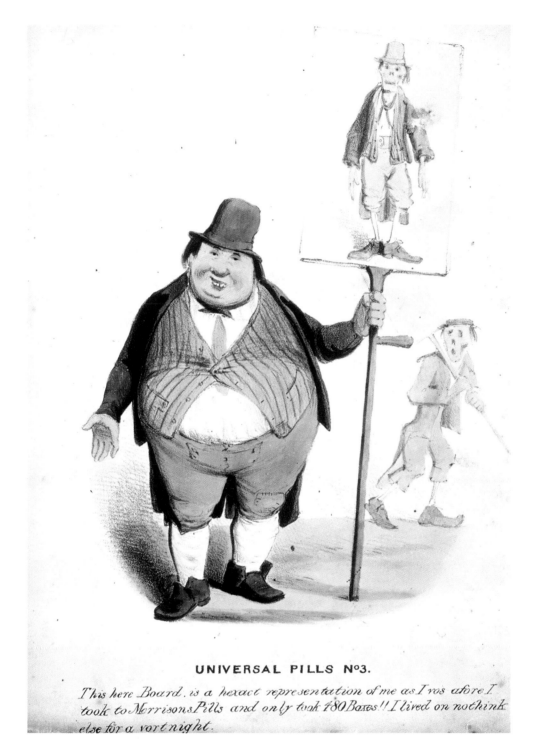

UNIVERSAL PILLS Nº3.

This here Board. is a hexact representation of me as I vos afore I took to Morrisons Pills and only took 480 Boxes!! I lived on nothink else for a vortnight.

The miraculous effect of just 480 boxes of Morison's Universal Pills. Coloured lithograph.

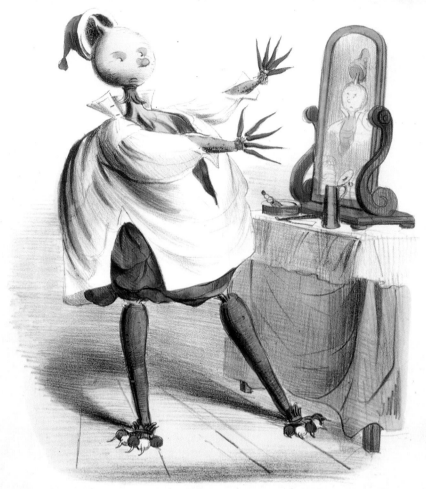

London Pub.d by O Hodgson 111 Fleet Street.

WONDERFUL EFFECT OF MORRISONS VEGETABLE PILLS

They told me if I took 1000 pills at night I should be quite another thing in the morning

Another unexpected result of over-indulgence in Morison's Pills. Coloured lithograph.

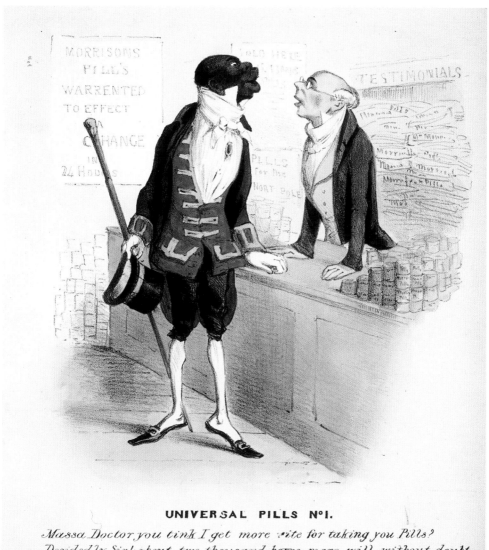

An unscrupulous shopkeeper ascribing unlikely powers to Morison's Universal Pills

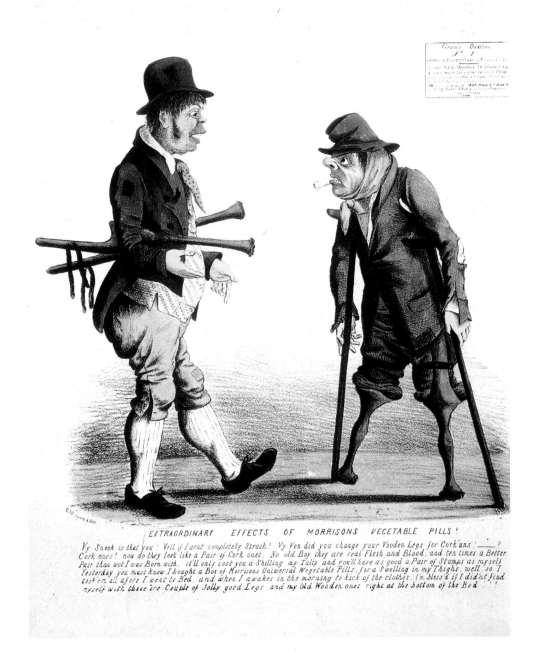

A tramp excitedly rells how Morison's Pills made his missing legs grow back. Coloured lithograph by C.J. Grant, 1834.

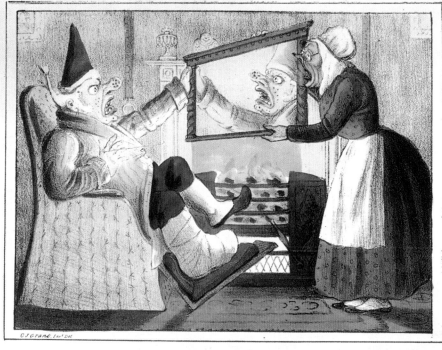

Another unwary user of Morison's Universal Pills is dismayed to discover grass growing out of his skin. Coloured lithograph by C.J. Grant, 1835.

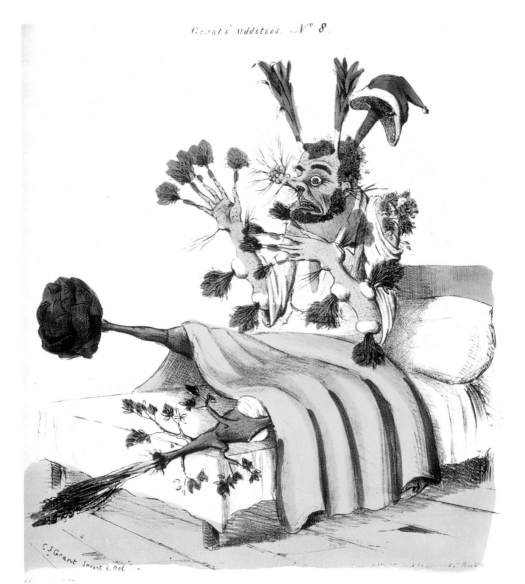

C.J.Grant Invent & Del.

SINGULAR EFFECTS OF THE UNIVERSAL _VEGETABLE_ PILLS ON A GREEN GROCER 'A FACT'

Who Green'un like was order'd to live for the space of one Month upon _Vegetable_ Diet & to Take during that time 132 Boxes of _Vegetable_ Pills for the Cure of a Gangreen. & being caught in a Shower of Rain in the Green Fields in the evening of the 1st of April last was put to Bed 'midst _Shooting_ pains & in the Morning presented the above Phenomenon of a Moving Kitchen Garden !!!

Query _ Is he not one of the _Productive_ Classes.

Perhaps the most spectacular mishap of the lot, this user of Universal Pills wakes up to find he has become a kitchen garden. Coloured lithograph by C.J. Grant, 1831.

giving sanction to specific chemical operations – acids and alkalis, for instance. Nevertheless, general physicians dragged their heels about developing specifics – precisely because they had a reputation for being quackish: as Coleridge remarked early in the nineteenth century: 'The study of specific medicines is too much disregarded now. To doubt the hunting after specifics is a mark of ignorance and weakness in medicine, yet the neglect of them is proof also of immaturity; for in fact all medicines will be found specific in the perfection of the science.'[30] Flanked with both panaceas and specifics, quacks could contend that their own drugs would cure all, even when the patient had already been damaged by disease and by other, inept practitioners. His own medicines for the pox, so Case claimed, cured even when patients were 'almost spoiled and undone by others'.[31]

But lest all such proofs of efficacy were not sufficiently convincing, they also advanced a standard rhetoric of subsidiary arguments on behalf of their own preparations. I shall examine some of these here, and others, in greater detail, in the next chapter.

There was, of course, the appeal to the pocket; this had a particular slant. On the whole, pre-modern quacks did not make their prime selling point the cheapness of their own preparations, arguing that here was health for sale at rock-bottom prices. Just how significant was competitive pricing – absolute and relative – in making or breaking products at this stage in the development of consumer-oriented capitalism? Nostrum-mongers certainly seem to have assumed that potential buyers could afford, and would be prepared to fork out sums in shillings rather than pence. Does this betray an assumption that those in quest of health should be prepared to pay the price? Was there a certain prestige in expense – did a highish price suggest that the medicine in question was indeed valuable? Was there a prejudice against cut-price health?

More prominent in the advertising than cheapness *tout court* were reassurances to buyers that they were getting a lot for their money – indeed, value for money. Many emphasized the large quantity one's outlay would purchase: a full pint bottle, or twenty-four or thirty-six pills. Case, like many others, sold his pills at three dozen for three shillings, a symbolic penny a pill. If pills were to be taken one or two at a time, a couple of times a day, than a tin of pills represented perhaps a week's medicine for a few shillings. To us, used to buying or being dispensed fifty or a hundred pills at a time, this does not sound many. But pre-modern regular physicians commonly prescribed, and apothecaries dispensed, medicines in far smaller numbers of doses – sometimes merely a single dose or a day's supply at a time, the rationale being the need for a modification of medicine or dosage almost every day. Such daily dispensing could prove enormously costly. To get a goodly parcel of medicine from a quack seemed more economical, even a bargain.

Moreover, obtaining a substantial quantity was specially important for those about to go on their travels, voyage overseas, or return to rural solitude. Quacks were not slow to appeal to the foresight of buyers, who would think it prudent to stock up in anticipation of future need. For such customers, they repeatedly stressed how their own preparations had quite extraordinary keeping properties. Quacks regularly claimed their pills would stay fresh and active for years, as would even their medicines if kept in tightly stoppered bottles. John Case boasted that his pills 'will keep good some years, whereby they may be beneficial to such as live in the Country or to Sea-men that Travel to Foreign Parts'.[32] The Universal Scorbutick Pills, it was similarly claimed, were 'durable in full vertue many years, a most necessary provision for all Country Inhabitants, Travellers, Souldiers, Seamen, Planters &'.[33] The implied contrast was with the boluses and electuaries of regular pharmacy – soft pills and syrups, intended to be taken within a couple of days of being made up. It was thus quacks who turned medication into a 'consumer durable', and who underlined the convenience and thrift thereby embodied.

Not least, quacks claimed their own medicines worked more easily, with less dislocation to the system and fewer side-effects than orthodox medicine. In an age in which drugs were standardly nauseous, and purges often so heroic as to operate fifteen or twenty times, this – if true – may by itself have been a welcome relief. But there was a further, more subtle, benefit. For quacks often claimed that – by contrast to regular therapeutic purges and vomits, where one would be forced to take some days' bed-rest while being physicked – with their own medicines, it was possible to continue about one's trade. Case claimed his pills worked 'without hindrance of business'. This, we may surmise, may have been the last thing the patient actually needed. But in a precarious economy, before sickness insurance, in which being off work would have spelt financial disaster to many, the rather more leisurely assumptions of Greek and humanist medicine could have no attractions to common people.

Whether or not quack medicines did much good, they showed sensitivity to customer demand (a demand they were partly instrumental in creating in the first place). Pre-modern quackery did not seek to create alternative understandings of health and disease: it battened on to those already existing. But it did effectively exploit those perceptions in mobilizing markets for its preparations.

6   Quacks and sex

Why don't they review and praise 'Solomon's Guide to Health'. It is better
sense – and as much poetry – as Johnny Keats.
Lord Byron, *Letters and Journals*

Rival readings of the sexual history of England during the long eighteenth century confront us. One scholarly tradition sees the age between the Restoration of 'Old Rowley' and the point – usually left rather indeterminate – when 'Victorianism before Victoria' set in as a golden age of sexual liberty, after the shackles of Puritan 'thou shalt notism' had been cast off, and before Bowdlerism and Grundyism drove sensuality underground, to fester for the benefit of later Freudian psychopathological analyses.

Another, more recent, revisionist outlook offers a darker picture: on the one hand, a more ferocious male libertinism, leading to intensified exploitation of vulnerable servant women, teenage prostitutes, and so forth; on the other, the excitation of new sexual fears, especially anxieties about masturbation (mainly in young males), about puberty in teenage girls, about nymphomania, hysteria, enervation – all these fears being intensified by the irrefutable sanction of disease.

Both pictures have their truths. The mistake is to present them as polar opposites, or as mutually incompatible, rather than as concomitants. Abundant first-hand evidence shows that the Georgian sexual economy was public and permissive in its fashions in dress, its street life, gossip, and, not least, its burgeoning printed erotica. The point is confirmed by its popular medico-sexual literature. In much-reprinted treatises for popular consumption, such as *Arisotle's Master-Piece*, the keynote fell not upon the blessings of chastity or sexual restraint, but upon the joys of sex, so long as they were experienced under appropriate moral, personal and medical circumstances. Plenty of quack medical writings promised to restore the old and jaded to the peak of sexual energy, excitement, and bloom. The underlying assumption of Georgian medico-sexual writings is that heterosexual erotic activity is, and ought to be desirable, pleasurable, normal, and healthy.

Indeed, it was a culture that set great store by erotic appearance. All manner of cosmetic and medical preparations were marketed for heightening sexual attractiveness. Some, such as hair-restorers, were targeted at both sexes. A 'Gentlewoman' at the Blew Ball in little Kerby Street, 'hath a most Excellent and Wonderful Art to make the Hair grow wherever it be wanting, though there had been none before (as she hath already done to the admiration of several)'. For her part, Sarah Cornelius de Heusde promised, most obligingly, to 'make the Hair to fall out, where it is too much, and make it grow, where it is too little'. Stephen Draper, who sold cosmetics guaranteed to remove 'Scurf, Morphew, Tan', replacing them with a complexion of a 'lovely colour', also boasted, 'You may have Hair taken from the Forehead, Lips, Chin or any other Part'.[1]

Products were also marketed, such as David Peronnet's Universal Dentrifrice, for whitening, polishing, and cleansing the teeth. As Christine Hillam has demonstrated, many itinerant dentists made a lucrative living in the provinces throughout the Georgian age; mere pulling of teeth remained, of course, the bread and butter of their trade, but the more up-market of them liked to publicize themselves as adroit in cosmetic dentistry (straightening teeth, replacing those extracted or broken with dentures made of ivory, etc.), so as to improve the face (toothlessness aged people dreadfully). Thus, one of the many late seventeenth-century 'High German Doctors' boasted his skills at setting in 'Artificial Teeth as if they were natural'.[2]

Not least, cleanliness, John Wesley's second greatest virtue, was expedited by all kinds of brand-name soaps, washes, milks, oils, and cleansers. These did not merely remove dirt but skin impurities, too. One product was puffed as the 'Only Delicate Beautifying Cream For Gentlemen and Ladies', which took away 'Redness, Pimples, Roughness, Worms, Morphew, Scurf, Sunburn, Freckles, Wrinkles, Pits of the Small Pox'.[3]

But if, as we have seen, some items were 'unisex', most beauty preparations were targeted at glamorizing the ladies. As part of a profound and ambiguous transformation in the social status and power (or, possibly, impotence) of women, being female was becoming equated with new criteria of 'femininity'; increasingly treated as sex objects, women found they were expected to conform to eroticized norms in their appearance. By consequence, the market was flooded with preparations claiming to cleanse women's skin, improve the complexion, remove or conceal spots, expunge scurf and other blemishes, and rid them of facial hair and body odour. Waters, fragrances, oils, and essences all promised to improve the appearance, put pink in the cheeks and a sparkle in the eye, obliterate facial lines, mask rank odours, and restore the bloom of youth (the 'young look' came into fashion amongst the late-Georgians, though – by contrast to the twentieth century – it did not lead to a preoccupation with slimming preparations).

Quasi-medical commercial preparations thus contributed to the selling of sex. Many also conveyed the promise of fecundity. Amongst the constant refrains in quack bills during the long eighteenth century was the promise to cure female infertility (it was typically assumed that women were to blame). Sometimes, the proprietor was a man (for example, Dr Stephen Draper, the man-midwife), and sometimes a woman's name headed the advertisement: the product and the by-line seem much the same, in any case. Addressing themselves to the ladies, they promised to remove 'female obstructions', and to procure, or renew menstruation. When teenage girls were the target, this meant attacking the 'green sickness' (chlorosis), a supposed disorder of adolescent girls, symptomatized by a lack-lustre complexion, listlessness, poor skin colour, want of appetite, weakness, moodiness, or downright melancholy, and either delay in the menarche or amenorrhoea (itself often regarded as the source of all other symptoms). In the case of older women, such preparations promised to 'restore the courses'.

Should we here be reading between the lines? For one way of 'removing obstructions' or 'restoring the terms' is by procuring abortion. Were all the advertisements promising to remove obstructions, in truth, selling not aids to fertility but abortifacients? – and, indeed, were they read and used as such? Certainly, some medicines for women delivered explicit warnings that they were not to be taken by women 'with child' – surely a pretty broad hint as to their covert purpose. And, likewise, what do we make of Samuel Solomon's claim, in respect of his Balm of Gilead, that 'ladies at any time of life may by this medicine, be freed from one of the most afflicting disorders incident to the sex, and at a certain period, it is most highly useful?'[4]

But certain preparations for women's diseases genuinely seem to have been targeted at ladies wishing to conceive and be fruitful rather than those seeking to terminate pregnancy. Thus Cornelius à Tilbourg touted 'a great Secret to help Conception; likewise a powerful Medicine to prevent Miscarriage, although you have Miscarried 5 or 6 times successively'. Similarly, 'A person that hath travelled abroad in the World hath got the knowledge of a great Secret, to cure BARRENNESS', adding (perhaps trading on the inevitable snigger) that he has 'made use of for many years with very great success'. He promised to take no payment till the woman conceived, and then only half, reserving the rest for when she was successfully brought to bed (a ploy, one supposes, to ensure her continued custom). Stephen Draper, having unctuously warned women to 'Beware of Cheating Mechanick Mountebanks', claimed to have medicines to 'prevent Abortion'.[5]

So there are good reasons for taking at least some quack fertility preparations at their word. And why not? After all, Georgian men and women subscribed alike to the medical commonplace that the fecund woman was the healthy woman (producing babies was one of many healthy forms of evacuation), great ignominy was attached to the wife who failed to produce heirs (or workhands), and barren women commonly visited spas and drank medicinal waters in the hope of conceiving. A 'Doctor of Physick' advertising 'The Private Cure', played upon the common association between women's diseases in general and barrenness in particular, by promising to be able to cure all at a stroke, including 'Fits of the Mother, Vapours rising up to the Throat, Passions or Tremblings of the Heart, Obstructions, Convulsions, Green Sickness, Weakness, and Pains of the Back, [He also] makes Fruitful, takes away the cause of Barrenness or impotence in men or Women, which secret preserves youth and prolongs life'.[6] Maybe there was little market as yet for terminating unwanted pregnancies. It is noteworthy that none of the nostrums advertised during the long eighteenth century appears to have boasted, or even hinted at, contraceptive properties. Likewise, none of the 'advertising physicians' of the late seventeenth century was selling condoms or other sexual prophylactics.

Venereal disease

Thus one facet of Georgian culture associated sexuality with health, happiness, beauty, and fertility, and quack medicine pledged to promote these ends. Yet there was, as already noted, a darker side. For the claims of the medicine-mongers and operators in the century after the Restoration reveal one disease type recurring far more commonly than any other: venereal disease. Even in a respectable magazine such as the *Female Tatler*, the most common advertisements were for venereal-disease cures.

Usually, there was no beating about the bush. One bill arrested the reader with the headline: 'An Herculeon Antidote Against the POX' (the public-spirited advertiser promised that so as not to 'give Incouragement to vice' he would not breathe a word about

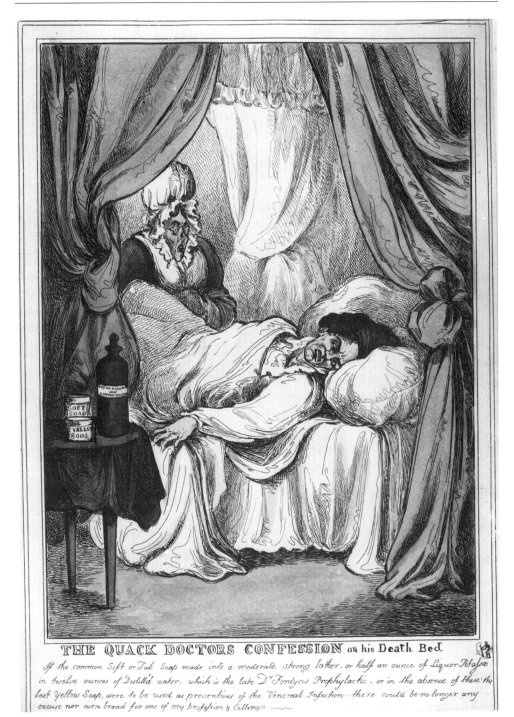

THE QUACK DOCTORS CONFESSION on his Death Bed

If the common Soft or Tub Soap made into a moderate strong lather. or half an ounce of Liquor Potasses in twelve ounces of Distilld water. which is the late D.ʳ Fordyces Prophylactic, or in the absence of these the best Yellow Soap, were to be used as preventives of the Venereal Infection. there could be no longer any excuse nor even bread for one of my profession & Calling

A dying unscrupulous medical practitioner confesses the error of his ways (and advertises Dr Fordyce's Prophylactic against venereal disease). Coloured etching by W. Heath.

the ingredients used in his remedy). Another bill, put about by John Case, announced in bold type, 'A Most Infallible, and Sure Cheap Secret Safe and Speedy Cure for a Clap', and 'Dr Rivers' headed one of his posters 'The True Symptoms of a Clap or Pox with its Cure', stating that he was available for consultations at the Golden Ball in Three King's Court on Ludgate Hill, where he had 'a light at the door in an evening'. In similar vein a bill headed 'Venus Deceiv'd, or An Account of the Seat, and Nature of a Clap' sold a cure, a mere seven doses of which would do the trick (a hint, surely, of a magic number?).[7]

Venereal disorders were widely called the 'alamode disease', and certain cures attained a wry public celebrity – for example, Velno's Vegetable Syrup and Leake's Pills, which both figured prominently, alongside empty port bottles and dice, in a satirical cartoon of the Prince Regent, 'A Voluptuary Under the Horrors of Digestion', produced by Gillray in 1792. Jokey or self-consciously euphemistic language was often employed in quack venereal-disease advertisements, presumably to minimize the apparent moral gravity of contracting the disorder. Those poxed or clapped had been 'sporting in the garden of Venus'; or (as James à Tilbourg put it) they were the 'children of Venus', who had 'anchored in a Strange Harbour' (this and other maritime metaphors indicate the occupation of the expected clientele for such nostrums).

Most quack clap-cures paraded their virtues in similar terms. Typical was a bill posted by a 'High German Doctor', who claimed that he:

> cureth in an Extraordinary, and most easy manner, the Morbus Gallicus or French POX with all its Symptoms (as the Gonorrhoea or Running of the Reins, Shankers, Buboes, or swellings in the Groin), pain in the Head, Arms, Shoulders and Legs, or Ulcers in the Mouth, Throat, Scabs, Itch, and breaking out over the whole Body, after a new and easy method, although you have had it several years, and have been Fluxt several times, and almost spoiled by others, and given over as incurable; he can cure you both surely and safely, without either Fluxing or Mercury, or any Danger at all; he has cured abundants when left off by other Doctors as incurable; and therefore for the satisfaction of those who have been Sporting in the Garden of VENUS, and instead of Pleasure have met with a CLAP or Running of the Reins; he promises to Cure them in 6 or 7 days time, or else desires nothing for his pains, which is as much as to say NO CURE NO MONEY.[8]

Note the salient features. We sense, for one thing, an atmosphere of 'anxiety making' – indeed, trading on fear. Anyone experiencing unexplained pains in the head, arms, shoulders, etc., might well be led to conclude – probably quite needlessly – from perusing this advertisement that he was poxed. This possibility was reinforced by the fact that various quacks explained that 'the Running of the Reins' (a urethral discharge) was not always 'got by women [that is, caught through having sex with an infected woman] as some think'.[9] Of course, this claim would provide a perfect excuse for those who were truly clapped; for the underlying implication is that (following traditional medical theory) someone might perfectly easily become clapped as the result of legitimate conjugal sex, if the act were performed too frequently, or too lustily, or at the wrong season, or when not in the pink of health (or, of course, if one's partner were unfaithful). Yet the consequence of floating such a view was that the potential pool of people who might be persuaded, by the advertising, that they were infected was widened.

And it may have been further augmented, thanks to the fact that venereal infections seemed to share many similar symptoms with 'scurvy'. As discussed in the previous chapter, scurvy was widely associated with running sores, ulcerated skin, and other signs of 'rottenness'. In fact, quack publicity openly traded on the elision of the two disorders, talking occasionally of the pox as 'the French Scurvy'. Quack doctors may thus have convinced many who were merely suffering from non-specific skin disorders that they were venereally infected – with particularly sad results if the poor wretch then underwent courses of quack treatment, which truly destroyed his health. The figure of the syphilophobe, fearful of every little twinge in the back, and convinced his nose was daily disappearing, looms large in the medical anecdotes of the time.

If quack venereal-disease publicity thus fomented fear, it also exploited hope. For, as we saw in the bill quoted at length above, grand promises were proffered, even to those poxed many years back, who had already undergone courses of treatment, and been 'given over as incurable'. Even such a person was vouchsafed a speedy cure. Above all, easy and painless cures were promised, without fluxing or the need for mercury. Precisely this claim formed the piece de resistance of all quack venereal-disease nostrums. Thus a 'Graduate Physician' reassured sufferers that 'I flux no one, let them be never so bad, or give any Mercureal Medicine'. In the same vein, a certain 'J. C. Physician', invited 'all who have slipp'd between the thighs of Venus' and ended up poxed, to try his pill, which would cure 'without the Tiresomeness of Physick, or multitude of purging, in a few days'.[10]

Thus the swiftness of the cure was important, too. A surgeon living 'without Temple Bar in St Clements Little Church Yard next door to the Sign of the Black Lion' had succeeded (thanks to 'practical Study and Twenty years travels in most Countries of the Universe') to 'attain to a Medicine that Infallibly Cures the Running of the Reins in Ten Days Time'. The preparation could also be used quasi-prophylactically, to get the 'poisonous Steem' from the body, after 'Copulating with a suspicious Bedfellow' – though, in advancing this, the author naturally covered himself by saying under no circumstances did he wish 'to give encouragement to vice'.[11] Avoiding time off work was likewise important. Thus Anthony Bellon claimed to cure the French pox 'without obliging his Patients to keep their Chambers, nor leaving their daily Occupations'.[12]

The claim to cure the pox without recourse to mercury was cardinal to all quack therapies. By the latter part of the seventeenth century, the standard – though, as Bynum has shown, hardly universal – treatment for syphilis amongst regular practitioners was mercury, often applied both internally and externally, and accompanied with bathing, steaming, and sweating. The treatment would 'flux' the patient: powerful evacuations, perspiration, and copious salivation (often a couple of quarts of saliva a day) would be produced, designed to force out the fever. The therapy was often lengthy, difficult, and unpleasant. It would require the patient being laid up; offensive side-effects resulted, including swelling of the gums, aching joints, and a

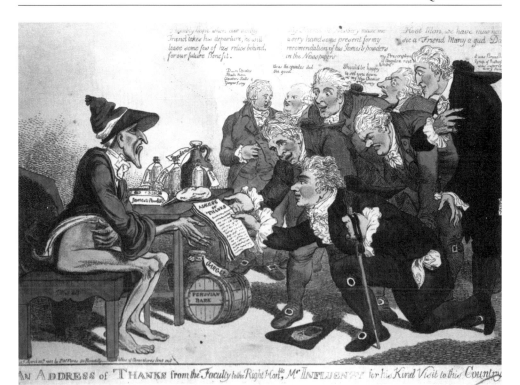

Physicians expressing thanks to 'Mr Influenza' while arguing the efficacy of different medicinal ingredients. Coloured etching attributed to Temple West, 1803.

fetid smell. Not surprisingly, it was a most unpopular treatment; anyone crying up an alternative found eager listeners.

Almost to a man and woman, quack venereal-disease doctors repudiated mercury. They contended that it did not work, and boasted effective alternatives. Thus G. Dean, a 'chymical physician', offered: 'Speedy and Absolute Cure for the French Pox, without Fluxing, or Confinement, or the use of any Poysonous Mercurial Remedies, also the Relicts of the same Disease not well Cured, are totally Extirpated, and all Injuries sustained by Mercury where the Parts or Faculties are not Perished, faithfully Repaired with the Blessing of God.'[13] Another bill claimed to cure syphilis where mercury had failed, even in patients already 'damnified by poisonous Medicines'.[14] Quacks commonly argued that mercury often made bad worse, by turning a mere 'clap' (gonorrhoea) into a full-blown 'pox' (syphilis). Here they traded upon the commonly-held belief that there was only a single venereal disease, the clap and the pox being respectively mild and serious forms of it. They also alluded by inference to the widespread fear that harsh and depletive treatment – here with mercury – could exacerbate the very condition it was meant to be curing. Contemporaries accepted the principle that fevers needed to be treated by 'lowering' and 'depletion'; yet they also feared that excessive lowering would undermine the constitution utterly.

Quacks offered alternatives. Insofar as these were not mere frauds, mere coloured, sugared water, they were probably based upon guaiacum, sassafras, and sarsaparilla –

vegetable extracts that held a minority following amongst the regulars and actually possess a certain therapeutic value. With such treatments, patients would appear to improve – thus accounting for the riposte of John Marten, the surgeon, that so many who had undergone quack 'cures' had had their condition merely cosmetically cleared up. (Quacks replied 'you too' to the regulars.)

In their appeals to the public, quacks underlined the personal undesirability, no less than the inefficacy, of mercury treatment. For one thing, mercury incapacitated. By contrast, their nostrums could be taken as people went about their business: there was no need for bed rest or a special regime of life. (Though if patients absolutely needed, or preferred, bed treatment, most quacks also undertook to find them secret lodgings, and could provide bathhouses for sweating.)

A second point followed. Mercury treatment was inevitably conspicuous. Even in the event that the sores, rashes, and chancres of syphilis could be concealed, mercury treatment itself marked one out – above all, by its fever and salivation, but also by swollen gums, loose teeth, and the fetid smell exuded. Even if the cure were not worse than the disease, it was certainly more visible.

Quacks claimed, by contrast, that their cures were a form of invisible mending. Not a soul – not even one's bedfellow – need know that one were undergoing what would, in the fullest sense, be a 'secret treatment'. Thus a 'physician' at Clerkenwell Green promised to cure 'the French Pox and Running of the Reins' 'by easie and speedy means, without keeping house, thereby to discover their distemper, or hinder business' . He even pledged to take 'No money till perfectly well'. James à Tilbourg similarly claimed to cure poxed people 'so private that the Wife shall not know whether her Husband be cured of that distemper, nor the Man of his own wife, nor none of their relations shall take any notice of their Cure'.[115] James Spinke likewise contended that his venereal preparations 'cure with such Privacy that those you are constantly in Company with shall not suspect it'.[16]

Moreover, quacks claimed that their cures would effectively dispel all visible signs of ever having been poxed. A 'Physician of Many Years Experience' undertook to get rid of all 'Scars, Pustulaes, Spots, Ulcers of the Mouth or Throat', doing it with 'great secrecie'.[17]

Quack venereal-disease cures thus exemplify one further appeal of the commercial practitioner: secrecy. The covert, or even sometimes quite explicit message of the quack doctor was that the venereally infected person would naturally wish to avoid having to broach the matter to a regular doctor. It would be embarrassing enough to have to inform the family physician; worse still, through the physician, his servants, or the apothecary, tittle-tattle was bound to leak out into the wider world, to one's spouse or neighbours (a reasonable fear, for the scandal recorded in many contemporary diaries proves that physicians blabbed about their patients).

Quack bills pandered in many ways to the patient's obvious desire for confidentiality, indeed furtiveness. Many late-Stuart empirics appear to have dwelt in seedy, out-of-the-way, backstreet lodgings (possibly because they were often on the move, or because their finances were precarious). If this was a necessity, it was turned into a virtue by emphasizing that such addresses were shielded from the public gaze, and so could be visited without discovery. Sometimes bills stressed how their chambers could be approached via alleys, passage-ways, or back-doors. Gilbert Anderson's bill told readers that his dwelling had two entrances, one of them advantageously 'private in a court' ('you may enter which way you please'). Likewise, the bill headed 'Venus Deceiv'd' informed reader; that they could approach the practitioner's house without the need to ask anyone the way, even after dark, for: 'There is a Lamp lighted at his door in an Evening, by which he may be readily found in the Night time without Enquiry.'[18] Venereal-disease quacks often emphasized that they kept late hours (sometimes as late as ten o'clock at night), thereby allowing rendezvous under cover of darkness; many noted the kind of lamp, or the number of candles to be seen at the window. (Such cloak-and-dagger tactics were not unknown, of course, with regular doctors too, for example, William Hunter.)

Despite all these elaborate precautions, customers still might prefer not to run the risk of a personal visit. In that case, various expedients were possible. Some empirics offered to make house calls. Others were happy to be consulted by post (as, of course, were regulars). Thus the 'Excellent Physician' who sailed under the flag, 'Nothing Without God', informed the public that, if so consulted, he would send to the venereally infected 'such proper medicines that they may Cure themselves, to the Admiration of the Patient'.[19] Confidential letters could be sent, as, indeed, could medicines themselves, with total safety and confidentiality by the routine carrier service, for patients living outside the City. Not least, doctors urged patients to send urine samples, care of a servant, who could then return with the appropriate medicines. 'Many are bashful', wrote a 'True Friend to the Publick': if that applied to you, 'send a servant'.[20]

These arrangements were all summarized by a 'Physician of Many Years Experience', who undertook personally to 'come and visit' venereal patients, if 'through Business or Bashfulness', they could not see him. Or they could even send 'but a Note of their Distemper'.[21] What is noteworthy is that such a notoriously 'public' form of medicine could represent itself, thanks to its impersonality, as by far the most 'private' form of practice – a privacy achieved, not through the confidentiality of private practice but through the anonymity of the medical market-place.

As Bynum has emphasized, venereal disease remained throughout the eighteenth and nineteenth centuries a fertile seedbed for quackish practices (performed no less by doctors who in many respects were impeccably regular) because it was shameful: secret diseases bred secret remedies. It is thus a field of medicine in which it would be more than usually historically misleading to draw hard-and-fast divides between orthodox and quack. Where would we fit for example the Oxford graduate, Gilbert Kennedy? Kennedy was to all appearances a regular practitioner, except for the fact that he marketed Kennedy's Lisbon Diet Drink for clearing up venereal infections – Boswell was one of many famous people who bought it at the high price of half a guinea a bottle (two bottles were to be drunk a day).

Another example is John Marten, the regular surgeon and venereal-disease specialist. Read one way, his *Treatise… of the Venereal Disease* (1708) was perhaps the lengthiest expose and denunciation of the villainy of clap quackery. Marten presents himself as resigned to spending his life picking up the pieces after gullible patients who, hoping for short-cut cures on the cheap from charlatans, had in reality made their original disease ten times worse. Yet Marten's own book is a comprehensive work of self-advertisement, his boasts being no less grandiloquent than those of the quacks he vilifies; and he himself was a prime target of Spinke's *Quackery Unmask'd*.

Sex and the Enlightenment

The tradition of quackery blossoming in the late seventeenth century thus treated sex as a relatively straightforward system of desires. It offered beauty preparations to heighten female sex appeal, and pick-me-ups to rejuvenate rakes and roués. And it dealt no less with its own consequences, purveying pills to the poxed. Those traditions persisted throughout the subsequent century.

Yet the age of the Enlightenment also enticed sex away from coitus into culture, or, in other words, shifted the focus from sex to sexuality in ways that proved pregnant with potential, not least for quackery. Above all, an influential current emphasized that sexual desire must be treated not simply as a given – a biological, physiological, and pathological drive – but as a psycho-social variable. Sexuality, many Enlightenment thinkers argued, was inseparable from sensibility, and hence was a function both of the nervous system and of the imagination. The head, no less than the genitals, was the organ of libido; indeed, the nerves mediated between them.

Sexuality was thus a state of mind. With this view, abundant opportunities unfolded for quack doctors to set themselves up as the 'sexperts' of their age, precisely because of the special insights their own trade gave them into the techniques of seduction. Crudely put, if to the Enlightenment mind, the secret of sexual power lay in arts of persuasion, who better equipped than quacks to teach that art? It is no accident that many of the crack quacks of the century – not least Cagliostro and John 'Chevalier' Taylor – dropped broad hints about their own prowess as seducers, in tandem to their medical capacities, almost as if the one stood as collateral for the other. In the disgracing of Mesmer in Paris, the implicit assumption that his séances must be a threat to female honour carried great weight.

The avatar of this late-Enlightenment fusion of quackery and sexuality was James Graham, whose medico-sexual theories encapsulated many of the key convictions of the English Enlightenment, and who, for a brief time, proved a major cultural catalyst. The broad outlines of Graham's life are well known, though partly by hearsay, for primary evidence is scanty. Born a saddler's son in Edinburgh in the starcrossed year of the '45, he studied medicine (as did his brother William) at his home university under Monro *primus*, Black, Whytt, and Cullen, though never (contrary to his own claims) graduating. In 1770, he married and settled in Pontefract, subsequently migrating to America. There, subsidized by Shelley's grandfather, he practised physic, specializing as an oculist and aurist, met Benjamin Franklin, and became an enthusiast for medical electricity. Travels in Europe were followed in the late 1770s by medical practice in Bristol and, above all, fashionable Bath, where he won quality patients such as the historian and essayist, Catherine Macaulay (who was to marry his brother), and Georgiana, Duchess of Devonshire. Success encouraged him to try his fortune in London. Opening his 'Temple of Health' (the 'Templum Aesculapio Sacrum') in 1780 at the fashionable Adelphi, just off the Strand, he combined lectures and multimedia spectacle with a practice privileging electrical therapy. In this Valhalla of health and fertility, he first unveiled his Celestial Bed, hired out at £50 a night as a specific against impotence and sterility.

Graham shortly quit the Adelphi (probably because of debts), removing to the less salubrious Pall Mall, where repeated delivery of what he called his 'libidinous' lectures on generation kept him in the public gaze. Forced to sell up in 1783 by his creditors – he passed some time in Newgate – Graham put his doctrines and electrical cures on the road. Shedding his phantasmagorical pyrotechnics, Graham modified his views and his style in the 1780s. He called himself 'born again', preaching an ardent if idiosyncratic evangelical Christianity, which wedded passionate defence of the divinity of Christ as Redeemer (against rational dissenters and Unitarians such as Joseph Priestley) to a holistic, hylozoic cosmology glorifying the spiritual unity of the Creation. He adopted the style: 'the Servant of the Lord O.W.L. [O Wonderful Love]. Recanting his earlier commitment to cures by artificial electricity (for example, ones based upon sparks from Leyden jars), he grew ardent for medical simplicity, grounded upon the healing power of Nature and trusting to the therapeutic properties of elements such as water and air.

And, most flamboyantly, aided by a bevy of lightly clad 'goddesses of health', he championed the omni-curative properties of mud-baths and had himself repeatedly buried fakir-like, naked, for days on end, and fasting all the while. (He found 'fresh, icy, cold earth brought from the top of Hampstead Hill' best; though even a turf strapped to the chest, he insisted, was better than nothing for busy folks.) 'I was present at one of his lectures upon the benefits arising from earth bathing (as he called it)', reported the gossip, Henry Angelo, after seeing an exhibition of Grahamian mud-bathing in Panton Street, where there gathered:

> a crowded audience of men [and] many ladies… to listen to his delicate
> lectures. In the centre of the room was a pile of earth, in the middle of which
> was a pit where a stool was placed: we waited some time, when much
> impatience was manifested, and after repeated calls, 'Doctor, Doctor!' he
> actually made his appearance *en chemise*. After making his bow he seated
> himself on the stool; when two men with shovels began to place the mound
> in the cavity: as it approached to the pit of the stomach he kept lifting up his
> shirt and at last took it entirely off, the earth being up to his chin and the
> doctor being left *in puris naturalibus*. He then began his lecture, expiating on
> the excellent qualities of the Earth Bath, how invigorating etc., quite enough
> to call up the chaste blushes of the modest ladies.[22]

In course of time, Graham grew monomaniacal, turning into a vaudeville Messiah; his latter-day Christian behaviour – stripping off in the street and giving his clothes to the poor – led some to call him mad. What old age may have had in store was pre-empted by his sudden death (allegedly by then insane) in Edinburgh, in 1794.

Graham, in the judgement of an anonymous *British Medical Journal* author early this century, was 'one of the most impudent quacks that ever lived'. Labelling him a charlatan (and sometimes a madman too, or, as Macalpine and Hunter put it, a luminary of the 'lunatic fringe'), historians have emphasized only the bizarre and supposedly exploitative features of his presentations. Of course, he made his living by selling his sexual opinions in the marketplace. He was, no doubt, a dazzling and egotistical exhibitionist. No less sure than John Wesley that he was a man of destiny, he termed his performances an 'essential service to the public health', and recognized no distinction between his personal prophetic mission and the public revolution in health he propagandized. Indeed, he projected himself as a charismatic enlightened despot over the body natural: 'By air, by magnetism, by musical sounds, by subtile, cordial and balsamic medicines and chemical energy and-by positive and negative electricity arbitrarily used, I have, as it were, an absolute command over the health, functions and diseases of the human body.'[23]

As with other Georgian self-made entrepreneurs and star performers, Graham had to puff his own public presence, and hyperbole was his stock-in-trade; yet he also displayed talents as jester, clown, and coxcomb – he would even refer to himself as 'eccentric'. His medico-scientific writings boast his powers and bulge with 'unsolicited' testimonials from those snatched from death's door. He was hardly being therapeutically modest when he claimed that his cures, techniques, and treatments were 'miraculous' and 'infallible'. His London premises – the 'Temple of Health and the Temple of Hymen' – were, of course, shrines for the sick, but they doubled as lecture-theatres, pleasure-domes, and grottoes of mystery, to which the curious polite would be admitted on payment of a trifling entrance fee. How far were these Aladdin's caves, bejewelled with scientific apparatus and instruments, baits for Graham's bread-and-butter medical practice? or vice versa? We cannot say (next to nothing survives about his finances). Graham certainly promoted his premises through saturation newspaper advertising in the most ravishing (and self-parodic?) vein:

> TEMPLE OF HEALTH AND HYMEN, PALL-MALL
> near the King's Palace
> IF there be one human being, rich or poor, male, female, or of the doubtful gender, in or near this great metropolis of the world, who has not had the good fortune and the happiness of hearing the celebrated Lecture, and of seeing the grand Celestial State Bed, the magnificent Electrical Apparatus, and the supremely brilliant and Unique Decorations of this magical edifice – of this inchanting Elysian Palace! – where wit and mirth, love and beauty – all that can delight the soul, and all that can ravish the senses, will hold their court, THIS, and EVE.RY EVENING this week in chaste and joyous assemblage! let them now come forth, or for ever afterwards let them blame themselves, and bewail their irremediable misfortune.[24]

In a substantial pamphlet, Graham evoked the illusionist sensory brew, mingling sounds, smells and sights, bewitching the visitor on entry into this fairyland of statues, symbols and devices, scenic and scientific apparatus, pillars, lamps, gorgeous drapes, paintings, shrines, 'medical music', glass and mirrors, all permeated with the ethos of

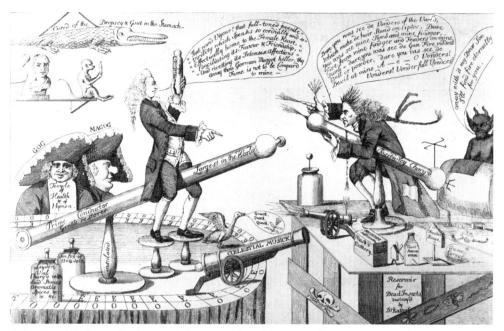

'The Quacks': James Graham and Gustavus Katterfelto. [British Museum satirical print 6325]

Minerva, Vesta, the Phoenix, etc. If Graham may be believed, the *bon ton* (or, as he himself styled them in his advertisements, 'The Adepts! The Cognoscenti! *et les Amateurs des delices exquises de Venus*') flocked to his events. 'There have been for the three last evenings past an overflow of at least nine hundred ladies and gentlemen', claimed one of his vast number of newspaper insertions.

Were figures Graham's forte? When Horace Walpole attended, the chaste and joyous assemblage numbered a choice eighteen, and he for one was disappointed with the trumpery. And, as with his contemporary, Katterfelto – the two quacks spar up against each other in a contemporary cartoon – the novelty soon wore off. Graham had to slash his admission prices and then finally dispose of his magic toyshop and up stumps in 1783.

Yet he seems to have been in considerable demand as a medical practitioner – he supposedly treated over 200 patients a day, and his exhibitions were the talk of the town, at least, for a season. Frederick Reynolds, who lived just behind the Temple, wrote, 'daily, he [Graham] attracted overflowing audiences'. Henry Angelo, the leading fencing-master, agreed: 'I remember', he wrote, 'the carriages drawing up next to the door of this modern Paphos, with crowds of gaping sparks on each side, to discover who were the visitors, but the ladies' faces were covered, all going incog'. Amongst the competing shows of London, Graham's Temple appealed to radical chic coteries craving the outré and the risqué. For this the Prussian officer J.W. von Archenholtz complimented him on his: 'perfect knowledge of the human heart, the success which attended his experiment proves that he has calculated with judgement. He has too much sense to be suspected of being a dupe to the occult science which he professed and must therefore be classed in the list of cunning and politic adventurers. [...] Nothing indeed is more superb than his Temple.'

Similar testimony to Graham's ability to tap the late-Enlightenment appetite for vicarious eroticism, mystery and sensation, illusion and equivocation, comes from the contemporary *Correspondance secrète*:

> Garlands, mirrors, crystals, gilt and silver ornaments are scattered about it with profusion, so that from all parts they reflect a dazzling light. Music precedes each lecture, from 5 o'clock till 7, when Dr. Graham presents himself vested in Doctor's robes. On the instant there followed a silence which is interrupted only at the end of the lecture by an electric shock given to the whole audience by means of conductors hidden under the cushions with which all the seats are covered. Whilst some jest at the astonishment of the others, a 'spirit' is seen to emerge from under the floor of the room; it presents the appearance of a man of gigantic stature, thin and haggard, who, without uttering a word, hands the Doctor a bottle of liquor which, after having been shown to the company, is carried off by the spirit. To this strange apparition succeeds a pretty woman under the form of the Goddess of Music, who, after singing six pieces, vanishes in her turn. Dr. Graham having finished his lecture, the audience breaks up without daring to express regret for the six guineas expended on so extraordinary a spectacle. Before the sittings the Doctor makes a public offer to dissipate melancholy and mitigate extravagant gaiety. In a word, it is electricity communicated by magnetized baths which for some months has made the reputation of Dr. Graham.[25]

Graham resists being categorized solely as an impresario, or as a fanatic; he was both, and it is through this double vision that we must approach the object which won him his notoriety, contemporary and present: in the most private part of the Temple, there stood the Celestial Bed. Graham apostrophized it thus:

> The Grand Celestial Bed, whose magical influences are now celebrated from pole to pole and from the rising to the setting of the sun, is 12 ft. long by 9 ft. wide, supported by forty pillars of brilliant glass of the most exquisitive workmanship, in richly variegated colours. The super-celestial dome of the bed, which contains the odoriferous, balmy and ethereal spices, odours and essences, which is the grand reservoir of those reviving invigorating influences which are exhaled by the breath of the music and by the exhilarating force of electrical fire, is covered on the other side with brilliant panes of looking-glass.
>
> On the utmost summit of the dome are placed two exquisite figures of Cupid and Psyche, with a figure of Hymen behind, with his torch flaming with electrical fire in one hand and with the other, supporting a celestial crown, sparkling over a pair of living turtle doves, on a little bed of roses.

The other elegant group of figures which sport on the top of the dome, having each of them musical instruments in their hands, which by the most expensive mechanism, breathe forth sound corresponding to their instruments, flutes, guitars, violins, clarinets, trumpets, horns, oboes, kettle drums, etc.

At the head of the bed appears sparkling with electrical fire a great first commandment: 'BE FRUITFUL, MULTIPLY AND REPLENISH THE EARTH'. Under that is an elegant sweet-toned organ in front of which is a fine landscape of moving figures, priest and bride's procession entering the Temple of Hymen.

The chief principle of my Celestial Bed is produced by artificial lodestones. About 15 cwt. of compound magnets are continually pouring forth in an everflowing circle. The bed is constructed with a double frame, which moves on an axis or pivot and can be converted into an inclined plane.[26]

The bed was presented to the late-Georgian fashionable world as a fertility shrine, available to couples on a nightly basis:

> Should pregnancy at any time not happily ensue [i.e., that is from the regular course of conjugal love] I have the most astonishing method to recommend which will infallibly produce a genial and happy issue, I mean my Celestial or Magnetico-electrico bed, which is the first and only ever in the world: it is placed in a spacious room to the right of my orchestra which produces the Celestial fire and the vivifying influence: this brilliant Celestial Bed is supported by six massive brass pillars with Saxon blue and purple satin, perfumed with Arabian spices in the style of those in the Seraglio of a Grand Turk. Any gentleman and his lady desirous of progeny, and wishing to spend an evening in the Celestial apartment, which coition may, on compliment of a £50 bank note, be permitted to partake of the heavenly joys it affords by causing immediate conception, accompanied by the soft music. Superior ecstasy which the parties enjoy in the Celestial Bed is really astonishing and never before thought of in this world: the barren must certainly become fruitful when they are powerfully agitated in the delights of love.[27]

The Celestial Bed was Graham's much-bruited *chef d'oeuvre*. He clearly intended it as a source of income, since he charged £50 a night for its use. It provided him with vast publicity, and was the subject of smutty lampoons such as *The Celestial Beds* (1781), and *Il Convito Amoroso* (1782) – this latter probably a self-satire by Graham himself, trading on the assumption that all publicity is good publicity – which depicted jaded couples flocking in, as if to a new ark, to repopulate the species.

Was the bed used, as contemporaries smirked, for debauch and prostitution? There is no evidence for this. Graham himself insisted that the bed was not for voluptuaries but for couples desiring children – an echo of a theme discussed earlier in this chapter – being designed to overcome flaccidity or barrenness by 'an electrical stroke or two'; and, he hoped, it would work towards the 'propagating of Beings rational, and far stronger and more beautiful in mental as well as in bodily endowments, than the present puny, feeble, and nonsensical race of probationary mortals, which crawl, and fret, and politely play at cutting one another's throats for nothing at all, on most parts of this terraqueous globe'. There was already a plethora of resorts to which the smart set could repair for amorous adventure (for example, Mrs Cornelys's Pantheon in Oxford Street) and bagnios and classy brothels aplenty where attractive bed-mates were to be had (Casanova found one paid up to six guineas). Hence it is unlikely that Graham's high-minded sentiments about sexual rejuvenation served merely as a façade for libertinism or commercial sex. In fact, we have no direct knowledge of what went on between the sheets of the Bed (although Angelo implausibly confides that 'many a nobleman paid Graham £500 to draw the curtains').

The activating principles of the Bed – according to Graham – were magnetism and 'electrical fire'. Magneto-electricity had come into vogue from the mid-eighteenth century, and was shortly to be indelibly stamped on the public mind by Mesmer's animal magnetism (though mesmerism reached England too late to influence Graham's Bed). In the context of his sexology, two aspects of Graham's use of electricity are worth dwelling on.

First, the 'brilliant' and 'celestial' forces of electricity were not just gimmicks casually associated with the Bed, but were integral to Graham's general medical armamentarium and practice, quite independently of his advocacy of them to treat sexual debility. Case histories from Bath and Bristol in the late 1770s show Graham offering electrical treatments for a spectrum of conditions, from the modish 'nervous diseases' to fevers, rheumatism, gout, and especially deafness and noises in the head. His galvanic therapy made use of a magnetic throne and relied on the influence of a so-called all-pervasive, superfine, electrical fluid, rather than specifically on shocks – which he later adamantly repudiated. Furthermore, he sold a range of 'electrical' medicaments: the 'Electrical Aether', the 'Nervous Aetherial Balsam', and the 'Imperial Pills', claiming that each distilled the envigorating powers of subtle, milky, thrilling, electrical fluids. In other words, were we tempted to see Graham's Celestial Bed therapy *merely* as a stroke of soft-porn opportunism, we should first remember that electrical therapy was integral to his overall medical doctrines and practice, and was, in any case, widely promoted by orthodox as well as quackish practitioners in the last quarter of the eighteenth century.

The second point is that Graham was not simply a minor British Mesmer. His approach significantly differed. Mesmer and his disciples sought scientific acceptance, and so mesmerism became a coherent body of alternative popular science into the nineteenth century. But not Graham, whose pitch was far more individual, and concerned with directly evangelizing the people. No carefully reasoned, experimentally supported, law-grounded natural philosophy of the physiological powers of electricity backed his descriptions of the Celestial Bed, which were written entirely in tremulous, glittering superlatives. His published accounts of magneto-electrical healing amount to

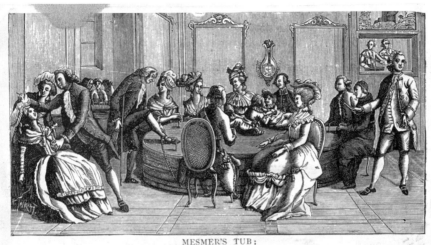

MESMER'S TUB;
Or, a Faithful Representation of the Operations of Animal Magnetism.

The following is a translation of the original description accompanying the above curious old print, which is of especial interest at the present day, when mesmerism has been advanced to the dignity of a science : " Mr. Mesmer, M.D., of the Medical Faculty of Vienna, Austria, is the sole inventor of animal magnetism. This method of curing a number of ailments (such as paralysis, gout, scorbute, and accidental deafness) consists in the application, by Mr. Mesmer, of a fluid or agent, which he administers occasionally through one of his fingers—or else by means of an iron rod—to those who come to seek his aid. He uses also a large tub, to which are fixed pieces of cord which the patients tie round their limbs, or iron hooks which they apply to that part of the body in which they suffer ; the patients, especially women, have fits, which bring about their recovery. The magnetizers (those to whom Mr. Mesmer has confided his secret, and numbering at least one hundred among the gentlemen of the Court) place their hands upon the ailing parts and rub them, thereby aiding the influence of the cords and hooks. There is a tub for the poor twice a week, and music is played in the entrance-hall to cheer the patients. People of all sorts and conditions flock to this celebrated physician, from Field Marshals to artisans. It is a scene to move the coldest heart to see men who have attained the highest honours in society magnetizing aged paupers. As to Mr. Mesmer, he is the picture of benevolence, of a serious disposition, and speaks little, seeming always to be absorbed in profound reflections."

A large gathering of patients and assistants to Mesmer's animal magnetism therapy, showing use of the special tub at his clinic. Wood engraving by H. Thiriat.

little more than a string of 'before and after' anecdotes, listing patients' symptoms, the inanities of orthodox physic, and his own successes. As a healer and a propagandist, Graham was a loner, who, despite his orthodox Edinburgh medical training, had remarkably little contact with the medico-scientific establishment. His ideas died with him: there was no 'Grahamism'. Mesmer craved professional acceptance, Graham popular acclaim.

Graham shared with Mesmer, however, a commitment to the physical and physiological reality of his healing practice, linked to a powerful insight into the powers of the psyche. Mesmer claimed that 'animal magnetism' was an authentic, Newtonian subtle fluid whose action determined health and disease. Yet he also had profound insight into abnormal psychology, becoming increasingly conscious that he was confronting essentially psychosomatic and nervous conditions, and treating them with sympathetic, psycho-therapeutic techniques.

Mesmer was adroit at stage-managing the collective drama and simmering hysteria of group therapy (comparison with Wesley might not be far-fetched), drawing upon traditions of sympathetic healing. Indeed, Mesmer himself increasingly cast off his technological crutches, realizing he could do without his *baquets* brimful of electricity, operating instead through personal mystique and the eye. The destiny of mesmerism, after all, lay in the psychiatric use of hypnotism.

Graham similarly possessed insight into the psychology of impotence and sexual performance. As with other physicians, his practice had made him acutely aware of the psychology of malaise and recovery, and specifically of 'the influence of imagination in the affairs of love'. He was to argue the importance of 'strong impressions' in stimulating the libido (for example, people became aroused, he noted, through watching animals copulate), and the dampening effects of routinized sex. He shrewdly saw that his Celestial Bed would kindle the flames of desire partly by creating heightened ambience and expectations, through attention to lighting, textures, colours, decor, and soft music.

Yet his own therapeutics gave pride of place to somatic cause and effect, and he betrayed no sign of treating his own medical apparatus and medicines as mere stage-prop placebos, effective only through suggestion. For all his egomania, Graham did not cast himself in the role of a medium or psychic healer, a 'stroker' in the tradition of Valentine Greatrakes; he always (one might say) shielded his personality behind his technology and drugs. Unlike the great John Hunter, or a medically informed layman such as Laurence Sterne, he did not argue that the roots of sexual difficulties lay primarily in the individual mind – or, as we might say, in the unconscious.

Graham's advice for restoring virility, by contrast, gave immediate priority to the physical, and broader attention to the social. He recognized that many of his patients were low-spirited, but his case histories of cures give no indication that he ever consciously set out to deploy psychological healing strategies, or saw the aetiology of his patients' complaints in individual psycho-biographies. Unlike the mesmerists, Graham did not practise group therapy or stage cathartic seances; his performances remained lectures, not 'conversions'. The conventional boundaries of performer and audience were not turned upside down. Nor did he develop private psycho-sexual therapy, and there is no evidence that – unlike Simon Forman before him, or many psychoanalysts nowadays – he became sexually involved with his patients. What he offered those with sexual problems was an environment and a mechanical fix: a magnetic bed, atmosphere, anonymity, and above all, electrical fire.

We may rightly see Graham as a wizard showman flourishing in the lubricious twilight-world of sex aids. Yet he was neither a pander nor a pornographer, nor even a simple 'sexploiter', for his sexual apparatus and therapies were part and parcel of a wider medical theory and practice. In any case, he claimed his displays were models of propriety: 'Dr GRAHAM desires most respectfully to assure the Nobility and Gentry, especially the Ladies, that everything is conducted at the Temple of Hymen with that decency and decorum which cannot fail effectually to silence envious, ignorant or malevolent tongues.'[28]

What exactly, then, did Graham think of sex? And how did his (quackish) sexual thinking relate to contemporary biomedical beliefs? As mentioned at the opening of this chapter, sex was freely and extensively discussed in eighteenth-century medical writings aimed both at professional and at lay audiences, and there was a wide range of approaches. Prominent was the tradition of practical help offered in such popular advice works as Ebenezer Sibly's *Medical Mirror* (1794) and the evergreen favourite *Aristotle's Master-Piece* (1690 onwards), focusing on sexual education, genital functions and malaises, discussing perennial problems (for example, how to anticipate the gender of a baby), and offering common-sense tips (for example, parsnips were a good cure for impotence, ragwort combated the green sickness).

At the opposite extreme were comprehensive naturalistic pan-sexual philosophies such as that developed by the prominent regular physician, Dr Erasmus Darwin, in his *Zoonomia* (1794-96) and *The Temple of Nature* (1803). In these works, sexual activity was conceptualized within a utilitarian psycho-physiology of pleasure maximization; the psychopathology of everyday life, for example the experience of beauty, was explained as having sexual origins, and erotic drives were postulated as the dynamo of an evolutionary process of cosmic development, being 'Nature's masterpiece'.

A further strand of sexual thought, biological and organic if not always strictly medical, was linked to the sentimental movement, finding its most explicit expression in the psycho-physical suggestiveness and double entendres of Laurence Sterne. This sought to perfect sensuality by civilizing it. The senses were regarded as the springs of action, and each was eroticized. The refinement of feeling brought about by the pursuit of politeness rendered sexual responses more thrilling, more exquisitely erotic.

The meaning with which Graham imbued sexuality, however, though drawing upon all of these, was somewhat differently orientated. For him, the key to sex was health, to be construed both biologically and socially. His primary concern was to specify under what conditions the sexual drive would function best: in other words, contribute most to, and least threaten organic well-being. Though this had a psychological dimension, Graham principally thought of sex in a hygienic-organic context. For him, the touchstone of general well-being was healthy eroticism – indeed, the drive to propagate the species. Nurturing the urge to procreate, multiply, and perpetuate mankind forms the core concern of his *Lecture on the Generation, Increase and Improvement of the Human Species*, and is a theme handled more broadly in his later, more cosmological writings, where he conjures a vision of the entire economy of Nature endlessly renewing itself, teeming with self-sustaining and self-perpetuating forms of life. 'Gentlemen', Graham would confide to his audiences, 'the most important business of everything in the animal creation, is to propagate the number of its species; this is an object of the greatest consequences, so great, that the attention of the philosopher and men of science have [sic] been directed to consider with care, and endeavour to find out the real cause of generation.'[29]

The healthy creature is the sexual creature, and sexual energy the acid-test of bodily well-being: or, put most directly, 'The genitals are the true pulse, and infallible barometer of health'. In furthering this goal of strength through joy, his remit, he claimed, was 'the health, beauty, vigour, happiness and security of the human species, and… the happy prolongation of human life'. 'The Propagation of the human species is the subject of our attention.'

Sexual instinct and its gratification ought, thus, to be an unproblematic, natural urge for men – and equally for women, for Graham regarded women as no less libidinous: 'Were we to be made acquainted with the real sentiments of the sex', he insisted, 'even the chastest, coldest, most reserved, and least amorously complexioned woman in the world, we would find her to be precisely of the same taste, with the bishop's lady, who very frankly declared that, for her part, she liked to have a GOOD THING in the house, or in the bed by her, whether she made use of it or not.' But, when he looked around him,

Graham saw a nation catastrophically failing, as he believed, to reproduce itself. Civilized man was an endangered species: 'We are told by political writers' – he may have had 'Estimate' Brown or Richard Price in mind – 'that the inhabitants of this island have decreased amazingly, and every succeeding generation becomes more and more weekly [*sic*]; tho' these are alarming circumstances, and call loudly for a remedy, yet it is totally neglected.' Graham's fears of depopulation, so shrilly expressed by contemporary moralists, primitivists, and 'country party' backbenchers, were, of course, grotesquely mistaken, and it is ironic that in little more than a decade Malthus would prove no less terrified of the superfecundity of the masses. The point, however, is that Graham's fears were not a cranky idiosyncrasy.

The failure of reproduction stemmed from the exhaustion of sexual drives; and this in turn was rooted in decrepit personal and, hence, social health. Doom lay ahead, for 'the degeneracy and imbecility of body and mind, so prevalent in this country', he predicted, 'not only destroys the state, but likewise the peace and happiness of individuals; for no man can have felicity in the hymeneal state when his wife is barren. Indeed, health and children are as necessary to the prosperity of mankind, as the genial rays of the sun are to enliven and cherish the fragrant plants.'

The strategy of Graham's sexology was, therefore, to recoup individual and, more fundamentally, social health, by maximizing libido, and thereby contribute to restocking the nation. The nub of the problem, as he saw it, was that modern, civilized, fast-lane lifestyles were at odds with wholesome sex. In Graham's view this was not – as in the Blake-Freud diagnosis – because free expression of personal sexuality was necessarily repressed in the name of civilization and culture, property, prosperity and propriety. Graham did not demand some Romantic kind of individual sexual liberation or free-love. Far from it: he called for social mores that treated desire with less laxity and indifference, arguing that sex could be healthy only within marriage and – precisely reversing the views expressed earlier in the century by Bernard Mandeville – that sexual well-being could be enhanced at a stroke by the banning of conventional licentiousness: 'The first step towards the encouraging of matrimony, would be to suppress all public prostitution'.

The nub of the matter was that contemporary society was crippling sexuality because it made people sick, feeble, and emasculated. By this, Graham did not primarily mean sick in the head or sick at heart, but rather physically degenerate, the puny brood of 'luxury, folly and dissipation'. Graham believed libido was on the wane because the nation was unfit, sexual appetite was flagging because other appetites went uncurbed. People gourmandised and guzzled poisonous and foreign tea, coffee, and spiritous liquors, sometimes mistakenly believing these were aphrodisiacs. They kept late hours, indulging in 'midnight racketing', stifled themselves in stuffy rooms, and slept on feather beds, which destroyed their muscle tone. Decadent living sapped sexual appetites, but also resulted, when conception did – albeit rarely – take place, in sickly and malformed offspring. Luxury was not spared Graham's lash:

> It is incumbent on us to restore that manly firmness and vigour, which,
> from the depravity of human nature, by means of luxury and dissipation,

has for more than a century been lost: this has brought on diseases which have enervated and debilitated the human race. The great author of our being, has, by the strongest ties, bound us to temperance and sobriety: but we, regardless of that authority or our own peace and felicity, have brought on diseases, and are so interwoven in our constitutions, which renders us totally unfit for the noble of fice of producing a vigorous and healthy offspring.[30]

Clean and decent living, by contrast, following the 'plain and simple laws of nature', promised good health, sexual energy, and sturdy offspring. Like Erasmus Darwin, Graham believed that paying due honour to Venus required abandoning Bacchus – and hot beverages as well (cold milk and water were more tonic). Along the lines advocated earlier in the century by George Cheyne, he advocated a strict regimen and a frugal food intake. He preferred macrobiotics to meat – carcasses were all too often rotten and adulterated, whereas vegetables were cleaner, and 'all flesh is grass' – and valued the raw above the cooked (raw eggs did possess aphrodisiac properties). Graham required a bracing atmosphere, open windows, fresh air, hard beds, and early hours, and adherence to the Wesleyan golden rule of cleanliness: 'bathing every night and morning, if not the whole body and limbs, at least the genitalia and fundament, with very cold water' A key reason for sexual indifference – 'mark me!' – he instructed his audience – was that men were turned off by female filth and stench: Graham explained that gentlemen preferred whores to their wives, because whores kept themselves cleaner. He set no store by traditional (indeed, quack) cosmetics and aphrodisiacs, deploring cantharides in particular, but he urged repeated bathing of the genitals in cold water as a stimulant. Above all, Graham argued that the tranquillity of the family provided the ideal milieu for rapturous coupling: 'Domestic music, gentlemen! little family concerts, and especially singing together, or in turn, trifling as these may appear to some, I strongly recommend', he told his listeners, 'and still more strongly, regular worship, and sentimental, philosophical, and religious conversations and intercourses. For, gentlemen, after the souls of an amiable couple have been softened, harmonized, illumined, and filled with approving peace, by duties and amusements so rational and delightful, when they return to an early bed, sober, serene and healthful! their bodies and their souls rush sweetly together! with the fullest, purest, intensest, and most celestial transports!'

Healthy sexuality would thus arise spontaneously from simple social habits. But it also required self-discipline. Graham passionately believed that copulation begun at too raw an age ('early venery'), or over-indulged in old age, or too frequently, all weakened performance and stamina, and so were short-sighted sacrifices to sensuality. His goal was to 'exalt and prolong the pleasure of the marriage bed'.

Graham was one of many moralists whipping up a horror of masturbation. He execrated self-abuse because it was the enemy of generation, wasting semen and sapping vigour. For he powerfully endorsed the biomedical theory that saw semen as an elixir, the principle of universal vitality, a 'true and inconceivably powerful stimulus', an 'exquisitely penetrating seminal liquor', almost the world-soul: 'The seminal principle, or luminous, ever-active balsam of life, is the grand staff, strength, all-animating vital source of principle of the beauty, vigour, and serenity, both of body and of mind.'

Though denying the doctrinaire preformationist embryological view that the 'type' of future generations lay exclusively in 'homunculi' contained in the semen, Graham thought that the seminal fluid carried the 'vivifying elementary fire', which enlivened the foetus. As the sacred torch-bearer of vitality, it was a precious liquor, whose waste was entropic, spelling danger and desolation: 'though nature be very fond of the species, yet she bears no hatred to the individual, wherefore though she be in raptures during the discharge of this matter, out of an intention to preserve the kind, yet when that is past, she grows sad for the loss of it, as well as for the damage done to the individual.' Just as semen was not to be squandered by masturbation, so similar misfortunes were also to be avoided. Thus he advised men to bathe their genitals post coitum in cold water, to halt dribbling emissions.

In the interests of spermatic economy, Graham recommended severe sexual self-discipline, above all, to youth:

> The young man who lives in the world, soberly, regularly, usefully, and perfectly continently, without ever once having known what any seminal emission is till he arrives at his twenty-first – or even to his twenty-fifth year; and is married – that young man is a hero indeed – an Hercules – an Angel – a God! I had almost said, in point of health, strength, beauty, and brilliancy, of body and of mind; when compared to those poor creeping tremulous, pale, spindle-shanked wretched creatures who crawl upon the earth, spiriting, dribbling, and drawing off, alone, or with their vile unfortunate street trulls, or other mates, in what is called the natural way, at twelve, fourteen, sixteen or eighteen years of age; As for my part, gentlemen, if you will pardon this breach of politeness, I seriously declare, that had I my time to live over again, and were I possessed of the same knowledge I now have, I would be, I believe, thirty or forty years of age, before I would know any at all, from personal experience, about these matters.[31]

But the aged needed his advice no less: 'The frequent use of venereal pleasures is hurtful to all men whatever, but especially to such as are old.' Abstinence was to be recommended during menstruation and pregnancy (at such times, copulation was 'rank-lust'): 'Long and peaceful inter-regnums, gentlemen! at certain monthly and strawbed periods; and by all means two beds in the same room, or rather in the adjoining apartment.' Moderation was the watchword: 'There is no body so strong, that Venus is not able to weaken and overcome' .

Graham thus saw semen as an 'exquisitely penetrating', 'precious', and 'nutritious' liquor, the spirit of vitality. This view made up one facet of his visionary cosmology, in which the animating and vivifying powers of Nature all found expression in vital fluids, such as celestial fire, electricity, magnetism, and, of course semen. Graham believed a delicate balance had to be maintained. Enough semen had to be released for procreation, but sufficient had also to be held back for animating the male body:

> for believe me, gentlemen! that the procreation of the species, is but at most a secondary purpose of which nature prepared the seed: the chief use of this balmy – spiritous – vivifying essence, is after it has been thoroughly concocted and exalted in the seminal and generative organs, to be pumped up again or exhaled into the general system, and intimately blended and churned, as it were, with the blood and all the juices, bedewing every fibre, bracing and sheathing every nerve, and animating with light, strength and serenity, the whole frame! in order that all those secretions, circulations and absorptions, upon which good bodily health and celestial tranquility of mind depend, may be more properly carried on. For without a full and genial tide of this rich, vivyfying luminous principle, continually circulating in every part of the system, it is absolutely impossible that either man or woman can enjoy health, strength, spirits, or happiness.[32]

(Not surprisingly, he viewed the medicines he vended as in essence seminal, describing them as ethereal, balmy, and milky.)

Of course, Graham's identification of semen with the vital principle made his view of human biology viricentric, indeed phallocentric. Through being a sperm factory and bank, the male was the higher, more spiritual, and lively gender. It was of the essence of the female principle, by contrast, to be lower, earthy, womb-like, passive, and receptive. Partly for this reason, most of his advice was directed to men, recommending, for example, that they must choose good stock upon whom to breed: 'In the choice of a woman, passions of the mind are to be overlooked [that is inspected]. Hysteria, and all the said train of hysterical gloomy melancholy are carefully to be avoided'. Graham's 'viricultural' viewpoint on human reproduction proves once again to have chimed with his wider philosophy. In his anthropomorphic, organic, cosmology, Nature was understood through the complementarity of male-female dichotomies, of which the male was the more active and spiritual:

> I may be indulged with the liberty of drawing the whole of what I have said to one point of view, and farther to represent our World or System, as a Creature of an ambiguous nature, and as partaking of both Sexes. The higher part of our system, namely the Celestial, being active and masculine, the lower, or more gross elementary part, of the passive and feminine nature. As the globe of the earth then is the wondrous and capacious womb, in which the all-engendering seed of Heaven is eagerly received and faithfully kept for innumerable, most kind and most obvious purposes: – I may finally be allowed to remark, that as from the upper masculine part proceed the Light, Serenity, Life and Strength of our System, so, from the lower or female part, (as, alas! from too many other female parts) do issue fires and

Aetean or Vesuvian furors, corruptions, diseases, discords, desolation, and Death.[33]

Graham was, in many ways, *sui generis* and enigmatic. His sexology cannot simply be slotted into some general schema. But his ideas should not, as so often, be neglected as a farrago of slogans and postures slung together merely to create eye-catching, money-spinning, cheap thrills. For Graham's sexual ideas resonate with the convictions of the moderate Enlightenment. He had no truck with fundamentalist Calvinist or Evangelical devaluations of the pleasures of the flesh seen as sinful consequences of the Fall. But nor did he countenance the voluptuary's decadent erotomania, and that kind of priapic self-expression traditionally found in much libertine writing and dressed *en philosophe* in France between Diderot and de Sade. For Graham, Nature grants the body sexual pleasures in abundance, but Nature also requires objective norms of conduct and hygiene, whose rewards are health and happiness, but whose sanctions are disease and decay. For Graham, as for the *idéologues* in France, the discourse of health is nature's decalogue for ensuring a stable, family-based, physiologically sound community. The balance, in this discourse, between nature as instinct, and nature as normative – between asserting the physical 'naturalness' of libidinous sexuality and at the same time sermonizing and even legislating to restrain its misuse – is obviously a delicate one, comparable to the dilemmas of enforcing a Rousseauist notion of freedom.

Graham's views may also be seen as a late fusion of civic humanist-cum-country party *virtù* with a moral primitivism, cast into biomedical terms. Man's duty – religious, civic and moral – is to procreate; from the time of Malthus, right through to the eugenists, civic duty would increasingly reside in reining back wanton sexuality.

Sexual anxiety and the nervous system

Graham is an ambivalent figure, whose complexity is in many ways an epitome of both the quackery of the late Enlightenment and of the times themselves. Showman and doctor, moralist and entertainer, opinion-maker and yet carnival character, Graham throve on his capacity to conjure up an ambiguous, intriguing public persona.

Various other quacks of the second half of the eighteenth century also thrust themselves, their lives, and opinions into the limelight. They were each exhibitionists of a sort, in ways distinguishing them significantly from the run-of-the-mill quack of a century earlier. This new career profile was facilitated by the fact that, by the late eighteenth century, far more efficient publicity opportunities afforded themselves.

Graham and his ilk were performers prominent at least as much for what they said, did and wrote, and for the images they projected, as for the pills they vended. His attitudes towards sex defy easy pigeon-holing. He certainly promoted it. He also, however, consciously or not, sowed the seeds of fear: in his lectures denouncing degeneracy, the very failures of his own audience seemed to be being impugned. Above all, he was instrumental in magnifying one particular sexual fear, the dire consequences of self-abuse – a phobia which, if not precisely created by Georgian quacks, was at least largely publicized by them. If late seventeenth-century quacks cashed in on fears of venereal disease – fears they in part created – a century later, quacks stirred sexual anxieties no less, but by then the focus of the fears had largely changed.

In the late seventeenth century, the constitutional, ingrained disease most prominent in quack advertising was, as surveyed in chapter 5, scurvy; its specifically *sexual* analogue was venereal disease. Quack medicines claiming to cure the pox – such as Velno's Vegetable Syrup, Keyser's Pills, or Kennedy's Lisbon Diet Drink – remained common throughout the Georgian century.

By the second half of the eighteenth century, medical opinion, discarding the theory of the humours, was emphasizing the 'nervous' basis of disease in general, from minor and unspecific functional disorders, colic and palsy, up to outright insanity. The teachings of Edinburgh University professors – most particularly Robert Whytt and William Cullen – spread theories of neurotic disorders to their pupils, who, in turn, helped to familiarize them amongst the laity. As shown in earlier chapters, the quack preparations widely advertised in late-Georgian newspapers capitalized upon interest in the nerves.

As with scurvy's implied connections with syphilis and gonorrhoea, the nervous disorders became twinned in the public imagination with particular sorts of sexual malaise: typically ill-defined and unspecific in their nature but centering upon the secret vice.

How did these fears arise? Public hysteria about the evils of onanism, accused Thomas Beddoes, the late eighteenth-century Bristol physician, was the fault of the quacks, particularly denouncing the 'alarm engendered by quack advertisements'. Truth lay in his accusation. Thus Graham excited fears that masturbation posed a great threat to healthy sexuality. 'As to certain solitary practices or bad habits', he warned,

> which boys &c. ignorantly fall into at schools, &c. and which, if persisted in, infallibly cheque the growth, and debilitate the bodies, and it is to be feared, damn the souls of boys and girls, or of the young men and young women, whom the Devil or their vicious companions seduce into them. Let me solemnly assure them, in the sacred name of God! – of nature, – of truth, – and of happiness, – that every such selfish and solitary act, yea, even every act of fornication, or of amourous commerce between unmarried persons, is expressly forbidden by God, and is a stroke from the hammer of death and condemnation, to everything that virtuous, wise and human beings ought to cherish and hold sacred.[34]

Self-abuse was the evil of evils, he cautioned his lecture audience:

> Where I now speaking before an assembly of the young, profligate, or thoughtless of both sexes, instead of a manly, rational, and highly respectable audience! I would assure them in the name of Posterity! in the name of HEALTH AND HAPPINESS – in the name of GOD himself! I would assure them that every seminal emission out of nature's road – I must speak

plainly, gentlemen! every act of self-pollution! and even every repetition of natural venery, with even the loveliest of the sex, to which appalled or exhausted nature is whipped and spurred by lust, habit, or firey unnatural provocations; but especially every act of self-pollution; is an earthquake – a blast – a deadly paralytic stroke, to all the faculties of both soul and body! striking off an irrecoverable chip from the staff of life; blasting beauty! chilling, contradicting, and enfeebling body, mind and memory! cutting off many years from the natural term of their life! Rather than begin, or continue this vile, soul and body destroying practice – this rebellion against, and murdering of nature, I would advise young persons to anything [...] indeed, I would seriously advise them at once, to put an end to their existence! for this horridly unnatural – this infernal – this all-blasting practice of self-pollution, and drunkenness, are the inlet to, or the aggregate of all the vices and curses, of soul and body, of time and eternity – bound up in one damning – one more than diabolical bundle.[35]

Graham's outburst shows how – as Beddoes alleged – quacks helped create the panic over masturbation. Yet Beddoes's thrust was at best half-true. For regular doctors, no less than quacks, had played their part in creating the scare about self-abuse. The anonymous *Onania* (1710) – the first major pamphlet denouncing the vice, sin, and disease of masturbation – had been augmented by the *Onanism* of the ultra-respectable Swiss physician, Tissot, quickly translated into English in 1769, which seemed to attribute most lethal wasting diseases to masturbation. Indeed, Beddoes was guilty of a certain hypocrisy. For in his lengthy essay on the 'Grand source of unhealthiness in the male sex', he himself expatiated at enormous length, though in veiled language, upon the gross evils of premature sexual arousal and masturbation, which (he claimed, in tones resonant of Graham) 'must blast every hope of the enjoyment of health'.

Why the shrill denunciations of orthodox and quack doctors alike as to the evils of masturbation fell on a prepared soil is altogether a more difficult question. Scholars have tried to account for this new phobia in various ways. It has been suggested that the Georgian dread of auto-eroticism was a response to the prolongation of childhood and the intensification of parent-child affective relationships within the more domestically orientated family, accompanied by greater desire on the part of parents to protect their children from waywardness and vice by overseeing and suppressing juvenile sexuality. It has alternatively been argued that it was a rationalization of a bourgeois-capitalist ethos of 'saving' and avoiding – or deferring – 'spending'.

Quacks of the second half of the eighteenth century pandered to, and stirred up guilty associations in the public mind between nervous conditions and some root in sexual malpractices little more than darkly hinted at. Advertisements often mentioned nothing so vulgar as poxes and claps, however, but rather a malaise, or a web of them, far more insidious, dangerous and worrisome, implied through terms such as debility and exhaustion. Often a conspiracy of silence bound sufferer and quack together (compare the unmentionability of cancer in the twentieth century). The sufferer knew he must be suffering from the condition to which the quack was alluding; the quack, as it were,

Dr Brodum, an infamous medical practitioner and author of A Guide to Old Age or a Cure for the Indiscretions of Youth. *Stipple engraving by E.A. Ezekiel after G. Barry.*

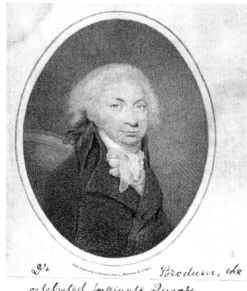

assumed for himself some credit for the polite restraint whereby he did not even need to embarrass sufferers with names.

Various late eighteenth-century quacks successfully fed off people's talent for convincing themselves that they were suffering from nervous disorders of sexual origin, and duly shameful: aside from Graham, the most prominent included Ebenezer Sibly, Edward Senate, William Brodum, and Samuel Solomon. Such men had much in common. They paraded their own orthodoxy. Graham, on occasions at least, emphasized his Edinburgh University training. Sibly trailed his University of St Andrews MD, and Brodum and Solomon their doctorates from Aberdeen, in front of the public's nose (all were legitimate, obtained through the regular process of purchase).

Rather as with regular physic, they also made the pill-vending side of their trade play second-fiddle in their self-presentations. Above all, this cohort of quacks principally aimed to sell their opinions, backed by the voice of science, scholarship, and authority. They pursued the printed healing word assiduously. Graham himself, in a great spurt in the early 1780s, published at least fourteen different pamphlets and short books; Sibly produced his full-length *Medical Mirror* (1792) and other publications besides; Senate brought out numerous promotional leaflets on the subject of premature old age (and how to overcome it); William Brodum produced a *Guide to Old Age* which went through multiple editions; and Samuel Solomon's *Guide to Health* proved a phenomenal success. Later editions of this 200-page book assured readers that it had gone through over sixty editions and sold more than 120,000 copies. Such figures may need to be taken with a pinch of salt, but the abundance of surviving copies with high edition numbers show that Solomon's claims were not mere pie in the sky.

Sibly pitched his works especially to the disorders of youth. He made much of the green sickness amongst adolescent girls, implying that physical debility and emotional waywardness were two sides of a single coin, and suggesting their liaison in the emergent sexual imagination (or even practices). Whereas an earlier tradition (evident, say, in Mandeville) had been disposed to take the jaunty view that the disorders of adolescence would melt away with sexual fulfilment in matrimony, Sibly was far more perturbed by the sexual malpractices – above all, masturbation – of adolescence itself, hinting that they might do long-term and almost ineradicable harm. Senate, for his part, looked from the other end of the ages of man, stressing how decrepitude was the fruit of the errors of youth, and offering the appropriate counter-acting medicines.

It was, however, William Brodum and Samuel Solomon who most effectively manipulated the secret sexual scares of the age of sensibility. Brodum, a one-time footman, published a *Guide to Old Age, or Cure for the Indiscretions of Youth*, which stressed the horrors of unspecific sexual disorders in a tone both lugubrious and insinuating. Without his book (he claimed in a blizzard of newspaper advertisements), both young and old offenders – and particularly sea-faring men on long voyages – would be utterly lost ('neither young persons, nor those of maturer years, should be a moment without having it in their possession'). This was because of the catastrophic consequences of 'the various disorders incident to mankind', which followed from 'irregular propensities in both sexes'. His book indicated 'the proper mode of relieif for a roster of distempers which included 'menstruation – chlorosis, scrofula, excess of libidinous indulgence – baneful effects of such indiscretions, especially among youth – Venereal disease'.[36]

The Liverpool quack Samuel Solomon produced an equivalent work, the *Guide to Health, or Advice to Both Sexes in Nervous and Consumptive Complaints Scurvy, Leprosy and Scrofula, and on A Certain Disease and Sexual Debility, in which is added An Address to Boys, Young Men, Parents, Tutors, and Guardians of Youth*, which supposedly reached its sixty-fourth edition by the early nineteenth century. Solomon built upon the association between nervous disorders, consumption (wasting conditions), and furtive sexual practices already forged in earlier anti-masturbation literature such as *Onania*.

But while Solomon collared offending members of the public, and left guilty readers in no doubt of the gravity of their sexual misdemeanours and the enormity of the consequences, he did so in a substantial book, which was infinitely varied, entertaining, learned, informative, diverting and intriguing. The *Guide to Health* was a cornucopia of classical mythology, anecdotes, warnings, tales of the trials of young love and of love-melancholy (Burton's *Anatomy of Melancholy* was pillaged for stories), advice as to the control of 'wild imaginations' and 'extravagant fancies', indexes of the symptoms of the nervous diseases consequent upon self-abuse (for example, 'the eyes are clouded'), and endless name-dropping of the heroes of medicine – Rhazes, Galen, Montanus, etc. All this was spliced with quotations from Shakespeare and random items of an improving nature – the true essence of a good prose style, etc. Above all, Solomon evoked the image, common in the age of sensibility or proto-romanticism, of the frustrated youth as his target reader, now pining and wasting away, now a volcano of erotic frustration, suffering melancholy, idleness, solitariness – and with fatal results. 'O blessed health', he apostrophized, quoting Sterne, 'thou art above all gold and treasure';[37] yet how often health was flung away in vice and folly!

Solomon was no fool. He hardly needed to tell his readers outright that they were suffering from these almost unmentionable sexual disorders, involving shocking symptoms such as 'involuntary emissions', back pains, weak memory, dejection, poor eyesight: he cannily treated this almost as a secret shared between his readers and himself. But he did need to make sufferers feel in good company – they were linked by association with the great names of history and literature – poets, writers, geniuses, heroes. And he left them in no doubt of their urgent duty to have immediate recourse to medicine... *his* medicine. In such conditions, he insisted, the 'patient must be comfortable and content to be ruled by his physician'. Above all, the sufferer had to come clean, face up to reality: Solomon orchestrated a kind of confession by proxy. 'How many are there', he boomed, applying great psychological leverage, 'that have perished because they dared not reveal the cause of their illness!' Thankfully many did: Solomon informs us of the mailbags of letters he had received from culprits confessing their sexual 'degeneracy' and 'depravation', and testifying to the power of his medicines and books in expediting recovery.

Immature and uncontrolled sexual desires were thus the roots of disease; excessive venery led to 'lassitude, weakness, numbness'; yet, at the other extreme, 'continued celibacy generally loads the glands, retards the circulation, and occasions fulness and stagnation in the vessels'. Worst still, celibacy led to bad habits, and eventually *habitués* became 'addicted to Onanism'.

Physiologically speaking, this was an evil because – for Solomon as for Tissot and Graham – it resulted in a 'waste of semen', whose consequence was constitutional weakness because 'this seminal liquor is a vast importance to the human frame'. And this, in turn, was well-nigh catastrophic, because such interconnected 'nervous and hypochondriacal complaints' resist 'all remedies' – 'except the famous and highly-exalted medicine, the Cordial Balm of Gilead'.

In the high-flown, self-regarding rhetoric of the late eighteenth century, Solomon liked to present himself in the guise of a medical philosopher, reflecting upon the human condition, rather than as nostrum-vendor. His sense of identity was complex. He chose to make almost romantic play of his marginality ('it is an incontrovertible fact', he boasted, 'that the most considerable improvements in medicine have been made by persons who were not regular and systematic professors of the art'), and to champion the paramountcy of 'experience'. Yet he also insisted that he was 'regularly graduated'.

The same ambiguity surrounded Solomon's preparations. On the one hand, he chose to represent his nostrum as a 'public medicine' available for the good of society at large. On the other, he explicitly championed free trade in medicines (it protected the public's right to choose: truth would prevail, he claimed, quoting Plato and Sydenham on his side), and paraded the sheer scale and success of his private enterprise: he claimed to lay out £5000 a year in advertisements, and to have sold 120,000 copies of his book. He was clearly an astute businessman. In his *An Account of the Balm of Gilead*, he offered a dozen bottles, normally priced at 10s 6d each, for just £5, thus offering a saving of £1 6s. Not least, he would send to any post office goods marked with a special sign, 'to insure inviolable secrecy'. Above all, Solomon's advertising is impressive for its sheer geographical spread. Thus the *Guide to Health* and the Balm of Gilead were even widely advertised in Scottish newspapers – a letter printed in one, by a Scottish wholesaler, ran:

'Sir, The cures effected in Scotland by your medicine, the Cordial Balm of Gilead in a variety of singular cases within my own knowledge, has rendered the sale thereof rapid beyond example, in this part of the island. I have now therefore to request you will lose no time in forwarding a very large supply by the first carrier. I shall take the opportunity of remitting you a draft for upwards of SEVENTY POUNDS in the course of a few posts... J. Baxter'. Solomon's medicines were big business. The large bottle of his balm cost a guinea, and he instructed that his medicines be taken 'Morning Noon and Night'.

Sex, we have seen, provided good business for quackery, because sexual diseases were widespread, secret and shameful. In its turn, quackery helped contribute to the culture of sexuality, and indeed sexology, by providing a lively focus for formulations on a subject upon which regular biomedical science was sometimes unwilling to speak.

7   The quarrel of the quacks

Quack medicine, as we have seen, was neither suppressed nor silenced in England. The public wanted to buy it; the state, increasingly disinclined to interfere in market regulation, preferred to tax rather than to ban it; the medical colleges lacked the power to force it out of existence, or even drive it underground – and, in any case, regular practitioners themselves were cashing in on commercial practices barely distinguishable from what was commonly denounced as quackery.

Thus quackery, rather like prostitution, was permitted to thrive as a necessary evil, a sop to human weakness. These were precisely the circumstances that led to its being anathematized so vociferously – by those who, claiming to represent the public interest, saw charlatanism rampant and everyone else to blame. The aim of this chapter is to lay bare the key themes ventilated in the polemics raging over quackery. Of course, it would be a mistake to assume that only quack medicine stirred up storms of controversy, the practice of regular medicine, on the contrary, being praised as all sweetness and light – just as it would be false to assume that regulars washed their dirty linen *in camera*: such a situation certainly could not obtain till after the founding of the General Medical Council in 1858. Far from it: the medical world of the long eighteenth century was a ferociously combative free-for-all in which regulars engaged in pamphlet wars, arraigning each other before the bar of public opinion, no less than they savaged the empirics.

Occasionally regulars even came to blows. Early in the eighteenth century, two of London's leading physicians, Richard Mead and John Woodward, apparently crossed swords in a duel (neither was injured; however, in a challenge between two practitioners in the Caribbean, both fell dead). Granville Sharp Pattison, the early nineteenth-century Glasgow surgeon, was similarly involved in several violent controversies culminating in pistols.

Usually, however, doctors confined themselves to wounding with words. The flashy world of spa medicine produced abundant vitriol, as in Bath, for instance, in the 'sulphur controversy' over the chemical analysis of the spa waters: Archibald Cleland, surgeon to the Bath Hospital, was dismissed from his post as a result of what he claimed – in a pamphlet appealing to the public – had been a vile conspiracy (he was accused of sexual malpractice) mounted against him by a cabal of local doctors, merely because he was an outsider. David Harley has elucidated how questions of poaching patients, traducing reputations, undercutting fees, and contesting priorities in medical discoveries all resulted in masses of mud being slung throughout the medical profession at this time. Doctors deplored the orgy of besmirching; but they participated in it, all the same. Such mutual vilification, William Hunter, doyen of medical teachers, told his students, was all an inevitable result of human nature and of professional 'emulation and contention'. Any anatomist worth his salt, Hunter contended, was bound to be 'impatient of unreasonable opposition and of encroachments upon his discoveries and his reputation'. By

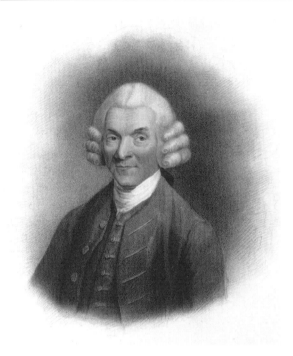

William Hunter. Coloured stipple engraving by B. Smith, 1817, after M. Houghton after M. Chamberlin.

consequence, 'there is scarce a considerable character in anatomy, that is not connected with some warm controversy'. Hunter himself was no exception. He feuded with almost all his contemporaries, and was not on speaking terms with his surgeon brother, John, for the last ten years of his life. Half a century later, the surgeon Thomas Wakley lanceted his own profession in the full-frontal glare of medical journalism. Public bloodletting was thus by no means confined to the quack end of the market.

Nor should we expect to find battle-lines drawn up in an orderly fashion between a thin red line of regulars on one side, and the barbarian hordes of medicasters on the other. Rather there was a mêlée, more like a Hobbesian *bellum omnium contra omnes*. Thus, if *esprit de corps* was pretty deficient amongst the regulars, there was none at all amongst the quacks, because what every irregular ached to do was to distance himself from the aspersion of being a quack, precisely by denouncing the vile race of charlatans. Sometimes quacks (like regulars) were literally involved in a fight to the death, to vindicate their honour as true physicians, as appears from this encounter recorded by Thomas Isham in the 1670s:

> Two quack doctors disputed with each other before the King of France as to which was the better physician, and to decide the point they tried which could kill the other. They drew lots to see who should begin, and after drawing, one gave poison to the other and told him to drink. He took the cup and drank it, afterwards he took his antidote and rubbed himself a little till he had recovered breath. He afterwards completely recovered and gave to the other a certain powder and told him to breathe it through his nostril. He immediately did so and died, the antidote being of no use. The King

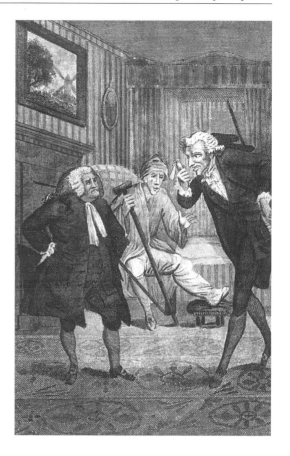

'The enraged Quacks'. Two medical practitioners arguing about opposing methods in front of a patient. Coloured engraving, 1787.

asked the quack what it was he gave him; he said, poison extracted from the most pestilential ulcers.[1]

Most quack poison, however, was merely verbal, and designed to slay only reputations.

The 'advertising professors' themselves displayed noble public spirit in alerting the world to the appalling evils of quackery. Thus, in the late seventeenth century, a flyer of Edward Grey's warned that through 'no Nation has been so fortunate in producing such Eminent Physicians as this Kingdom of ours', all the same, ''tis obvious to every Eye, that no Country was ever Pestered with so many ignorant Quacks and Empericks'. Indeed, he was ready with his own sociology (one of secularization and upward social mobility) to explain how this sorry state had come about: 'The Enthusiast in Divinity having no sooner acted his part, and had his Exit, but on the same Stage, from his Shop, enters the Enthusiast in Physick; Yesterday's Taylor, Heel-maker, Barber, Weaver, Rope-Dancer, &, Today, *per saltim*, a learn'd Doctor, able to instruct *Esculapius* himself.' This irrational state of affairs had induced him, dedicated as he was to the protection of the public, to venture into this 'publick way of Information' – his bill then went on to assure readers that he had a unique method of curing the pox without fluxing or mercurials, and so forth.[2]

This *plus royaliste que le roi* strategy was not unique to Grey. Thus a 'German doctor' in Petty France grumbled of 'pretenders' who ruined health by their 'irregular methods',

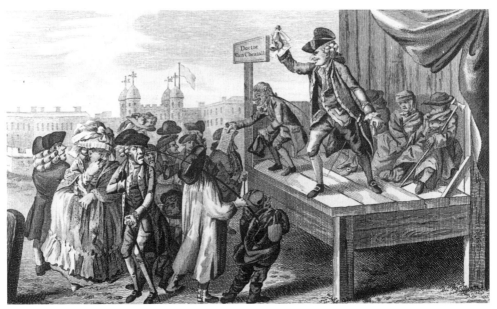

'Doctor Van Cheatall' performs his sales pitch to a suspicious crowd against a backdrop of the Tower of London. Etching, 1792.

rather as Salvator Winter lamented how the masses were 'Deceived by some ignorant Persons', who had the effrontery to counterfeit his 'Elixir Vitae'.

Commercial doctors plumed themselves upon their public service in exposing charlatans. Thus David Irish, in the course of a quack pamphlet puffing not only various nostrums but also his own private lunatic asylum, explained that quacks were the very scrapings of society. It was even common, he revealed, 'for the Servants of Deceased Physicians to Usurp the Name of Doctor; These make the Ignorant believe they know much, by reason they copied out their Masters Bills and Prescriptions.' No better was the 'crowd of Woman Doctors' who ought not 'to meddle with an Art far beyond a Feminine strength'. And even worse, if possible, were 'Mountebanks' who were just 'catterpillars', lacking even the skill 'to give a Drench to a Horse'. The poor would be crazy to allow themselves to be cheated out of their money by 'such strange Fopperies, foolish Pastimes and Jack-Pudding Tricks', concluded Irish, while trumpeting his own extraordinary powers ('I have cured several of the Palsie, who had lost the Use of their Limbs and Speech').[3]

John Pechey was another nostrum-monger itching to rescue the gullible from the 'innumerable mischiefs arising from Quacks, and their ill compounded and worse prepared Trash'. Of course, most such vermin were 'cobbling Doctors', outstanding only in 'skill in nonsense', whose medicines were brought by the herd. By contrast, the connoisseurs of his own preparations were 'people of Eminence [known] both for their Rank in the World and their Parts' – yet more evidence that quacks saw little advantage in cultivating an overtly demotic appeal. Another bill, 'A Caveat to the Unwary, or Venus Unveil'd', summed up this 'quack eats quack' line in a jingling cautionary tale: 'Beware of Quacks, Mercury and all such foes,/ Lest Need require a Supplemental Nose.'[4]

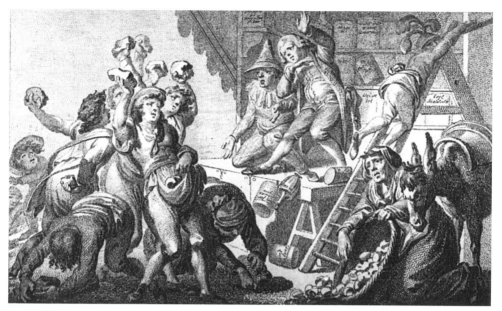

A travelling nostrum-vendor and his assistants are pelted with stones by an angry audience. Engraving by C.F. Stoelzei, 1798, after J. Schenau.

Accompanying such barrages against quacks and quackery in general, the 'advertising professors' frequently slaughtered individual rivals by name, mainly for stealing their products. Thus the vendor of the Elixir Magnum Stomachicum revealed, 'There is lately extant a Liquor called Tinctura Stomachica, or the Cordial Tincture, a Counterfeit of Mine, beware of it.' Likewise, the bill for the Water of Talk [that is, Talc] told readers to watch out for 'another Person, who has lately set forth Bills, Entituled, The Fountain of Beauties, who does pretend to something of this Nature, but nothing to the Purpose.'[5] The truth was that this rival had been 'taken in by me for sometime as my servant, till he thought he had gained experience enough then ran away in my Debt, and is now gone further distant to deceive others'.[6]

Scurvy-grass products, being in demand, were particularly subject to counterfeiting. Controversy started with a bill from Robert Bateman, headed 'Bateman's Hue and Cry after the Pretended Sieur de Vernantes, and his Counterfeit Spirit of Scurvey Grass, lately Shammed upon the World by one Clark, an Ale-Draper, near Temple-Bar'. Bateman was obviously a touchy – or, rather, a much-wronged – man, for he alleged that his True Spirits of Scurvey Grass had also been pirated by the 'Billingsgate-orator', Blagrave and pilfered by other 'Whistling Upstarts' besides, all notorious for their 'Fraud and Boldness'. When Blagrave responded, he became the butt of another blast from Bateman, entitled 'A Gentle Dose for the FOOL Turn'd Physician, or A Brief Reply to Blagrave's Ravings', which expostulated that it was hardly more fruitful to argue against Blagrave than to 'Syllogize to an Oyster wench'. Blagrave's bills contained nothing but 'Slander, Lies, false English, Nonsense, and Impertinence'. This 'impudent Quack Doctor' might claim to have travelled in 'Terra incognita', but in reality, his peregrinations amounted to little more than 'a Ramble through Berkshire' – 'like all Ignorant Quacks', Blagrave lied to 'amuse the world'. Others also pilloried the pirates. The advertisement for Dr Anderson's Scots Pills warned against counterfeits produced by 'broken Merchants, ignorant Tradesmen, and scandalous Persons'. Only one maker had authentically inherited the late Gilbert Anderson's business and recipe, and she was 'Isabella Inglish'.

If counterfeiting was one sharp practice that altruistic bill-writers exposed before the world (it was itself, of course, a sign of the ill-defined state of product proprietorship in early modern capitalist manufacturing), another was the phoney testimonial. Don't believe other people's attestations, Dr Pernot told his readers: they were all a farrago of fictions, made up of the 'names of Persons, some of whom have above 30 to 40 years since been deceased, and the rest no where to be found'.[7] Yet another fraudulent practice was adulteration. Thus Theophilus Buckworth laid bare the 'wicked designes of Lownds and Piercy', who were making substandard, counterfeit lozenges. Such a rogue was Lownds, Buckworth revealed, that he would even sell 'Brick-bats' parcelled up as medicines if he could do so at a profit. These evil cheats were furthermore slandering Buckworth by suggesting he had a criminal record.[8]

The indictment against quacks

We might thus see it as ironic that there was no honour amongst thieves, and that quack operators rehearsed, with great *ad hominem* panache, all the arguments directed against themselves, thus apparently sparing regulars the trouble. In reality, however, orthodox practitioners did not let the 'swarms of pseudo-medici' off the hook. As Thomson argued in his *Family Physician*, in a section headed 'Of Empirics': '[medicine] is infested by a race of ignorant and shameless empirics, who are daily tampering with the public credulity, to the destruction of numbers of lives. It may safely be affirmed, that a very considerable part of the annual deaths in the capital and its vicinity,… are occasioned by the profligate temerity of these unprincipled impostors'.[9] Quacks were lashed and lashed again, but the attack was highly stereotyped. Quacks were ignorant impostors (regulars claimed), mushrooming up from the dunghill of society. Thus, Adair revealed, Joshua Ward started off his career as a footman; Walker (proprietor of the Jesuit Drops) had been a porter; Myersbach, the uroscopist, was a failed rough-rider; Sir John Hill had started as a linen-draper; and Turlington (of Turlington's Balsam) had been a ship's master.

Not surprisingly, in view of their medical ignorance, their cures did not work – or worked too well! 'Many persons have been destroyed by quack drugs', revealed the sardonic Adair, 'but dead men tell no tales.'[10] Along similar lines, William Buchan warned the public about the perils of quack vermifuges, which contained dangerous concentrations of mercury. A woman bought one, took it, drank cold water, whereupon 'she immediately swelled and died that very day, with all the symptoms of having been poisoned'.[11] William Heberden similarly reflected upon the plethora of such proprietary vermifuges: 'we have the misfortune to have innumerable remedies for the worms: this

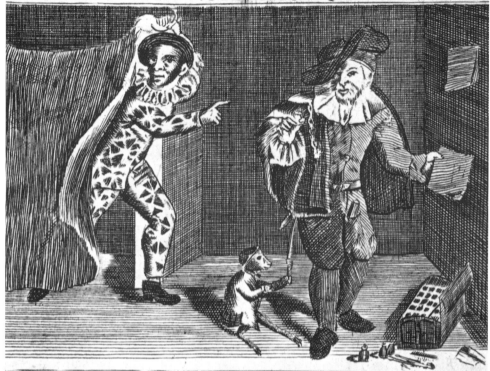

The Infallible MOUNTEBANK or Quack Doctor

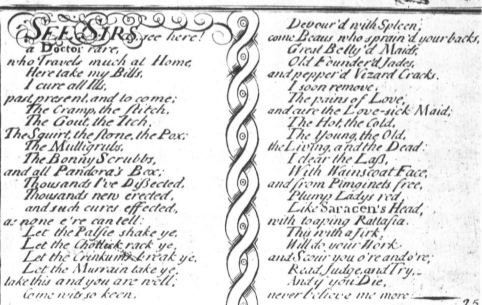

SEE SIRS, see here!
a Doctor rare,
who Travels much at Home,
Here take my Bills,
I cure all Ills,
past, present, and to come;
The Cramp, the Stitch,
The Gout, the Itch,
The Squirt, the Stone, the Pox;
The Mulligruts,
The Bonny Scrubbs,
and all Pandora's Box;
Thousands I've Dissected,
Thousands new erected,
and such cures effected,
as none e're can tell:
Let the Palsie shake ye,
Let the Chollick rack ye,
Let the Crinkums break ye,
Let the Murrain take ye,
take this and you are well;
Come wits so keen.

Devour'd with Spleen;
come Beaus who sprain'd your backs,
Great Belly'd Maids,
Old Founder'd Jades,
and pepper'd Vizard Cracks.
I soon remove,
The pains of Love,
and cure the Love-sick Maid;
The Hot, the Cold,
The Young, the Old,
the Living, and the Dead;
I clear the Lass,
With Wainscoat Face,
and from Pimginets free,
Plump Ladys red,
Like Saracen's Head,
with toaping Rattafia.
This with a firk,
Will do your Work,
and Scour you o're and o're;
Read, Judge, and Try,
And y'you Die,
never believe me more.

25

Hans Buling, a travelling medicine salesman, professes to cure all ills. Engraving.

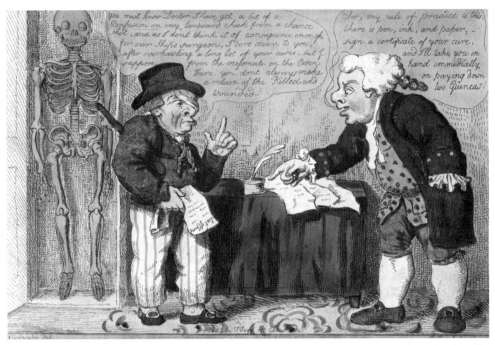

A quack doctor requests a testimony to his cure before treating a wounded sailor. Coloured etching by I. Cruikshank, 1807, after G.M. Woodward.

being pretty generally a good sign, that we have not one, upon which we can with certainty depend.'[12] Regulars commonly alleged that quacks made irresponsible use of mercury (which, because of its spectacular purgative qualities, certainly did 'work'): 'Mercury... has long been the chief ingredient in quack remedies', noted Thomas Trotter, 'It is thus vended under the form of tincture, drop, powder, pill.'[13]

In any case, regulars argued, those quack medicines that did work had simply been filched from regular practice. Thus, revealed Adair, Ward's medicine was common 'solution of sublimate'; Norton's Drops were ordinary 'sublimate mercury'; Daffy's Elixir was just 'tincture of senna'; Barrett's Pills were 'extract of hemlock and wolfs bane'; Stoughton's Drops were 'stomachic tincture'; Godfrey's Cordial was 'sassafras, syrup and opium'; Norris's and Spilsbury's drops were 'antimonial wine'. All quack medicines, Adair judged, were routine variations upon mercury, antimony, and opium, for example, Velnos' syrup comprised sublimate mercury plus gum arabic, honey, and syrup. When a physician heard of stupendous cures worked by a quack patent remedy, Adair reported: 'he is always disappointed when, on obtaining a copy, he finds it to be a thing known to every apothecary's apprentice, or such a collection of useless rubbish, as cannot avail more in the cure of a disease than bread pills, sheep's dung or powder of post.'[14]

In short, quackery was a con. For instance, empirics invented their testimonials: 'look into almost whatever newspaper you please', challenged Thomas Beddoes, 'you will find reverend names, dangling by dozens, to the tail of frauds at half a guinea the bottle.'

John Lambe, an infamous quack and magician, who was killed by an angry mob in London. Engraving, 1823.

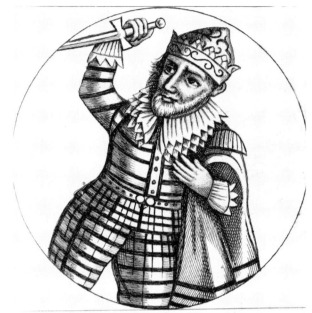

John Lambe, alias D:Lambe,
A Quack and reputed Conjuror.
Killed in the Streets of London by a Mob.

The quack doctor had the rare privilege of being 'his own historian', reflected Beddoes, 'and publishes in every pamphlet and newspaper cases of cures never performed.'[15] Overall, therefore, quack medicine was just bad medicine.

Naturally, quacks did not take such charges lying down. The typical response was the deflective: 'who? me?'. Quacks reiterated the evils of quackery but denied the charges applied to themselves. Thus, for instance, the bill announcing 'There is lately come to London, an Italian Doctor', made a point of insisting that the author had 'never [been] any stage Quack or Mountebank' – though he was 'very successful in the Speedy Cures of these following Distempers', etc. A guerrilla war of assertion, denial, and counter-assertion developed. Thus the proprietor of the Universal Scorbutick Pills pre-empted the usual charge of ignorance by claiming, instead, that he was 'an eminent Physician', who had practised on people of 'Honour and Quality'.[16]

Quacks tried to make the regulars' attacks rebound. Empirics were accused of being know-nothings. True, some would respond, they had not had a university education. But who would want one? Were not the lectures of the schools all tinkling theory and vacuous verbiage? They had instead graduated in the University of Life, gaining vastly valuable practical experience. Thus in the mid-eighteenth century, Ralph Heathcote defended James' Powders against detractors: physicians decried them as no better than an empirical remedy, Heathcote noted, but was not that a point in their favour? – for experience proved that they worked.

Along similar lines, the advertisement for Clark's Compound Spirits of Scurvey-Grass contended that practical experience must be the ultimate yardstick in medicine: 'every Tree is known by its fruit'. What counted were not abstractions but 'great Effects'

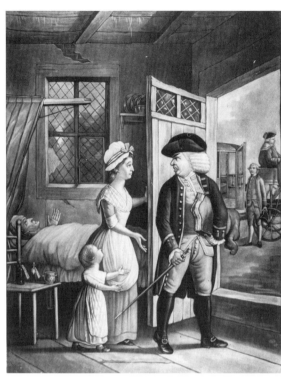

A greedy medical practitioner demanding a leg of bacon as payment from a poor family. Mezzotint.

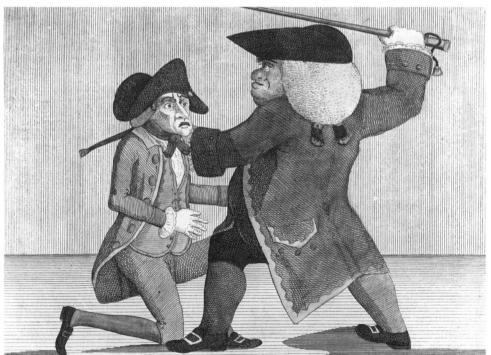

Dᴿ SALTINBANCO ᴀᴘᴘʟʏɪɴɢ ʜɪꜱ ʟᴀꜱᴛ. DRESSING ꜰᴏʀ ʜɪꜱ PATIENT'S ɴᴏɴPAYMENT.

Doctor Saltinbanco assaults a client for non-payment. Coloured etching.

– to which end, the author appended a string of spectacular cures, with authenticating testimonials. Physicians might scoff, John Case warned his readers, pre-empting criticism, but the acid test was the personal first-hand experience of the people:

> Dear Country-men, I pray you be so wise,
> When Men sack Bite him, believe not their Lyes,
> But go see him, believe your own Eyes.
> Then he will say you are Honest and Kind
> Try before you Judge, and speak as you find.[17]

Quacks recognized that counterattack was the best form of defence. They were often accused of lacking book-learning and familiarity with ancient languages. But, riposted John Spinke, in truth the boot was upon the other foot: it was his accuser-in-chief, the surgeon, John Marten, who was a tyro at Latin. Spinke must have enjoyed titling his book *Quackery Unmask'd*, claiming that the true quack was, after all, his surgeon rival, whose hypocritical tirade amounted to nothing other than 'one large quack bill'.

Indeed, many quacks went on to the offensive. Cornelius à Tilbourg warned the public not to 'tarry... too long till you are spoiled by other Practitioners', for that way 'it will be worse to be cured'. Luckily, so great was his skill that even when dealing with 'such as have been tampering with other Practitioners' – notwithstanding 'they have been sweated, Fluxed, and lanced by other Doctors' – he would 'certainly reduce [them] to their former health'.[18]

Neither were they slow to accuse their regular cousins of enormities. Thus John Pechey indicted the Collegians of profiteering. He, by contrast, would treat the parish poor free, and generally charge but a shilling for advice. Other quacks made much of the public service they were doing by smashing the physicians' fee cartel. A certain J. Russel informed the public that he was 'publishing' precisely because he was concerned for the plight of those 'that cannot go to the Charge of Fees, and are not able to pay for such costly Courses of Physick as is commonly used in Practice'.[19] Many quacks emphasized that, unlike physicians, they did not have the gall to charge for advice, desiring payment solely for medicines (which, of course, put them on a par with the apothecary).

Quack drugs

One area of controversy flared in particular: the claims for quack drugs. Quack therapeutics relied especially heavily upon medication. Adair mockingly suggested that quacks were implementing Falstaff's 'Turn Disease into a Commodity'. Certainly, they were turning cure to commodity.

Nevertheless, their promotion of pharmacological cures left them open to attack, in three ways in particular. First, critics assailed their habit of secrecy: clandestine remedies were sure to be dangerous, fraudulent, or worthless. Quacks, however, saw little need to be apologetic about secrecy. Indeed, they brazenly attempted to make capital out of the allure of mystery. Thus a Dutch physician had come to England to sell 'an Excellent secret'. In a culture in which secret societies and associations had powerful cachet – freemasonry was expanding fast – and which widely believed that religious, scientific, mystical and erotic wisdom had been handed down from Antiquity cloaked in coded symbols to prevent its profanation amongst the vulgar, the very notion of secrecy had a guaranteed mystique.

Moreover, it stood to reason that a secret remedy must be something special and extraordinary – particularly if it had been obtained at staggering expense (as was typically claimed) from some expiring adept thousands of miles away.

What is more, its vendor was by definition the sole possessor. Thus the recipe for the 'Princess Powder' had once been privy to old M. Ranet, the Paris apothecary; he left the recipe exclusively to his son, who alone knew how to pound these beauty powders. If such secrets were to exist, who dared to miss out on them?

Patenting – although nominally making a nostrum an open secret – could serve as a further device whereby, to all intents and purposes, a secret was protected, for the specifications required by law were lax. The patented medicine carried the additional kudos of passing, as it were, as a state-endorsed official secret. Regulars were not slow to lodge patents of their own, for instance, the leading Restoration scientist, Nehemiah Grew, with his Epsom Salts, excellent for colic, worms, and indigestion.

Quack medicines took two forms, both of which drew howls of protest. On the one hand, there was the panacea. Cure-alls were, of course, hopelessly vulnerable to the accusation that the very idea that one single medicine could cure all the ailments under the sun was moonshine. 'An universal remedy', argued Willich, 'or one that possesses healing powers for the cure of all diseases', was, in fact, a 'nonentity, the existence of which is physically impossible, as the mere idea of it involves a direct contradiction.' Fortunately, he claimed, it was an idea 'losing ground every day, even among the vulgar, and has long been exploded in those classes of society which are not influenced by prejudice or tinctured with fanaticism.'[20]

No less absurd, regulars claimed, was the quacks' promotion of nostrums and specifics, trading upon the idea that every ill had its pill. Despite a superficial attractiveness, the notion must equally be a chimera, regulars argued: since diseases acted upon the system in general, so too must truly effective medicines. How could a single medicine cure the same illness in every patient, because one particular disease typically manifested itself through distinct symptoms in different patients, just as, conversely, identical symptoms could be the sign of disparate diseases. Thus, concluded William Buchan, nostrums were a vestige of the magical mentality: the masses believed in nostrums because 'they are used more like charms'.

The public way of practice

The very marrow of the regulars' attack on quackery, however, lay in denunciations of what was often known as the 'publick way of practice'. Through hawking their goods in the marketplace, quacks were downgrading medicine from its true standing as a noble art or science into a vulgar traffic, like selling trinkets.

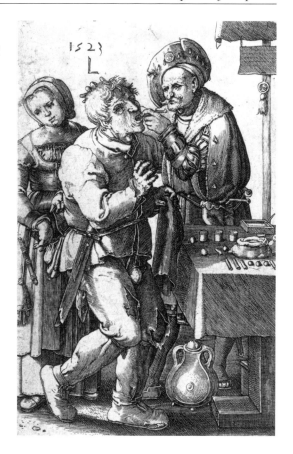

A tooth-drawer extracting a tooth from a standing patient, who is being pickpocketed by a woman. Line engraving by L. van Leyden, 1523.

Quacks, of course, had answers to this. They knew a certain defensiveness about their way of practice was in order. Thus a 'Graduate Physician' said in his billet that 'I request a favourable Construction upon this Publick Way of Practice', being aware, he told readers, that he 'would have to adventure the Censure of some'. Yet how was this to be avoided, given that he wished to promote a medicine 'which may be of so great use to many'?[21] More deprecating still was the rigmarole of the author of The Most Excellent Universal Pill, who quite openly admitted that: 'The Vast number of Bills which are daily distributed about the Streets and the multitude of Pretenders to Physical Cures (which it may be supposed) they never did nor can do; has rendered this way of exposing Medicines to Sale, not only Contemptible, but almost unprofitable, which might reasonably discourage a Man, who is neither a Fool, nor a Physician, from meddling in this kind.'[22] Yet, so anxious was he to promote the public good, that nothing could restrain him from maximizing his publicity.

Many, on the other hand, vindicated 'public practice' aggressively, by playing creatively and even punningly upon the connotations – positive and negative – of the public-private axis. Above all, they contended, it was absolutely in the public interest for them to advertise their wares and services. For one thing, many doctors had newly arrived from abroad, or at least were new to town: what other way did the public have to learn of their presence? Without thus issuing a 'Printed Paper', Elizabeth Maris claimed, she might 'for some Years have remained unknown to you, and so

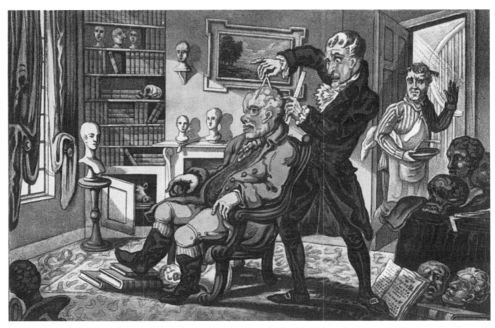

Doctor Spurzheim in his consulting room measuring the head of a rather peculiar looking patient. A bemused barber looks on. Coloured aquatint by J. Kennerly, 1816, after R. Cocking.

consequently incapable of imploying that Talent which Heaven hath bestow'd on me'.[23] It was a common line. 'Gentlemen and Ladies', wrote a button-holing 'German Surgeon', 'who (being a Stranger here) am oblig'd to Publish Bills, therefore I must beg Pardon of the Publick if I do not express my self so well as others.' Likewise, a surgeon from 'without Temple Bar' assured readers that he had travelled beyond England so long to get experience, that as a consequence, he was a stranger in his own country: 'this is the cause of publishing a Bill, which is become so customary, a body can hardly be known (without the loss of a great deal of time) without it'.[24] Advertising, in other words, was just good business practice.

Conversely, many sick people were new to London: how, except through advertising, were they to seek out doctors? As Thomas Saffold versified the matter:

> Some envious Men being griev'd may say
> What need Bills thus still be given away?
> Answer, New People come to London every day.
> Believing Solomons Advice is right,
> I will do what I do with all my might.
> Also unless an English proverb lies,
> Practice brings experience and makes wise.
> Experimental knowledge I protest,
> In lawful arts and science is the best,
> Instead of Finis, Saffold ends with Rest.[25]

Moreover, how could it possibly be in the public interest to deny the maximum airing to remedies that outstripped all rivals and would spare mankind from disease and death? Thus John Pechey accounted for his own way of publicity by claiming that his medicine was 'of such great Virtue, that it ought not to be concealed, when so many Dangerous and Stopping Medicines are daily used for the French Disease.'[26] To behave otherwise would be the depths of selfishness. J.T., vendor of a Pilula Imperialis vel Sospitalis, naturally disclaimed any self-aggrandizing motives for publicly touting his goods, but assured his gentle readers that he had yielded to the 'important solicitations of several friends and gentlemen', who had appealed to his overriding sense of public responsibility. 'As we are not altogether born for ourselves I have exposed these my medicines to the Publick, for the benefit of those who labour under that unhappy distemper, the POX.'[27]

The most considered defence of 'public practice' was advanced in a bill addressed 'To the Judicious and Discreet Reader'. This engaged in historical mythologizing. Time was, it claimed, when medicine had been an honourable profession, and physicians had indeed developed and publicized medicines in their own name. Such times were past and the occupation had fallen into the hands of a breed of doctors who were no better than mercenary tradesmen, becoming 'a vulgar business'. Not surprisingly, therefore, the true professors of medicine had felt obliged to stand up against vile commercialism, 'for fear of scandal'. This was an understandable reaction, yet it was an over-reaction nevertheless, for it had abandoned the public domain to hucksters. Therefore, it was crucial that doctors of good will – such as himself – should eagerly cultivate the public arena: 'Publishing of Medicines thus shamefully defamed by ignorant pretenders, must be restored into esteem by the learned, which will prove most advantageous to the people; and it is their interest to incourage skilful experienced Artists that they may not lock up their rare inventions and fortunate experiments, confining them within the narrow compass of a private practice; but rather that they expose their Arcanum to publick use, that all who stand in need may partake thereof.' Fortunately, this was already happening, and good physicians were now 'reviving the primitive practice'. This must benefit healing. For true public medicine, supplied through publicity, would ensure that 'the meanest of the people may purchase the best of Medicines... Those who will not undergo, or cannot bear the charge of a course of Physick, may receive great relief by a single Medicine.' In turn, this would create desirable competition. 'Physicians then will be stimulated to out vye and excell each other in the rarity and excellency of their Remedies, being to undergo a publick Tryal'; thereby new specifics will be developed, 'known and conveyed through the Nation': 'These publick great advantages as great reasons being considered, the learned Physician need not be ashamed to publish an extraordinary Medicine of his own designment and elaboration (although ignorant bold fellows have abused the Custom) for if Physicians must shun all that they do, then must they leave their practice too.' Nobody complained, the author reflected, when a preacher published a sermon; so what could be wrong with publishing a nostrum? 'If a Treatise of Anatomy, &c be laudable, why not a discourse of discovery of an incomparable Medicine?'[28] Here, we see the quack struggling to win the moral high ground, by demonstrating that the public practitioner was the public-spirited practitioner.

Rather more opportunist was the line taken by the proprietor of the Universal Scorbutick Pills. The advertising physician was able to make contact with the anonymous public, a technique for ensuring cures 'with great Secrecie'.[29]

Quackery contextualized

There was thus animated thrust-and-parry over the claims of the quacks, some of it *ad hominem*, some concerning particular facets of their practice. But certain commentators cast their eyes and minds more widely over its evils. Prominent amongst these was the Bristol physician, Thomas Beddoes. For Beddoes, writing around the beginning of the nineteenth century, 'destruction and disgrace from unauthorized intruders into medical practice' was an unmitigated national scandal: 'consumption-doctresses, cancer-curers, mechanics professing to treat divers disorders' and so forth were all proliferating. In short, he judged, 'this profession is overrun with quacks'. An egregious imposter such as Samuel Solomon, he reflected, has 'as much confidence' – implying both effrontery and public credibility – 'as almost all the fellows of the three royal colleges put together'.[30]

Yet Beddoes's conclusion was 'Physician, heal thyself'. What right had regulars to grouse about quacks when doctors were themselves indulging in barely-veiled if not bare-faced quackery? So many MDs had poured out pamphlets, commending this, or damning that mineral water, spa, or bath, in publications that were 'merely a diffuse quack bill'. Regulars were no strangers to the arts of self-publicizing. Alluding to Farquhar's *Recruiting Officer*, Beddoes envisaged the beginner in practice drawing upon his own 'Sergeant Kite in petticoats' – his pretty wife – to advertise his arrival by giving dinners and putting invitations about – all in all, asked Beddoes, was there really much difference between 'us and our bastard brethren' – 'are all our artifices to be accounted pious?' So long as regulars and apothecaries colluded in loading the public with unnecessary visits and gallons of superfluous medicines to cure often semi-fictitious diseases, quackery would thrive.

Beddoes had a point. Regular doctors were quite candid about the need to mimic quack tactics to build up business. Thus Erasmus Darwin advised a young practitioner, trying to launch a practice:

> use at first all means to get acquainted with the people of all ranks. At first a parcel of blue and red glasses at the windows might gain part of the retail business on market days, and thus get acquaintance with that class of people. I remember Mr Green, of Lichfield, who is now growing very old, once told me his retail business, by means of his show-shop and many-coloured window, produced him £100 a year. Secondly, I remember a very foolish, garrulous apothecary at Cannock, who had great business without any knowledge or even art, except that he persuaded people he kept good drugs; and this he accomplished by only one stratagem, and that was by boring every person who was so unfortunate as to step into his shop with the goodness of his drugs. "Here's a fine piece of assafoetida, smell of this valarian, taste this album graecum. Dr Fungus says he never saw such a fine piece in his life.[31]

Thomas Beddoes. Pencil drawing after E. Bird.

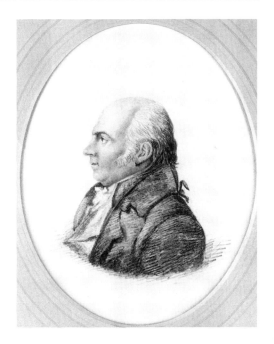

Of course, a veil of decency had to be thrown over this self-publicizing: 'Dr K—-d, I think, supported his business by perpetual boasting, like a Charlatan; this does for a blackguard character, but ill suits a more polished or modest man.'

Darwin's junior contemporary, the American Benjamin Rush, also believed physicians must take a leaf out of the quacks' book in order to succeed in medicine. Departing on his travels, the medical student, John Foulke, was sent 'a few hints' by Rush to help him to win friends, influence people, and learn the ways of the world. Amongst other things he was advised that he must 'Converse freely with quacks of every class and sex, such as oculists, aurists, dentists, corn cutters, cancer doctors, etc. etc. You cannot conceive how much a physician with a liberal mind may profit from a few casual and secret visits to these people.' Rush also advised the young practitioner to make himself prominent in other ways, not least: 'Go regularly to some place of worship. A physician cannot be a bigot. Worship with Mohamitans rather than stay at home on Sundays.'[32]

Beddoes, as we have seen, thus execrated quackery, but suggested – and with reason – that many pillars of orthodoxy were, in fact, quacks in masquerade. Rather like Wakley a generation later, Beddoes feared that the malpractices of the regulars supplied *carte blanche* to the abuses of the quacks: the proliferation of quackery was thus made the occasion for medical reform.

James Makittrick Adair, the fashionable Bath doctor, was another hammer of the quacks; unlike Beddoes, however, he believed prime blame for the perpetuation of the evils of quackery was to be laid at the door of the laity, with their foolish pretensions to medical know-how.

Quackery, Adair believed, was epidemic: everywhere there were 'barbers and medicasters', engaging in all kinds of malpractice. But medical quackery was merely

The QUACK - DOCTOR Outwitted.

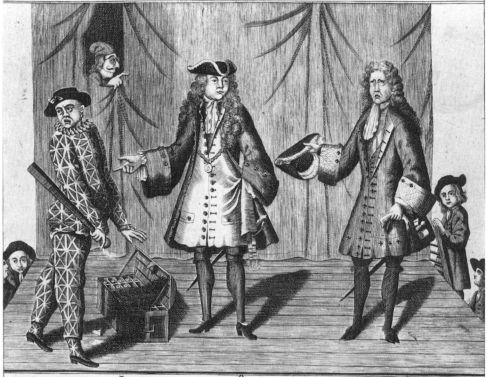

The Devil did complain he was not well _ _ _ _ _
And would go take some Physick out of Hell, _ _ _ _ _
To Brittain, France and Spain with speed he got, _ _ _ _
Where all refus'd him he did burn so hot. _ _ _ _ _ _
In haste he then to Germany did hye, _ _ _ _ _ _ _
The cunning of a Quack-Doctor to try ; _ _ _ _ _ _
Where in a Market-place upon a Stage, _ _ _ _ _ _
He found a Fellow could all Griefs afswage : _ _ _ _ _
Doctor (quoth he) I want some of thy Skill, _ _ _ _
For I do find I am exceeding ill, _ _ _ _ _ _ _
And any thing for ease I will indure ; _ _ _ _ _ _
What! wilt thou undertake my pain to cure ? _ _ _ _
If thou canst ease the Malady I have , _ _ _ _ _ _
Thou shall have Gold, even what thy self will crave :
Gentleman, (said this Doctor to the Devil.) _ _ _ _ _ _
Upon my Life I'll rid you of this Evil. _ _ _ _ _ _
Make unto me those Griefs you have but known, _
And with the curing them let me alone . _ _ _ _ _ _

Why Sir (quoth he) my Head with Horns doth ake, _ _ _
My Brains like Brimstone doth Tobacco take ; _ _ _
My Eyes are full of ever-burning Fire, _ _ _ _ _ _ _
My Tongue a drap of Water doth desire ; _ _ _ _ _
About my Heart doth crawling Serpents creep, _ _ _
And I can neither Eat, nor Drink, nor Sleep; _ _ _ _ _
There's no Diseases whatsoe're they be, _ _ _ _ _ _
But I have all of them impos'd on me ; _ _ _ _ _ _ _
All Torments that the Tongue of Man can name, _ _ _
Within, without, in a continual Flame. _ _ _ _ _ _
Quoth the Quack-Doctor , I will under take _ _ _ _ _ _
A sound Man of you in a Month to make . _ _ _ _ _
Wilt please your Worship, show me where you dwell ? _
Marry (quoth he) my Chamber is in Hell. _ _ _ _ _ _
Thy Charges in thy Journey I will bear, _ _ _ _ _ _
And I'll prefer thee to the Devil there : _ _ _ _ _ _
With speed get up, I'll take thee on my back , _ _ _
The World may spare thee and in Hell we lack . _ _ _

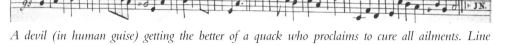

A devil (in human guise) getting the better of a quack who proclaims to cure all ailments. Line engraving by S. Nicholls.

symptomatic of a wider malaise: 'In all departments of life, quackery prevails. Hence we have Imperial quacks, (as the present Emperor has experienced to his cost); legislative quacks, who tamper with political constitutions which they do not understand; philosophical, ethical, critical and religious quacks.'[33] What was special about Georgian medical quackery was that it had become utterly embroiled in the whirl of fashion, luxury, and 'artificial wants' – that syndrome of social sickness sketched in George Cheyne's *English Malady* (1733). When fashion is king, the distinctions between truth and falsehood dissolve away, language is destabilized, and medicine reduced to questions of taste, choice, opinion, and noise. In such circumstances, quackery was sanctioned by the assurance of 'Lady and Gentlemen doctors' that they knew best when it came to medicine, and that it was their right to select nostrums for treating others as well as themselves.

This proved disastrous. Thus consumer choice gave people a taste for buying nostrums; but excessive recourse to 'salts, magnesia, rhubarb', and so forth served only to vitiate their constitutions, thereby leading people to require ever more medicines: 'I am entirely convinced that Anderson's pills, and James's Analeptic Pills (now the fashionable remedy) have been more destructive to his Majesty's subjects than even the havock of war.'[34]

For Adair, quackery thus reigned thanks to a particular alliance. On the one hand, there flourished 'the sordid and selfish race of nostrum-mongers'; on the other, foolish 'Lady and Gentlemen doctors' confident of their ability to serve as their own doctors, acting on the empiricist, individualist grounds that 'as they understand their own constitutions, they are best qualified to determine what is fit for them'. Such people were for ever thumbing over the latest 'dispensatories and practical compilations', becoming infatuated with such books as *Aristotle's Master-piece*, *Culpeper's Midwifery*, *Salmon's Practice of Physick* and *Every Man his own Physician*', and installing in their closet 'a medicine chest, generally the refuse of a druggists shop'. Both such sets of ignoramuses – indeed, 'all pretenders to such distinction – are, in the just sense of the term, QUACKS'. They were mutually sustaining, parties to a *folie à deux*.

Indeed, the situation was even worse than met the eye. For one thing, many quack medicines were habit-forming: 'This is peculiarly the case with rhubarb, magnesia, Anderson's and James' Analeptic Pills etc., the first dose creating a necessity for a second, and so on.' For another, quack doctors and these lay 'experts' between them had cooked up a bogus philosophy about swallowing medicines by way of 'prevention'. 'Knavish quacks' furthermore exploited people's moods when sick, as they lurched from fickleness to desperation. Moreover, in this age of heightened sensibility, people increasingly fancied themselves sick, and so suffered from hypochondria and other 'imaginary diseases'. All such factors conspired to create drug dependency.

But in such harmful developments, Adair, like Beddoes, thought the medical profession far from blameless (indeed, he might well have pointed an incriminating finger at Beddoes himself!). For 'one principal cause of the prevalence of quackery is the illiberal manner in which medical men often treat each other, for the base purpose of establishing a reputation on the ruin of that of a rival.' Professional backbiting undermined public confidence.

Bad was made worse when regulars published popular tracts such as William Buchan's *Domestic Medicine*; these were manna to the hypochondriac, while encouraging the sick to think they could safely dispense with regular medical attendance. Not least, regulars had grown soft on quackery. Though it was 'the duty of every physician to discountenance empirical practice', nevertheless, in these corrupt times, quackery was 'not very strenuously discouraged by physicians'. It was all very well to adopt the lofty maxim 'SI VULGUS DECIPI VULT, DECIPIATUR', yet it pained Adair to see how far physicians actually pandered to fashionable quackery. Many regulars prescribed quack remedies because they 'concede to the whims and prejudices of patients or their connexions'; while, worse still, regulars compounded the offence by compounding nostrums – such as the fever powders of Dr Robert James – a man 'so careless in dosing the medicine' that 'he left the care of it to an old woman' – or Dr Kennedy, whose Lisbon Diet Drink was a farrago of droppings and sweepings, in which only guaiacum, sarsaparilla, and mezereon were active ingredients.

The English legislature was equally culpable, because of its 'sordid and shameful practice of giving [quacks] patents'. They ordered these things better in France. Louis XVI had made short shrift with Mesmer, and 'the legislators in almost every civilized society have considered quacks as pests, and have therefore enacted penal laws for the suppression of quackery.' In England, by contrast, mountebanks were merely taxed: was mulcting the way to deal with murderers? Rather, it was high time to 'suppress the nostrum mongers'; if Parliament acted as resolutely as had Louis XVI with Mesmer, it 'must effectually suppress quackery'. As it was, quacks were in the driving seat, because, in a society governed by opinion, their appalling effrontery commandeered all the greatest organs of opinion.

Quackery and authority

Underpinning the entire attack by regulars upon quackery was the assumption, implicit or explicit, that orthodox medicine was authorized to arbitrate upon matters medical. The weight of tradition, numbers, and the law gave some plausibility to such claims. Yet sustaining them was no cut-and-dried matter, as emerged whenever quacks contested the taken-for-granted status of their assailants. This became especially apparent in the dog-fight waged in the 1770s between John Coakley Lettsom, one of the most eminent London physicians, and Theodor Myersbach, a German quack.

For a time at least, Myersbach was a prominent London personage. His clientele included David Garrick, who assured his friend, Ralph Lodge, 'I feel myself at this moment better for your recommendation of Dr Mierbach' [*sic*].[35] According to public gossip, at one stage Myersbach was pulling in 'about one thousand guineas a month' in fees. Dr Myersbach – his doctorate was purchased from Erfurt – specialized in uroscopy. He had – at least, so enemies claimed – started life in Germany as a lowly post-office clerk, then had migrated to Amsterdam, and, failing there, had moved on to London, where he contemplated becoming a rider at Angelo's equestrian circus (he was judged too short). Impoverished, he boned up on the palaver of urine-casting, despite being medically ignorant. Pro-Myersbach sources never denied the accuracy of this pedigree. Rather, they riposted: so what? The notion that a man's humble background should disqualify him from exercising medical skills smacked of disgraceful elitism.

Urine-casting, as mentioned above in chapter 5, had been a reputable diagnostic procedure from Antiquity, through the Middle Ages and beyond; indeed, a man gazing at

Hans Buling, a travelling nostrum-monger, with his performing monkey. Engraving after M. Laroon.

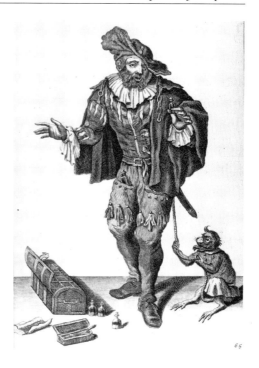

65

the urine flask became a cliché image of the doctor in paintings and prose alike. Scrutinizing urine made good sense within humoral medicine, which stressed how the body's fluids were crucial to health, and which relied heavily upon evaluations for diagnosis.

Yet during the sixteenth and seventeenth centuries, urine-casting fell under a cloud as irrational and magical, and exclusive reliance upon urine-gazing for diagnostic purposes became the hallmark of a sub-species of empirics. Uroscopy declined, though certain 'pisse prophets' continued to make a living in more remote regions right through the eighteenth century (John Byng came across rural Myersbachs on his travels). For faith in urine-casting evidently lived on amongst the people long after the faculty abandoned it. For example, the story circulated that a cobbler's wife brought the great Dr John Radcliffe some of her husband's urine for diagnosis. The exasperated physician responded in kind by presenting her with a sample of his own urine, so that her husband could make him a pair of shoes. Certainly, when Myersbach set up in London he found no shortage of customers who had faith in the ancient art.

He quickly built up a practice distinguished for quality no less than quantity – so much so that detractors implied that he exploited titled hypochondriacs ('Lady Hysteria, Lady Credulous, Lady Innoffensive [*sic*], Lady Widow-Weed, the Hon. Miss Pregnant and many others').[36] Authentic fashionable clients included the Duke and Duchess of Richmond, Lord Archer, Lord Hawke, and Lady Harrington. And his testimonials came from bankers, goldsmiths, attorneys, clergymen, and army and naval officers. He kept a spacious house in Berwick Street, Soho – then a smart address – and his fees indicate an affluent clientele, for he charged half a guinea for a consultation and several shillings more for medicines. Of course, if, as Lettsom alleged, Myersbach actually saw 'two hundred votaries a day', he must also have had a mass of lower-class customers for whom his charges were correspondingly lower.

Why did sick members of the polite and propertied classes go to Myersbach? Did they have a positive faith in uroscopy itself? Or – as seems more likely – was it that the better class of customer typically visited Myersbach as a last resort, after regulars had failed to achieve cure or relief, or, as one pamphlet put it, when 'on the brink of the grave [when] all hope is gone.'[37] This was certainly so with David Garrick, who had long suffered excruciating pain with gout and kidney disorders. Myersbach's drugs may also account for his popularity. One was a brandy and opium cocktail, doubtless an effective knock-out analgesic.

How did Myersbach perform? Clients would either attend in person, bringing a flask of urine, or, if too ill to move, a urine sample would be brought on their behalf by a servant or relative. Myersbach would scrutinize their water. He boasted that on the basis of that inspection only, and without questioning or other forms of interrogation, he could judge their sex, age, and life story.

Detractors, of course, regarded him a rank fraud, and denounced his diagnostic procedures as balderdash spiced with trickery. Myersbach could create this illusion of preternatural prophetic powers (enemies alleged) because his servants and porters were expert at striking up casual conversation with sufferers while they were waiting in the anterooms: patients would prattle on about the details of their condition, and that information would speedily be conveyed to Myersbach himself in time for the consultation. In the case of eminent clients, who made advance appointments, the delay would allow Myersbach's servants plenty of opportunity to gather information through discreet local enquiries.

To expose all this knavery, Myersbach's detractors sent along their friends as stool-pigeons, carrying with them flasks of cow's urine which they pretended belonged to their wives, and thus allowing him to dig his own grave by his absurd prognoses. One such expose of Myersbach's boloney appeared in the *Gazetteer* newspaper for 26 August 1776:

> Being thus introduced, I stepped forward and presented the sagacious Doctor with my vial, which contained no other than the urine of a young gelding. He looked at it with much seeming attention, and turning round, enquired whose water it was. Instead of giving him a direct answer to the question, I told him I came from my wife: this response, which by no means would have been deemed satisfactory to a cautious physician, well satisfied this water-doctor, who, very significantly shaking his head, and drawing up his shoulders, cried, with a kind of transport at his intuitive knowledge, Oh! I did think it was a Lady's water – it be no good – she be very bad – Upon which the following conversation and particulars ensued.
> *Patient*: What do you think is her complaint, Doctor?
> *Doctor*: It be, Sir, – it be a disorder in her womb – her womb – her – her womb be somewhat affected – she have a pain across her loins – she be very bad – I do see she be very bad.
> *Patient*: The water seems very clear, Doctor, doesn't it?
> *Doctor*: Ah! Ah! It look so to you: but I do see – I do see a slime upon the

kidneys she be very sick at the stomach – she have a pain in her head, and in her limbs. – Has she had many children?

Patient: Two, Doctor.

Doctor: Her pains in labour be very bad – be they not?

Patient: Why, Doctor, I think all women say labour-pains be very bad: I cannot speak from experience.

Doctor: No! No! No – your wife's temper be much affected by her disorder – it make her very peevish – very fretful – passionate – every little thing – (here he paused, and gazed once more on the gelding's urine, and turning round, cried) every little thing, I see, puts her in a passion – Does it not?

Patient: Why, Doctor, she is as most women are, not always in the best humour.

Doctor: Ah! Ah! There you do see – I did say so; she has had this complaint – yes, she has had this complaint these three years – I do perceive dat – and she always be coughing.

This last piece of presumption, in attempting to ascertain the precise time in which he supposed my wife to have been seized with these several chimerical disorders operated too powerfully on my passions to admit my remaining any longer the auditor of such ridiculous conjectures: and therefore requested him (in order to maintain the deception) to give me a prescription, which he did. I then gave him half a guinea; for which he returned me a most servile, unmeaning cringe, with a God Almighty, he grant I may do your wife good, namely, the gelding.[38]

Myersbach had a further diagnostic technique. He professed to gauge the site and type of disorder by allowing his hands to hover quivering over the patient's body, moving them around until, experiencing the right rapport, he would cry, in his broken English: 'It is here, it is here'. Doubtless, many patients were impressed by this 'magic'. But his opponents exposed it as just another trick. By running his hands fast enough over a sufficient expanse of the body, and by keeping up a non-stop patter interlarded with 'It is here, it is here', he would sooner or later get it right, befuddling the dazed client into believing that he'd hit upon the spot through arcane skills. Moreover, his diagnoses themselves were couched in a farrago of pseudo-technical jargon. Female patients would be told they had a 'disorder of the womb' – a diagnosis so vague as to have a fair chance of ringing true; and 'sick in the stomach', 'slime in the blood', or 'slime in the kidneys' were further favourite meaningless diagnoses.

Having made his diagnosis, Myersbach then wrote out a prescription to be made up by his own apothecary. When he embarked upon investigating the 'Urinarian', John Coakley Lettsom began to collect his prescriptions, to ascertain whether he was – as Lettsom suspected – poisoning his patients. Lettsom discovered that Myersbach's 'green drops', 'sweet mixture', 'silver pills', 'red powder', and so forth kept fairly close to the official pharmacopoeia, but were dispensed randomly and recklessly. Many of the preparations were innocuous anodynes (such as water in which toasted bread had been steeped), but others were potent and potentially harmful, some containing heavy concentrations of opium, and others solutions of sugar of lead (lead acetate); both temporarily quell internal pains, but compound intestinal disorders if taken repeatedly.

Indeed, it was through the effects of such drugs that Myersbach first attracted hostile attention. Having been permitted to practise for two or three years in peace, without interference from the Royal College of Physicians, Myersbach met with Lettsom's gaze when the latter found patients coming to him with iatrogenic disorders which, with a little detective work, he traced to the medicines prescribed by Myersbach. Always passionate in the cause of righteousness, Lettsom privately investigated Myersbach's activities, by taking testimony from his patients and planting friends as clients. He launched into print with a public denunciation entitled *Observations Preparatory to the Use of Dr Myersbach's Medicines, in which the Efficacy of Certain German Prescriptions… is Ascertained by Fact and by Experience*. This forty-two-page pamphlet appeared in two editions in 1776, the first anonymous (though it was an open secret that Lettsom was the author), the second acknowledged. Moreover, through much of 1776, Lettsom also sent volleys of letters and insertions to the London newspapers, in particular the *Gazetteer*, the *Morning Chronicle*, and the *Public Ledger*, exposing the quack. Lettsom's attack received support from other quarters. Two other pamphlets were published in the same year. One – *An Essay on the Inspection of the Urine, Shewing the Impossibility of Being Acquainted with the Diseases Incident to the Human Body, by the Inspection Only*, published under the heading 'By a physician' – was brief and content mainly to ridicule urine-casting as an almost worthless diagnostic test. The other – *The New Method of Curing Diseases by Inspecting the Urine Explained: as Practiced by the German Doctor. Intended for the Serious Perusal of Physicians, Surgeons, Apothecaries, and the Public in General* – was more substantial, exposing Myersbach for a fraud. The irony is that by using the authority of medicine to destroy the quack, Lettsom laid himself open to accusations of being an arch-defender of those very excrescences of oligarchy and monopoly which he himself, as a reformist physician, decried.

A wearisome war of words was waged in the press from 1776 into early 1777 – running to well over 100 items, most repetitive and vituperative. The substance of the case made by Lettsom and his allies was that Myersbach was an ignorant and incompetent fraud. Lettsom had some special trump cards up his sleeve, as when Myersbach's apothecary's assistant, Haussman, defected and testified to Lettsom that Myersbach was medically illiterate and a swindler. Lettsom spelt out at length, in his pamphlets and in the press, horror stories of patients whose health had been ruined by Myersbach's vile ministrations, for instance:

> JANE REILY. of St. Mary at Hill, applied to Dr. Myersbach, with a vial of urine, on the 21st of May 1776, and was told by him that she had a disorder in her womb. At that time she laboured under a dysentery, which induced her to ask him, if her purging arose from the disorder in the womb? The Doctor avoided answering this question, by saying, that he could soon cure her; and gave her the silver pills. In a fortnight afterwards, the patient again applied, and told the Doctor that the purging was augmented, and her strength and constitution were greatly impaired; he assured her, however, she was getting better: and added, that he now perceived by her urine, that there were little kemels in the womb which he would soon remove. He then gave her the green drops, the red powder, and the sweet drops: but after attending three

months, the kernels which Doctor Myersbach discovered in the womb were not removed, and her real disorder, which was a dysentery, continued, with additional violence, when I saw her on the 25th of September.[39]

Lettsom drew two main conclusions. On the one hand, such episodes proved the evils of medical 'empiricism'; indeed, 'the history of empiricism affords no parallel of deception so general as that which actuated the votaries of this impostor for upwards of two years'. Who could tell, he added, just how many patients had been 'murdered by empiricks'?[40] The only safeguard for the public was to put themselves solely in the hands of regulars, those who had been through an authorized education and training and who, expert in anatomy and the animal economy, could make rational diagnoses.

This was especially important on account of his second bête noire, the hopeless gullibility of the English people. 'It has been an observation', he informed readers of the *Gazetteer*, 'no less true than common, that the English are the greatest dupes of novelty and deception under the sun': however gross the charlatanry, 'no people will swallow the bait with less reluctance than the English', who were in medical matters a 'weak people', infected by 'national folly and credulity', and especially the disease of 'Urinomania'. Lettsom's supporters concurred. 'To explain this matter more clearly and satisfactorily', opened the author of *The New Method of Curing Disease*:

> to investigate the cause of such absolute folly and madness in the people, is not difficult. Let us recollect the South Sea scheme and bottle conjurer, Elizabeth Canning's story, the Cock-lane ghost, and the knavish trick of Le Fevre, the reputed Doctor, for curing the gout, and many other such like impositions; not to mention the two lotteries, for the disposal of house and trinkets, which received parliamentary sanction; and for which the fortunate holders of prizes of five hundred pounds were offered by the honest projectors about sixty. Here are indisputable proofs, that not only the illiterate caught the alluring baits of designing artists; but the polite and well educated had implicit faith in doubtful schemes, or the most improbable fables.[41]

Thus leading physicians told the public they were fools: but was this wise? Lettsom was, it seems, following three contradictory strategies all at once. First, he was arguing the supreme authority of the regular medical profession; second, by laying his case before the public, he was inviting them to judge and vindicate that authority; but, third, he was telling the public they had no judgement. The paradoxes in this position were, not surprisingly, exploited to the full both by Myersbach's defenders and, it seems, by neutral bystanders without an axe to grind.

What was it but obfuscation (claimed Myersbach's vindicators) to attack the urinarian for his lack of regular medical training and degrees? For that created a fetish of forms, turning possession of skills in dead tongues such as Latin and Greek into a form of medical hocus-pocus. Neatly reversing the standard anti-quack thrust (which denounced quacks for being all words and no skills), the author of *The Impostor Detected* declared the boot was on the other foot: it was 'tools of the faculty', such as Lettsom, who out of self-interest

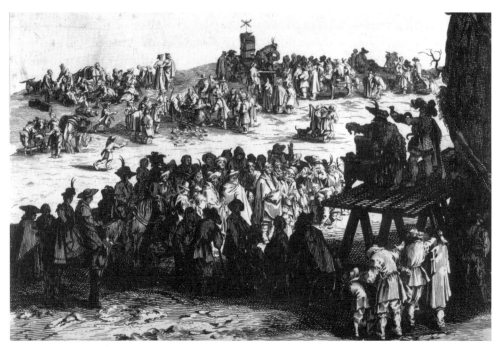

A popular medicine salesman sells his wares as part of a stage performance at the huge travelling fair knoen as the Fiera dell' Imprunetta. Etching by J. Callot.

were equating medical skills with magical words such as BA and MD. Myersbach's merit, the pamphleteer claimed, 'depends upon the knowledge of nature, and of things, and not of words;… To think otherwise, is to suppose every physician must be a magician; seeing medicines are incapable of healing, unless accompanied with the knowledge of the import of certain sounds, or the signification of words of certain languages, to which they have no relation, but what is given them by the arbitrary appointment of man.'[42]

Yet such recourse to the authority of arcane and exclusive knowledge was, of course, to be expected from physicians who made a fetish of their membership of closed societies such as the Royal Society and the College of Physicians, groups whose interest lay in setting the 'false dignity of the faculty', and 'low arts of a craft', and the 'private police of a corporation' above those real objects of true medicine, 'the life and health of the human species'. Thus (it was alleged) Lettsom was exposing his false colours, for 'the true dignity of the profession can never be supported by means that are irreconcileable with its true objects'.

Of course, medical mystagogy must be exposed, argued *The Impostor Detected*; but who was the true mystery-monger here? It was the Lettsomians who hid behind the facade of the faculty, with 'an affection of mystery in their writings, conversations, and whole demeanour; a shew of deep erudition and profound knowledge relating to their profession, discoverable to none but the adepts in the science, an air of absolute confidence in their own skill and abilities; and a deportment stately, solemn, and superlatively expressive of self-importance are among the arts they practice.' By such theatre, the faculty might thereby hope (argued the controversialist) to 'captivate the ignorant', but the great British public would not be taken in by this mummery.

Thus paper qualifications were, at best, a side-issue, at worst, yet another form of professional mystification. Medicine's acid test (argued Myersbach's camp) was: does it work? Which practitioners have the best track record? In other words, empiricism, far from being a threat to medical standards, was, in reality, their upholder. Elite physicians had wrapped and trapped themselves in systems and hypotheses, but these had proved hindrances to healing: 'The greatest obstacle to the improvement of the medical art, has been an inattention to its principal end and design, which is the convenience and happiness of life; to preserve health, to prolong life, and to cure diseases. But this most valuable object has been sacrificed to vanity and ostentation, and the acquisition of a fortune by craft, artifice, and mean adulation

Facts must take priority over theories, and the true empiric was the practitioner putting his trust not in systems but in that crucial tool of the advancement of learning – the experiment. For 'an attachment to novelty, however, is productive of some good, to systems and hypotheses none; the first from experiments communicates some real truths to the stock; the latter, are unproductive of any real knowledge.'

Thus the question the public must ask (argued Myersbach's defenders) was this: on whose side were the facts? Lettsom published his own case studies of patients sent to the grave by the urinarian's treatments. Myersbach's minions defended him in the same coin: 'to support that Dr. Myersbach is infallible would be to run into the contrary extreme and render one as deservedly ridiculous as Dr. Lettsom. His knowledge, as a physician (in the technical sense of the word) may be as slender as some of his enemies; but from many of the cases following, it is undeniably certain, that he has cured many which the faculty could not cure, and to deny it is to belye and affront the common sense of mankind. Here then is clear irrefragable proof that he has (in some cases at least) more skill, or nostrums, of greater medicinal virtues than they have any knowledge of.'

And if the issue was thus a matter of facts, and the public thus a competent judge, then Myersbach could present armfuls of testimonials from satisfied customers to match Lettsom's disaster stories. *The Impostor Detected* staged a parade of happy dients and their cases: 'A list of persons who have received benefit from Dr. MAYERBACH's [sic] advice and medicines, either in their own persons, families, or friends. The particular case referred to is denoted by the figure following the name. JOHN Willan, Esq; Mary-le Bon, Case 1. Thomas Limbery Sclater, Esq; Tangier Park, Hants, 2. Robert Johnson, Esq; Bath. Mr. Pybus, Banker, in New Bond Street. Mr. Parker, Glass manufacturer, Fleet Street, 5. Mr. Stephenson, Goldsmith, Ludgate Hill, 11. Mr. Wolfe, his acquaintance. Mr. Chinnery, Writing Master, Gough Square. [etc.]' And not only did the pamphleteer chronicle these and eleven other cases, but some of these patients then also wrote (presumably of their own volition) to the newspapers testifying to Myersbach's skill and integrity, as witness this letter from John Willan in the *Gazetteer*:

For the GAZETTEER
To Dr. COAKLEY LETTSOM.
WHEN I first entered upon a vindication of Dr. Mayersbach's character, which I saw wantonly and grossly attacked, by the pen of self-interested ill nature, I

had not the most distant thought of a personal altercation with you; but the shameful abuse, and glaring untruths you daily advance against the object of your envy, call aloud for the pen of truth to stand forth in the vindication of injured innocence. Where Dr. Mayersbach acquired his knowledge I will not pretend to determine; I have however the greatest right to say that he knows more than many of the most skilful of the faculty for he saved my life when they could not; and I might justly be thought the most ungrateful of wretches, if I should refuse to declare to the world that I owe my being entirely to his judgement as a physician; as a man I see him traduced, vilified and belied: excuse the expression, you call for it and you have it. I every day read the most glaring hlsehoods attested by your name: I therefore have a right to call you by the worst appellation which the promoter of untruths deserves. Your asserting, that Dr. Mayersbach made use of the preparation of lead in his prescriptions, is publicly confuted by the affidavits of the Doctor and Mr. Koch, before the Lord Mayor, which were inserted in the Gazetteer of Monday last. In the same paper you advance the most impudent and barefaced falsehood I ever met with. You there assure the public, that 'Lady H. sent a message last Tuesday to the Urinarian, desiring him never more to enter into her Ladyship's house.' Now I assure the public and pledge myself for the truth of what I say, that it is a palpable and direct falsehood, which I have it in my power to prove in one moment, to any one who has credulity enough to put the least confidence in Dr. Lettsom's infamous assertions, and chuse to have those erroneous opinions removed by self-evident convictions. A pamphlet which makes its appearance this day, will, I doubt not, afford the world sufficient proof of Dr Mayerbach's knowledge as a physician, and of the shameful intention of the prostituted pen of Dr. Lettsom. Mary le-bone, Oct. 17. JOHN WILLAN.[43]

Both Lettsom and Myersbach thus presented themselves as champions of the public good. But which was a reader of the public press to credit? With hindsight, we can feel pretty sure that Myersbach was a cheat, and no one doubts that Lettsom was a physician of the highest probity. But would a reader have discerned this? Lettsom hardly got the better of the argument. For one thing (as was pointed out in the *Gazetteer*), the whole controversy afforded Myersbach masses of free publicity: 'Doctor L. and the whole College may write against him, they'll only expand his fame, together with their own ignorance.' For another, Lettsom's own motives and conduct were questioned. If he really had the public interest at heart, why didn't he activate the College of Physicians' machinery for examining unlicensed practitioners? Such would have ensured public justice rather than a witch-hunt, and, had Myersbach been found guilty, his punishment would have afforded real protection to the public. Wasn't Lettsom's newspaper campaign, then, essentially an uncandid piece of self-advertisement and *ad hominem* vilification? As 'Amicus' put it in the *Gazetteer*:

To Dr. LETSOM.
In perusing the daily papers I have often observed the animadversions on

Myersbach's practice and impositions on the public; and without being an advocate for this outlandish water-conjurer, to give him no harder epithet, I would just hint, that if he is in truth deserving public censure, (which he very probably may be) would it not be more effectual; and withal be more convincing to the world, that Dr. Letsom possesses a pure generosity, and liberality of sentiments, if he were to bring a fair open accusation for malpractice before the Censors of the Colleg of Physicians, who solely, in their judicial capacity (when an accusation is brought before them, and not before) are by law appointed the competent judges of the practice of physic in London and seven miles around, with full power to fine, imprison, and coerce all detected unwarrantable practice, than to let the Gazetteer be the weekly channel of vague accusations against this (as Dr. Lettsom terms him) water-caster. This would be a convincing proof that Dr. Letsom was not aiming to build up his own fame upon the ruins of a more favoured opponent, but that the public welfare and safety were his aim and greatest ambition.[44]

Above all, the controversy brought to light the core contradiction in Lettsom's argument. If he chose to make a public appeal, the public had a right to decide for themselves; and here authority must make way for fact. As 'London Spy' put it: 'Will Doctor L. and his colleagues have the effrontery to attempt to disprove matters of fact by argument, and to insist the old gentleman who was thus surprisingly restored to health and seeming rejuvenescency, had, in fact, received no benefit at all, but was imposed upon by a 'plausible tale, and an application they call suitable,' which is destitute of all sense and meaning?' Or as another correspondent, presenting himself as a bewildered, disinterested bystander – summed up the dilemma:

> To the PRINTER of the GAZETTEER
> I have perused two late publications, the one by Dr. Lettsom, and the other is an answer to it. Dr. Lettsom asserts, and quotes the opinion of Dr. Heberden and others, that it is exceedingly difficult to judge diseases, by urine… He next states, though mostly in initials, several cases were Dr. Mayersbach gave a very erroneous account of disorders, and therefore insists on it that Dr. Mayersbach is ignorant of what he pretends. As I intend impartially to survey these publications, I shall take it for granted what he has asserted, and the cases he has stated to be strictly true. Dr. Lettsom's antagonist, to controvert the above, has published cases authenticated by the person's own names, that Dr. Mayersbach in their several disorders judged perfectly right by urine, though different from what the opinion of their former physicians had been. If I admit what Dr. Lettsom says to be true, must not I do the same here? What then is an impartial man to conclude? Facts are superior to opinion. Those well-authenticated cases clearly prove Dr. Mayersbach's skills in finding out disorders by urine, and Dr. Lettsom's, that in those cases he was mistaken; errare humanum est; saying himself a great part of this city crouded to have Dr. Mayersbach's advice, can it be

otherwise but what he must be sometimes out? Do not then Dr. Lettsom's own assertions prove Dr. Mayersbach a regular-bred physician, a great anatomist, and a very skilful man?

All mankind take medicines against inclination; pay physicians fees and apothecaries bills with reluctance. Whatever stress Dr. Lettsom lays upon the effect of tales once propagated, was not Dr. Mayersbach obliged to deceive every patient separately? He therefore must be of opinion that, contrary to their inclinations, Dr. Mayersbach had that art to deceive a great part of one of the greatest cities of the world. If my first conclusion be wrong, this must be right. Haussman's evidence is inadmissible: revenge occasions duels, and often murder.
Oct. 30, 1776 J.S.[45]

The paper war raged unabated for several months, ending, it seems, only when the editor of the *Gazetteer* declined to print any further contributions by Myersbach's leading defender (the 'London Spy') on account of his anonymity. This decision wears a certain arbitrary appearance – after all, many other insertions had been anonymous or pseudonymous, and for a long time Lettsom himself had used the pseudonym 'Cassius'. The author of *The Impostor Detected* hinted that behind-the-scenes pressure had been put on the editor by Lettsom's cronies.

But the controversy didn't end before it had escaped from the hands of the initial antagonists. For a kind of secondary debate sprang up, in which both parties fell under the lash of those deploring how the whole debate was bringing medicine into disrepute. Thus the *Public Ledger* for 30 September 1776 ran a long poem by 'Galen', whose burden was 'I think ye both quacks'. It consisted of a wrangle between Myersbach and Lettsom, the last section of which ran:

Dr. L. and Dr. M. talking confusedly together,

Pray, who are my betters?
 Why I am – yes, I Sir,
You mistake in good French, but in English you lie, Sir,
I appeal to this friend, I submit to another
Why thou Talk'est like a fool, neither one thing nor t'other.
I will and I won't, and you can't and you dare not.
Either this Judge or that Judge, by heav'n I care not:
He'll pronounce thee an ass, my good friend, never fear it,
If he proves you a fool, I'll be happy to hear it.

Friend says,
Gentlemen,
At a club once established,
for drinking and dining,
Two amazing great wits
were determined on shining

They contended,
who most like a blackguard could quarrel,
Who scolded the best
was to bear off the laurel.

They curs'd and talk'd
bawdry,
and shouted and thunder'd
And so equal their parts,
the spectators all wonder'd.

And the umpire himself,
who was fix'd on to hear'em.
Vow'd no Billingsgate whores,
Sirs, could ever come near'em.

With one it was art,
with the other 'twas nature,
But that both were such blackguards,
he never saw greater.

Now permit me to say,
that it's hard to determine
In a case that concerns,
Sirs, such physical vermin:

But I think ye both quacks,
who prescribe in the dark,
Sirs, By trusting to p--s p-----s,
and opium, and bark, Sirs.

GALEN[46]

'Galen' was then answered by 'Hippocrates' in the *Morning Chronicle* (9 October 1776), who, in a rather similar way, suggested that Lettsom and Myersbach were 'two chips of one log', like Tweedledum and Tweedledee.

What is particularly remarkable is that even Lettsom's colleagues seem to have recognized that his attacks were damaging both the case against Myersbach and the standing of regular medicine. The dignified Dr John Fothergill, who had earlier lent his support to Lettsom, even went so far as to publish an anonymous letter early in 1777, whose gist was 'a plague on both your houses'. In the context of the national war against the rebel American colonies, the mud-slinging must stop:

To the PRINTER of the GAZETTEER
At a time when the fate of this great empire is depending, and a contest of

such a magnitude as the world never saw is undecided,… It shocks me to think that a nation can be interesting itself about trifles, while their all is at stake, and that either public diversions or private quarrels, should fill up, as they do, the channels of public information. Let the two lawyers contend in Westminster-hall as long as they please. Let Mayersbach endeavour, like the scuttlefish, to hide himself in ink, and raise an army of credulous hypochondriacs in his defence; but do not let the public be pestered with such uninteresting combats. If Mayersbach has any thing to say against Dr. Lettsom let them fight in Warwick-lane.[47]

How should this affair be viewed? In the short run, it proved a victory for Lettsom, for under the glare of publicity, Myersbach upped stumps and returned to Germany. Nevertheless, he was soon back, and as Lettsom admitted, some thirty years later, he was: 'as much followed as previously to his emigration. The physician [Lettsom] who had taken so active a part against the enterprise was dissatisfied with the conduct of the College; he was likewise insulted by a numerous herd of anonymous writers in the public prints; and having become an object of their envy, he avoided further interference.'

Moreover, later in his career, Lettsom was to rediscover that vituperation in the public press was a doubtful technique for hounding quacks. In 1804, he launched a series of anti-quack exposés in the *Medical and Physical Journal*. The third of these pilloried Myersbach, by then dead. The fifth hurled a stream of abuse against the empiric Dr William Brodum, author (as discussed in chapter 6) of *A Guide to Old Age or a Cure for the Indiscretions of Youth*, and vendor of a Nervous Cordial. Lettsom dubbed Brodum an itinerant orange-seller, a renegade Jew, a footman, and a mountebank, and alleged that he had tricked Marischal College, Aberdeen, into giving him his MD. Brodum sued the *Journal*, and the upshot of much backstairs legal negotiations was that Lettsom was forced to issue a public recantation – which effectively served as a puff for Brodum and his Nervous Cordial – and to pay costs.

This spectacular war of words tells much of the shifting status of regular and quack medicine in the Georgian age. In the 1770s, the state and law were supine in the face of quackery; the Royal College of Physicians did nothing. Hence, a hammer of quacks like Lettsom had to appeal to the public through the pages of the press. But how could Lettsom simultaneously invoke professional authority while appealing to the public as judge and jury? The paradox was insoluble: if the public was to be invited to pass judgement on Myersbach, Lettsom's own credentials would also come under public scrutiny.

Moreover, if the public could be in a position to judge, it would judge by results, and so some form of empiricism must necessarily be ratified. The open world of late-Georgian medicine was not yet a comfortable place for the regulars in their attempts to crack down on quacks and assert professional authority.

8   Profession, fringe and quackery

The eighteenth century – that time when Hogarth could feature the 'Chevalier' Taylor, Sally Mapp, and 'Spot' Ward as a trio in an engraving entitled 'The Company of Undertakers' – has been widely judged by historians as the 'golden age of quackery'. It was, however, perhaps during the early decades of the nineteenth century that the cry that quackery was destroying the very vitals of the nation rose to a crescendo. We should, however, be cautious before accepting such wails of public-spirited anguish at face value. For they emanated from the medical profession, and were blows in tactical professional infighting; they perhaps tell us more about the politicization of medicine than of the fortunes of quackery itself.

From the late eighteenth century, ordinary regular practitioners – provincial apothecaries and small-town surgeons – began mounting an agitation for the reform of medicine, claiming such a move was urgent for the good both of the public and of the practitioners themselves. The sick were not receiving adequate medical care – too many went without proper medicine at all, or they received shabby treatment: the public had a right to demand that the profession should heal itself.

And indeed, as critics from within admitted, the profession itself was in bad shape, sapped from below by swarms of sharp operators – untrained druggists, irregulars, and itinerants, all making their pile – and rendered top-heavy by an oligarchy of elite physicians and surgeons, wielding power and making fortunes out of all proportion to their deserts. These twin evils were but two sides of the same coin. Reformers believed a new deal for ordinary general practitioners must be common cause with the crusade on behalf of the nation's health. They pledged to fight all these dragons, which they collectively labelled quackery.

The campaign to purge the Augean stables of quackery was spear-headed from the 1820s by the radical, Thomas Wakley, through his journal, the *Lancet*. A surgeon by training, and a vocal coroner, Wakley was no mincer of words or respecter of reputations: the Society of Apothecaries appeared in his pages as the 'Old Ladies' or 'Hags' of 'Rhubarb Hall'; the Corporation of Surgeons were the 'Bats'; and the College of Physicians was judged to be no less 'vile' than the Society of Apothecaries. Wakley vowed to rid the profession and the nation of the 'satanic system of quackery'. In his office of coroner, he particularly publicized inquests upon those who had died after taking proprietary medicines ('the cause of death to hundreds of their fellow creatures') – using such tragic victims as the excuse for a two-pronged campaign for the public suppression of quackery and the institution of a statutory medical coronership.

Wakley had no patience with quackery in the sense of profit-oriented commercial practice performed by the medically unqualified. The *Lancet* attacked this on a broad front. In its early years, it ran features revealing the ingredients of nostrums: Spilsbury's Antiscorbutic Drops, it was shown, were essentially antimony, Dalby's Carminative chiefly opium, Daffy's Elixir a composition of senna, Speediman's Pills were little other than aloes, and so forth; at best, the claims made for such drugs were wildly excessive. Public-spirited readers echoed Wakley's attempt to debunk quack nostrums. Thus a certain Edward Melville wrote to the editor (praised as 'always... the avowed enemy of every kind of empiricism'), demonstrating that a certain 'Specific Extract', sold as 'an infallible remedy for gonorrhoea', was compounded mainly of copaiba and opium, and hence utterly worthless.

Wakley also encouraged provincial readers to denounce egregious operators in their localities: they leapt at the opportunity. 'A surgeon apothecary' wrote from Newcastle eager to expose 'quackery in Northumberland', where its evils were predictably increasing, the worst of these 'illiterate fungi' being rural bone-setters, who practised to the 'injury of the regulars and the public'.[1] Another correspondent warned of the ignorance of Halifax quacks, especially a certain soidisant 'Dr Smith', who practised, like so many, under the pretence of being regularly qualified. This author typically laid the blame squarely on the shoulders of public benightedness – 'ignorance is the root of the evil' – contending that 'until people are more enlightened, and education is more general, legal measures to put down the evils and abuses,... are comparatively inefficacious'.[2]

Another reporter regaled readers with lurid details of the lethal infamies of 'Baron Spolasco', who operated around Swansea; and a certain Wiltshire worm empiric, the self-styled 'Doctor Reynolds Fowler', provided a focus of outrage the following year. Fowler, 'a strapping man with huge whiskers', kept a shop which served 'as his advertising sheet', but made most of his income in the itinerant way, advertising in the local newspapers. No sooner did he set up his pitch in the various local market-squares, but 'scores of his credulous followers disposed of their cash, if not their worms, in most copious streams'. The correspondent contributed to the by now familiar victim-blaming: the worm-doctor's customers were captivated by the 'sesquipedalia verba' and other 'clap trap' of this 'bastard doctor', being no less 'infatuated' than the devotees of 'Mad Thom' of Canterbury – the religious visionary who had recently led a desperate labourers' revolt in Kent.[3]

All such offenders were, however, small fry, and the *Lancet* did not shirk its duty of anathematizing the more notorious irregulars of the day. John St John Long, who practised from 41 Harley Street and claimed to cure consumption by the use of caustic blisters, was especially excoriated, both by Wakley and by his subalterns. 'Your Constant Reader MD' wrote from Plymouth in 1828 to share in the condemnation of Long, 'as you profess to expose quackery in all its forms'. Long was a bounder: in all his extravagant claims for his powers and cures he never mentioned failures, but exploited social snobbery to the hilt by constantly deferring to the 'authority of Lord this and Sir George that'. It was the last straw that he had been permitted space to put his case in the *Literary Gazette*.[4]

Wakley broadcast the efforts of doctors up and down the country to mobilize anti-quack opinion. He gave considerable footage to speeches and resolutions passed by various branches of the Provincial Medical and Surgical Association, the general practitioners' ginger group that became the British Medical Association. At one Shropshire meeting, a certain Dr Cowan, after denouncing the evils of 'medical empiricism', proceeded to advocate the desirability of 'suppressing it'. This brought to a head one of the most acute dilemmas reformers faced.

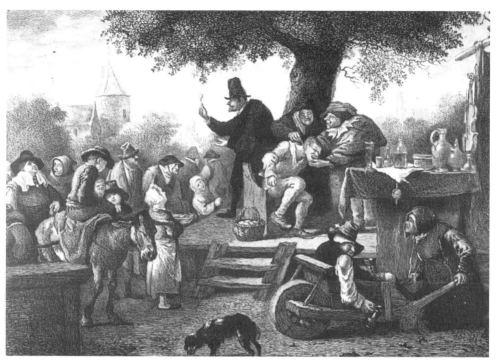

A rural scene with a tooth-drawer proudly displaying a tooth he has pulled on stage while his two companions treat a sick man. Etching after J. Steen (?).

Cowan outlined the options. Some doctors thought quackery such an egregious evil – a moral crime – that they petitioned Parliament to outlaw unqualified practice. Indeed, his own Society was pledged to 'suppressing quackery and protecting legally-qualified practitioners'. Others, however, doubted the wisdom of a coercion that must prove utterly unenforceable, counter-arguing that quackery would eventually wither away of its own accord, rather like witchcraft, as part of the march of mind. Cowan, however, had his doubts about vesting such hope in public enlightenment. For did not the masses 'evince a disposition to believe the most marvellous statements' – indeed, was not 'this credulity… a defect peculiar to human nature itself'? It was vain to expect quackery's quietus to come from the populace, for 'the mass of every nation will be found an easy prey to medical charlatanry'.[5] After all, had not the spread of literacy already increased the practice of dabbling in domestic medicine, an evil which arose from ideas culled from do-it-yourself health books?

Cowan's scepticism as to the possibility of improvement coming from the people was rounded off with a familiar onslaught against the corrupt corporations. Quackery would never be defeated so long as the 'culpable indifference of the chartered bodies' continued. The solution lay in a stronger, more united, better-qualified medical profession, whose shining virtue, expertise, and integrity would show quackery in its true colours. Cowan could already detect some traces of this millennium; for example, because more regulars were now prepared to operate on eyes, quack eye-surgeons were on the wane.

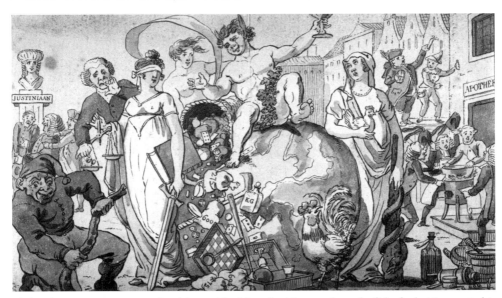

A drunken satyr cavorts atop the globe; to his right, physicians and quacks fight for legitimacy; to his left, the scales held by a blindfolded Justice are tipped by a lawyer's money. The picture is an allegory of the world of justice and health overturned into one of chance and greed. Colour etching after J. Smies, c.1800.

During the 1830s, Wakley mobilized a campaign – doubtless it helped sell his journal – to set up 'an ANTI-MEDICAL QUACKERY SOCIETY', whose prime task would be to educate the public, and, through petitioning Parliament, to work for the 'total suppression of the sale of stamped, patent, and secret medicines'. Wakley's tone was visionary, even at times messianic. 'The quacks, regular and irregular', were trembling, Wakley intimated.[6] The days were numbered for nostrums such as Morison's Vegetable Pills and no less Macleod's Bread Pills (which contained nothing but bread) vended by one of the physicians at London's St George's Hospital. Yet Wakley never wavered in his core message. The nation's love of dabbling in quackery would not cease until the medical profession revitalized itself. But that could not happen until quackery in high places within the profession was eliminated. And so 'a vigorous attack must be made at the commencement, in the ranks of the regulars' – for there was corruption in 'our Colleges and Companies', and medicine had languished too long amidst a 'frightful system of quackery which has been invented and sanctioned by our medical colleges'. Oligarchy, corruption, and nepotism all needed a drastic purge.[7]

The debate was joined by a certain 'H. H.', who insisted that he detested quackery as fiercely as any man, and was second to none in his zeal to 'promote the public welfare'. Yet the political goal of outlawing quackery was ill-conceived, because no consensus existed as to what manner of beast it was or how to demarcate it: 'if you cannot pretend to define where quackery begins, or where it ends, how is it possible for an Anti-Quackery Society to do any good?' Was it then surprising that 'all attempts hitherto made by the legislature to suppress or punish quackery have completely failed'? One

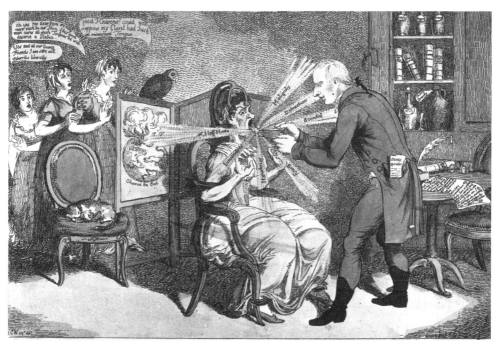

A satirical cartoon suggesting that Dr Perkins's magnetic tractors might be put to good use curing Ann Ford, a society lady, of her venomous tongue. Coloured etching by C. Williams, 1802.

could strive to discredit the quacks. Yet to achieve even this would require a revolution in attitudes both in the legislature and in public opinion at large. For 'the educated and highest class of persons in this country are decidedly the greatest patrons of quackery, and therefore it is that our College never dare to attempt to prosecute the regular Charlatan.' Consider, H. H. suggested, what the court would 'have said had we sent to prison the German Homoeopathist who was giving the millionth part of a grain of some indescribable compound to our most gracious Queen Adelaide?' The sanctions of the law were a sideshow; rather Parliament ought to promote a well-trained, respectable medical profession, and the 'public at large must be left at full liberty to judge for themselves, and place full confidence in whom they please'. Was 'H. H.' simply pouring a bucket of much-needed realism over the frenzied Wakley? Or did he have fish of his own to fry?[8]

The pages of the *Lancet* thus rang with denunciations of quackery – a 'hydra', a 'pest', a 'nefarious trade', a 'heartless and dangerous piece of deception'. 'If medical empiricism could be grasped and exhibited in all its plenitude of craft and villainy', thundered Henry Savage, 'the scales would fall from the eyes of the public, now so deluded and quack-ridden; with one voice its suppression would be demanded and the monstrous abomination would cease to exist.' There was no doubt about the doctors' duty: 'the duty of thus guarding the public against quackery is incumbent on every individual member of the medical profession'.[9] And yet – the perennial problem – the profession itself seemed the worst culprit. Despite the fact that quackery 'is diametrically opposed to the interests of medical science', most doctors nevertheless 'regard the subject with apathetic indifference'.

Not least, this was because top practitioners were up to the chin in quackish practices themselves. For instance, a *Lancet* correspondent pointed out that no less a luminary than Bransby Cooper, surgeon to Guy's Hospital, together with his colleague, Mr Green, had endorsed in the Globe a patent medicine marketed by one Franks – the advertisement was nothing other than 'illiterate trash'. Thus, concluded the irate correspondent, Green and Cooper 'give their names to the promulgation of a libel on the profession which they are sworn to uphold, and thereby become parties in the exhibition of a nostrum-vendor and heralds to the achievements of a quack'. And yet the London colleges did not lift a finger to discipline 'those who indubitably violate their oath'.[10] Not long later, the doyen of the early-Victorian obstetricians, Charles Locock, was the centre of a similar scandal, when protests were received that a patent medicine was being marketed in his name. He rather evasively responded that the name being used was in fact his father's, while side-stepping requests that he should publicly dissociate himself from the product.

In its occasional lighter moments, the *Lancet* allowed itself to reflect upon this Jonathan Wild world, in which the guardians of physic turned out to be but piddling quacks writ large. A song, entitled, 'Sound Chirurgical Knowledge', hammered home the point with devastating frankness:

> Away with all your stethoscopes, your stomach-pumps and tractors;
> Away ye little mountebanks, make room for greater actors!
> Here comes Sir Astley Cooper, Bart, Bill Buzzard, and Old Luddy,
> With bellies big, and purses deep, and brains cold, soft and muddy,
> With seven other learned pigs from London's Royal College,
> Who come to tell us when and where to purchase good 'sound knowledge';
> To show how learning, like the itch, prefers a northern station,
> And how thermometers become fit tests of education.
> 'Sound knowledge' says these cunning quacks, dwells only, on permission,
> With those to whom we grant a right to sell it by commission.[11]

It was thus a world of small-fry quacks and greater sharks, or 'cunning quacks'. Small wonder the *Lancet* was moved to insist in 1836, 'never have quacks, quackish doctrines, and quack medicines, exercised a greater influence over the minds and bodies of the people of this country, than they exert at the present epoch' – indeed, its 'fatality' was 'not exceeded by the cholera'. Wakley diagnosed the disease: 'The source of the existing evil is to be found in the odious, the exclusive conduct of our rotten and contemptible medical corporations'. The public saw their bloated, decaying carcasses: it was thus 'scarcely surprising' that they resorted to quacks.[12]

Quackery was undoubtedly flourishing at the accession of Queen Victoria – in every sense including the rather opportunistic blanket meaning commandeered by the *Lancet*. This state of affairs continued throughout her reign. Victorian chemists' and druggists' shops were crammed with a profusion of proprietary pills, powders, and potions. Street and station advertising hoardings, magazines, and newspapers blazoned the virtues of

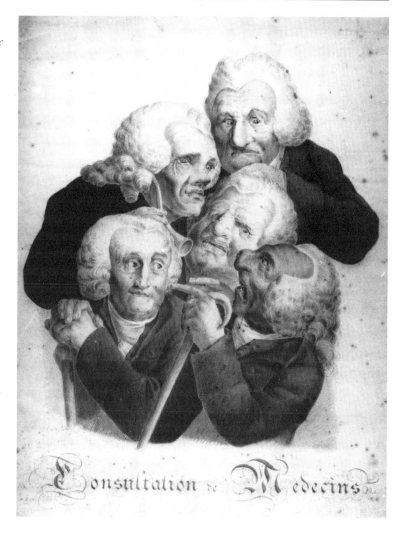

A nineteenth-century caricature of doctors in consultation. Coloured lithograph after L. Boilly, c.1823.

commercial medicines. With the help of new pill-rolling machines and other mass-production technology, James Morison, Thomas Holloway, and Thomas Beecham – they would have featured in the mid-Victorian remake of 'The Company of Undertakers' – were to market medicines throughout the globe on a scale that would have made 'Spot' Ward gape. At the beginning of the present century, the British Medical Association published two entire volumes, *Secret Remedies, what they cost and what they contain*, and its sequel, *More Secret Remedies*, exposing the worthlessness of well over three hundred popular proprietary medicines, from Absorbit Reducing Paste (a slimming preparation) to Zox (socks headache fast), and including such family favourites as Beecham's Pills and Owbridge's Lung Tonic.

No one has yet researched the business history of the many thousands of small-time irregular healers and medicine manufacturers operating in Victorian England; generalizations are thus premature and hazardous. Nevertheless, it appears well established that, though quackery continued to thrive, there were also important ways in which it also suffered eclipse. The remainder of this chapter will examine this gradual and partial edipse.

The fringe

Of all the quacks unmasked by Wakley in the *Lancet*, he hated none like James Morison. 'Murder by Morison's pills' was Wakley's lurid line in 1836, after a coroner's inquest had found that the deceased had been taking that particular nostrum. The *Lancet* teemed with condemnation of the arch-quack's 'life-destroying career', expressing horror at the public's endorsement of his claims, which could only be described as a 'hallucination of the human mind'. Wakley loathed Morison for being the most successful of his tribe – his 'poison is swallowed by bushels'. Mimicking the heads of the medical colleges, he swanked by being driven round in a carriage with a coronet on top and livery servants flanking. 'Nearly every country paper contains columns of advertisements, all puffing the wondrous efficacy of the 'Universal Pills' – and worse still, Morison's publicity was full of testimonials from certificated members of the medical profession. So successful was Morison that he even forced out of Wakley a rare compliment. Advocating his national Anti-Quackery Society, Wakley at one point argued that such an association could surely succeed, precisely because the 'King of the Quacks' had already organized a similar society – for selling his own products, of course – with spectacular success.

What was so special about Morison? James Morison was a businessman who had suffered ill health, tried any number of regular doctors and their remedies, without any benefit, and had despaired of physic. That was a familiar enough story: how many others had undergone precisely the same experience? Morison's response, however, made him different. For he came to despise the regular medical profession with a positively evangelical fervour, which provided him with the starting point for the total revolution in medicine he proclaimed. One of his publications has on the title-page the characteristic slogan, 'The old medical science is completely wrong'. (One wonders whether Wakley detested Morison in part because he had stolen his thunder, making Wakley's onslaught on the medical oligarchy look like a mere pinprick.)

Doctors were simply useless – Morison's own medical history proved that. They knew nothing about the true principles of health and disease. They tried to conceal their ignorance behind a fancy jargon larded with obscurities and neologisms, designed to dazzle the laity. It was time the parasitic restrictive practices of the faculty were exploded, once and for all. But doctors were not merely ignorant and mercenary: they were dangerous. Their polypharmacy and habits of heavy dosing (therein lay their profits), and, above all, their reckless indulgence in prescribing poisonous medicines – heavy metals and artificial chemicals – were little less than criminal.

So far, there was nothing especially original in Morison's battery. As we have seen, this was the standard language of mutual vilification between regulars and quacks down the ages: it even echoed Wakley in some respects. It was his positive prescriptions that made Morison novel. Drawing upon his understanding of his own recovery, Morison proposed a new set of institutes for medicine. Ten simple commandments encapsulated all there was to know about health and disease. The new decalogue contended:

1. The vital principle is contained in the blood.
2. Blood makes blood.
3. Everything in the body is derived from the blood.
4. All constitutions are radically the same.
5. All diseases arise from the impurity of the blood, or in other words, from acrimonious humours lodged in the body.
6. This humour which degenerates the blood has three sources, the maternine, the contagious and the personal.
7. Pain and disease have the same origin; and may therefore be considered synonymous terms.
8. Purgation by vegetables is the only effectual mode of eradicating disease.
9. The stomach and bowels cannot be purged too much.
10. From the intimate connection subsisting between the mind and the body, the health of the one must conduce to the serenity of the other.

In a nutshell, there was a single cause for all disease – bad blood – and a single therapy: heavy and frequent purgation, using vegetable laxatives. Morison produced the perfect purge, his Vegetable Universal pills. Available in two strengths (no. 1 and no. 2), these contained only natural products – aloes, jalap, colocynth, gamboge, cream of tartar, rhubarb, and myrrh. They would cure all diseases (not least, Morison insisted, cholera), and, if need be, could be taken in heroic quantities – up to thirty pills a day.

Morison was a quack of the old school, insofar as he made his living by marketing a nostrum. But he was also creating a new mould in a number of ways, each of which became indicative of future medical developments. More insistently, consistently, and persistently than earlier quacks, he taught the public to beware doctors, and to do so, not merely on pragmatic grounds, but on principle or as a point of faith. Professions were ramps, and the medical profession a racket for the expropriation of health. He taught that, though mystified by the medical profession, health care was simple. He repudiated orthodox physiology and disease theory, enunciating a radical alternative. He dinned into the public mind the inextricable association between his heterodox philosophy of health and his own nostrum. Previous nostrum-mongers had done little more than persuade the sick to buy their medicines, touted as secret panaceas. Morison wanted the public to take his pills because they believed in his philosophy. He wooed his age with a simple, attractive vision of healthy living that all consumers could understand.

Not least, Morison became a medical missionary, proselytizing his opinions. He was the first quack to exploit the nineteenth-century passion for organizations and institutions, establishing the so-called 'British College of Health'. Terming himself 'the Hygeist' – and through that name dissociating himself from the common quack practice of assuming the mantle of a doctor – he made the further innovation of publishing a magazine, the *Hygeian Journal*, and bombarding the public with any number of books and pamphlets besides. Unlike any Georgian quack, Morison attempted – and with enormous success – to turn the selling of health into a cause and a crusade.

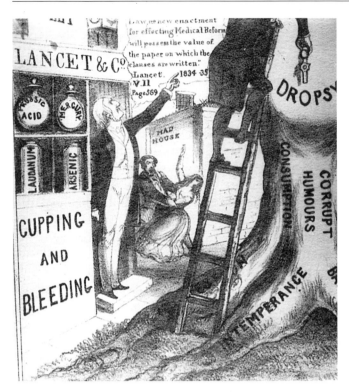

Two trees being cultivated by doctors. The top print shows the traditional (what Morison called the 'organic' method) as dictated by the reguoler medical profession embodied in the Lancet. The quoted comment about legal reform echoes the views of 'H.H.' (see pp.195-196). Below is shown the strength of a tree tended to with Morison's 'hygeist' method and framing his British College of Health.

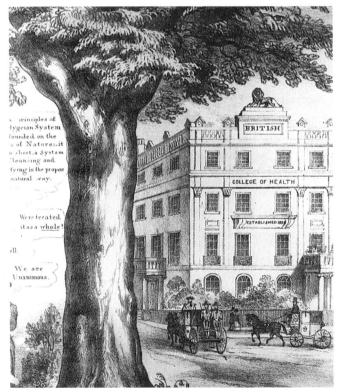

Zealot or fraud, Morison certainly was a businessman. He wanted converts to his creed, but he also craved customers for his pills. And, in turn, he paved the way for generations of health ideologues, men perhaps more genuinely idealistic, or at least less profit-oriented than himself, yet prepared to build upon his innovations in organization and on similar ideas of lay self-sufficiency and anti-professional animus. Of these new medical movements, gaining momentum particularly from the late 1830s and 1840s, there is no need to rehearse the details at length here, for they have been admirably investigated by Pickstone, Harrison, Barrow, Nicholls, Cooter, Brown, and others.

The early-Victorian age saw the flowering of a variety of medical movements: homoeopathy, naturopathy, hydropathy, medical botany (often called 'Thomsonian' medicine after Samuel Thomson, a leading American herbalist, or 'Coffinism' after Isaiah Coffin, one of his followers, active in England), phrenology, mesmerism (and its hybrid form, phreno-mesmerism), spiritualism, and so forth. Sometimes, these merged and married; sometimes, there were splinter movements; often, advocates were tinged with other philosophies, such as Behmenism, Swedenborgianism, or spiritualism. Comparably to Morison, all made their epistemological break with regular, allopathic medicine and dissociated themselves from the medical profession. Each argued in its own language that the entire system of regular medicine was radically wrong. Characteristically, they accused the orthodox of erroneously striving to destroy disease with poisonous drugs. Each of these movements proclaimed itself to be in possession of a more subtle understanding of the true nature of disease as an integral part of the active processes of Nature. Each offered a new plan of life based upon Nature's way and claimed to use more natural modes of healing – drawing upon herbs alone, or pure water, or (as with homoeopathy) infinitesimal quantities of the purest drugs. A common 'physical puritanism' set great store by temperance, moderation, and self-control.

All such movements built up sizeable followings amongst Victorian artisans and the petty bourgeoisie (thought not exclusively within those strata: homeopathy, for instance, had many middle-class and some noble adherents, while hydropathy was widely sampled by the intellectual aristocracy). The attractions are obvious. These medical philosophies put into practical form those high-minded individualist, self-reliant, anti-elitist, and even democratic sentiments that were becoming the hallmark of Victorian popular opinion. Each with its own particular nuance aimed to demystify and deprofessionalize health. Each appealed to popular distrust of corporate power and privilege; each gave vent to the widespread 'Romantic' disgust at urbanized, commercialized, mechanized living. Each professed to invest the individual with a new control over his own health as part of a wider culture of self-improvement and self-realization. He who tended his health, thereby improved his mind and ennobled his character.

Not least, such movements typically translated into medical terms that radical grassroots anger which in politics fuelled radicalism and in religion generated the dissidence of dissent. Medical heretics typically doubled as heretics in politics and faith as well; they also cultivated unorthodox lifestyles in other directions too, backing causes such as vegetarianism, Friendly Societies, co-operation, the savings movement, teetotalisim, self-education, and resistance to compulsory smallpox vaccination. Close links were forged with the 'New Life' aspirations of American communitarianism.

All such multifarious medical movements – not uncommonly engaged in mutual sectarian sniping – were incessantly execrated as quackery by the medical profession (it is not to deny, of course, that some regulars could see virtue in, say, hydropathy). But, if this was quackery, it was quackery with a difference, quackery of a kind previously only hinted at in this book. For one thing, in profound contrast to the tenor of earlier practice, which had clung to the regulars' coat-tails and bathed in their reflected glories, these movements chose to secede wholly from official medicine. In so doing, they chose to set themselves up in judgement upon the medical profession, rather as regular medicine had traditionally put quackery in the dock.

For another, these medical movements marked a break with the individual entrepreneurship of the classic quack from Case to Golbold. As the very names Thomsonianism or Coffinism testify, the charismatic leader could still be a force to contend with; and the sale of special medicines continued. All the same, purely commercial transactions formed a relatively muted part of the activities and attractions of these gatherings. By contrast, ideology, philosophy, and morality moved centre stage. These were movements that had designs on men's minds more than their pockets. Preferring the pamphlet to the pill, activists prided themselves on being the moral vanguard, expounding emancipatory doctrines upon health, advancing popular physiologies as a somatized religion of life, and holding out hope, both personal and social. Transcending the atomized consumer, these movements were made up of enthusiasts glad to share a common cause, participating in an uneasy but effective mixture of organization from above with practical grassroots self-help, which mirrored the organizations of cellular religion. The classic doctor/patient relationship (or the supplier/customer nexus) was displaced by aspirations to supportive mutual self-help in such bodies as the United Medico-Botanic Sick and Burial Society, founded in Leeds by the herbalist John Skelton, replete with rules and officers, but exuding a do-it-yourself ethos as an alternative to professionalism. Those involved would be activists more than patients. John Stevens, enthusiast for the Thomsonian system of medical botany, thus argued – and note the contrast with Wakley and his ilk – that the people knew best: 'the common sense of the people, when in possession of a true theory of medicine, will be found quite capable of curing all diseases to which they are subject'.[13]

All this, of course, amounts to the emergence of fringe medicine, an authentically populist medical creed, articulating the aspirations of the Victorian common people for self-determination, and repudiating the newly aggressive professional designs of the Victorian medical profession. If Georgian quackery has some loose affinities to the Wilkite political movement – in its opportunist if somewhat adventitious fusion of interests between an adventurer from above and a restless mass below – the Victorian fringe was more like the medical equivalent of Chartism: indeed, as Harrison has shown, many one-time Chartists turned to fringe medicine after the demise of that movement. The herbalist, John Skelton, thus advanced 'Six Propositions' of vegetable medicine, an unmistakable echo of the six points of the People's Charter.

It is not my argument that the emergence of alternative medicine of this kind in early-Victorian England replaced or ousted quackery. But by capturing the imaginations of substantial numbers of 'plebeian intellectuals' and 'independent spirits', and by laying

A practitioner of mesmerism using animal magnetism on a woman, who responds with convulsions. Wood engraving.

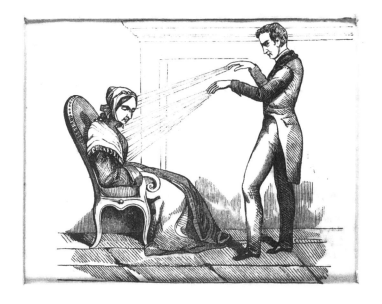

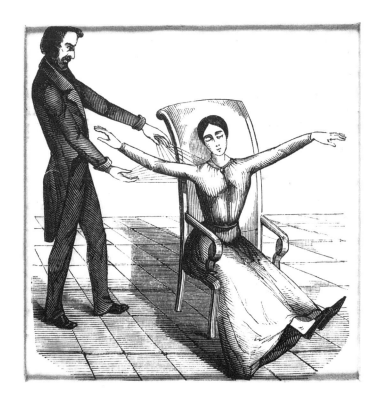

claim to the political dimensions of popular health care, the emergence of the fringe notably circumscribed the potential development of commercial quackery. It ensured that quacks were thereafter channelled into the routine business of marketing over-the-counter medicines. The possibilities opened up by the career of Morison for new directions in quackery were hijacked by the authentic appeal of populist healing cults.

Indeed, in other respects too, the Victorian age was to manufacture competition for the quacks and block off possible avenues of development. Highly significantly, state endorsement of regular medicine, thanks to the emergence of medical regulation – the great watershed was the setting up of the Medical Register in 1858 – stymied the traditional quack's dream of hobnobbing with the medicos. Above all, from mid-Victorian times, the quack doctor was progressively excluded by statute from holding any of the increasing number of official and salaried posts underwritten by the state – as Poor Law surgeons, public analysts, asylum physicians, consultants to insurance schemes, and the like. By contrast with the heyday of Sir William Read or the 'Chevalier' Taylor, the career options open for an unqualified practitioner shrank and became less enticing. The advantages of being a regular doctor consequently increased. Exclusion began to turn quacks into a caste apart.

And even in vending drugs, quacks felt the pinch. The passing and subsequent extension of food and drugs legislation, in particular the 1868 Pharmacy Act, and the emergence of prescription-only medicines combined to limit the range of really potent preparations that quacks could legally market. It is remarkable that the British Medical Association publications, *Secret Remedies* and *More Secret Remedies*, mentioned above, are revelations of the inertness of quack preparations rather than of their dangerousness. The traditional regulars' gibe, that sufferers bought nostrums because they were more potent than those medicines which prudent regulars thought it safe to administer, ceased to hold water.

In time, moreover, the larger manufacturing chemists serving the profession, companies such as Allen & Hanburys and Boots, forefronting high standards of purity and, eventually, developing traditions of laboratory research, upstaged the mere commercial nostrum-maker. Some, such as Beechams, successfully made the transition from empiricism to scientific pharmacy, but the example serves mainly to illustrate where the real profits have lain within the last century.

Trapped somewhat between the vast expansion of regular, professional medicine during the Victorian age and the emergence of a popular, attractive fringe, quackery became somewhat of a backwater and lost its erstwhile innovative role in British medicine. Time was when, in the developing free market economy, the individual quack could flower as an inventive entrepreneur, both selling his own individual persona and skills, and vending a commodity. Massive transformations – in medical professional organization, in state economic regulation, and in market capitalism itself – were reducing these possibilities to a shadow of their former selves.

Conclusion

It is, I hope, obvious by now which historical issues connected with the history of quackery this book has been attempting to tackle, and which it has shirked. It has not ventured a continuous chronological account of irregular medicine, nor has it delved into the prosopography of the quacks, or their business history, or the pharmacological and therapeutic aspects of their activities. These are fascinating fields, which largely remain to be researched. Rather, this book has focused upon a series of questions.

First, it has aimed to demystify the subject, disentangling the realities of irregular medicine from the verbal, ideological, and moralizing smokescreens behind which it has often been hidden.

'Treason doth never prosper. What's the reason?/ For if it prosper, none dare call it treason', rhymed the seventeenth-century wit. The history of quackery is perhaps illuminated by this epigram. Contemporaries and historians alike have had a similar pact to agree that quackery never prospers, for if and when it does, it becomes termed medicine instead – witness the fortunes of mercury as a specific against syphilis, the history of mesmerism and hypnotism, and the whole arena of medical specialism. But this is to be wise after the event; remove hindsight and it is evident quackery prospered, both in the immediately vulgar sense (quacks abounded, they did a good trade, and some grew rich and famous), but also in more complex ways. For some made real contributions to meeting the healing needs of the time, occasionally perhaps through genuine therapeutic and pharmacological innovation, sometimes simply by bringing medicine to the people, sometimes by cultivating areas of medical 'need' (real or putative), such as sex therapy, arguably neglected by regular medicine.

This book proceeded to explore (in chapter 2, above all) the 'conditions of existence' allowing quackery to survive and thrive. English quackery became a healthy plant – albeit a weed – in the seventeenth and eighteenth centuries because it was rooted in a favourable soil. Free market capitalism and the culture of consumerism helped provide both business opportunities and a common language shared by quacks and sick alike.

Even so, commanding authority was a battle that quack operators could never win often enough. This was not merely because they were not medically orthodox. It was because entrepreneurship itself in the emergent capitalist order created dilemmas for all vendors who were not personally known face-to-face by customers. The promotion of medicine as a merchandisable commodity had immense business advantages; but it posed severe problems of legitimization.

One tactic to resolve such difficulties lay in the rhetoric of conviction developed in quack advertising and publicity, as explored in chapter 4. Irregular medicine in the early modern era, I argued, found it strategically wise to ring the changes upon the images and idols of regular medicine and culture, and to claim to embody these in a superior form.

By way of contrast, major currents in unorthodox healing in the Victorian era preferred to present themselves as a dissenting tradition.

Examination of concepts of health and disease, and of therapeutic practice likewise suggested that pre-modern quacks tended to share, appropriate, or be parasitical upon the pillars of orthodoxy (one's choice of word betrays one's interpretative bias). A persistent polemical war was certainly waged between the champions of orthodoxy and the empirics. But this fact must not be allowed to mark the reality that, in pre-modern medicine, there was far greater convergence between the activities and attitudes of regulars and quacks than either side commonly allowed, or than historians have been primed to perceive.

We continue to speak of the history of regular practitioners as the history of a profession, thereby deploying concepts nursed by the profession itself. As a result, the business of medicine remains neglected. When the development of medical entrepreneurship finally receives its due share of attention, it will become clearer how far there truly were profound distinctions between the ways in which the 'typical' itinerant, and the 'typical' regular practitioner – both mythical beasts – drummed up custom and turned a penny; or whether the differences were as much matters of manner as of substance. Future socio-economic historians of medicine may find it profitable to examine the careers of quacks and regulars in tandem, rather than, as is traditional, distinctly in separate genres of study.

The same applies, it has been argued, to the history of patients and practitioners. We cannot begin to understand the enduring appeal of irregular healers unless we discard the stereotype of the quack's customers as 'gulls' and inquire instead as to how such people regarded the crowd of healers clamouring for their favours and the entire range of medicaments available.

To do so involves looking beyond medical history. The histories of consumer behaviour and material culture are now beginning to be developed. Drawing upon these, we must strive to obtain a better understanding of the impact of market capitalism. Not least it was shaping attitudes towards the body as a secular property, and health as a purchasable commodity. Such developments often discomfited the traditional humanist physician no less than they benefited the 'advertising professors'. Being so heavily dependent upon the market, quacks were forced to be specially adroit in exploiting these emergent attitudes.

Not least, we must not view the pre-modern commercial healers exclusively in a medical light. They were experts in showmanship, they drew upon the heritage of carnival, and understood the commercialization of entertainment no less than that of medicine. The history of quackery is thus comprehensible only in terms of the wider histories of the media, of the interplay between plebeian and patrician culture, and of attempts directed from above towards the 'reform of popular culture'. We must bear in mind the democratic intellect and democratic epistemologies, and the multifarious routes to individual identity and career opportunities opening in a capitalist, individualist culture. Only by understanding these dimensions of quack medicine shall we fully understand the contours of regular medicine, too.

Notes

Chapter one

1 Jonson, *Volpone*, p.50.

2 Ward, *London Spy*, pp.135-6.

3 King-Hele, *Doctor of Revolution*, p.195.

4 Thompson, *Quacks of Old London*, p.268.

5 Thompson, *Quacks of Old London*, pp.132f., 29

6 See Hambridge, 'Empiricomany', p.51.

7 Swainson, *Directions for the Use of Velno's Vegetable Syrup*, p.9.

8 See Paget, *John Hunter*, p.165. Newbery was a leading publisher and distributor of commercial medicines. Booksellers were major distributors of drugs.

9 Jenkins, *Observations*, p.112.

10 Davis, *Fear, Myth and History*.

11 Szasz, *Myth of Mental Illness*; Gilman, *Difference and Pathology*; Mayer, *Outsiders*.

12 Adair, *Essays on Fashionable Disorders*, p.75.

13 Smollett, *Launcelot Greaves*, p.79. For Smollett see Rousseau, *Tobias Smollett*; Hambridge, 'Empiricomany'.

14 Erasmus Darwin, *Zoonomia*, iv, p.152; quoted in King-Hele, *Essential Writings of Erasmus Darwin*, p.76.

15 Wadd, *Mems., Maxims and Memoirs*, p.66.

16 Hunter and Macalpine, *Three Hundred Years*, p.498.

17 lSouthey], Letters from England (London, 1814), p.284; quoted in Thompson, *Quacks of Old London*.

18 Agnew, 'Quackery', p.313.

19 Porter, 'William Hunter'.

Chapter two

1 British Library, *Collection of 185 Advertisements*, C112, f.9, 166.

2 Bagley (ed.), *Great Diurnal of Nicholas Blundell*, II, p.74.

3 Corry, *Satirical View of London*.

4 Beddoes, *Letter to Joseph Banks*, pp.10, 115.

5 *Gentleman'sMagazine*, IV, 1734, p.618.

6 *Collection of 185 Advertisements*, C112. f. 9, 436.

7 Adair, *Essays on Fashionable Disorders*.

8 Nicolson (ed.), *Conway Letters*, p.87.

9 Crellin, 'Dr James's Fever Powder'.

10 [Turner], *Modern Quacks*, 54.

11 Clowes, *Brief and Necessarie Treatise*, quoted in Webster, *Health, Medicine and Mortality*, pp.185-186.

12 Collection of 185 Advertisements, C112, f. 9, 125.

13 'Poplicola', *Gentleman's Magazine*, XVIII, 1748, p.346.

14 *Notes and Queries*, 7th series, 6 April 1889, p.273.

15 Norton (ed.), *Correspondence of Edward Gibbon*.

16 Marchand (ed.), *Byron's Letters and Journals*, IX, pp.75, 216.

17 Bessborough and Aspinall (eds), *Lady Bessborough*, p.40.

18 Lustig and Pottle (eds), *Boswell*, p.195.

19 Cozens-Hardy (ed.), *Diary of Sylas Neville*, p.24.

20 F. Darwin (ed.), *Life and Letters of Charles Darwin*, I, p.373.

21 Matthews (ed.), *Diary of Dudley Ryder*, p.288.

22 Hartshorne (ed.), *Memoirs of a Royal Chaplain*, p.299.

23 The *Festoon*.

Chapter three

1 Whitbread (ed.), *I Know My Own Heart*, p.292.

2 Galt, *Annals of the Parish*, p.57.

3 Vaisey (ed.), *Diary of Thomas Turner*, p.208.

4 *Ibid.*, p.11.

5 Tibble and Tibble (eds.), *Prose of John Clare*, pp.50-1.

6 Taylor, *History*

7 King, *Political and Literary Anecdotes*, p.131.

8 *Grub-Street Journal*, no. 293, 7 August 1735.

9 Nichols, *Literary Anecdotes*, Il, pp.383, 1812-15. Copies of Taylor's syllabuses exist in the British Library, Wellcome Institute Library, and Royal College of Surgeons' Library.

10 *A Parallel, between The late Celebrated Mr Pope, and Dr Taylor, Oculist to the King of Great Britain. With various Observations on the Proceedings of Dr Taylorfor nearly Twenty Years, not only in his Tour through these Kingdoms, but most parts of Europe. Address'd to the Gentlemen, the Ladies, the Clergy, and all of Literature and Distinction who would be acquainted with his Lectures, Operations, and Success. Wherein The Reasons of all, with many Advantages of a publick Concern from his Undertakings, are accurately and impartially consider'd. By a Physician. Invidia Siculi non inventere Tyranni Majus Tormentum. Hor.*, Printed for the Author, 1748.

11 Nichols, *Literary Anecdotes*, VIII, 400.

12 *The Operator: A Ballad Opera*, London, Printed for the Author, and sold by T. Payne, Bookseller, in Round Court in the Strand, opposite York Buildings, 1740. The description is in Coats, 'Chevalier Taylor', pp.161-2.

13 Barry, 'Publicity and the public good.'

14 *Collection of 185 Advertisements*, C112. f. 9, 6.

15 *Collection of 231 Advertisements*, 551. a, 32, 88.

16 *Collection of 185 Advertisements*, C112. f. 9, 37.

17 Hone, *Radcliffe*, p.71.

18 *Collection of 185 Advertisements*, C112. f. 9, 17.

19 *Collection of 231 Advertisements*, 551. a, 32, 128, 191.

20 *Collection of 185 Advertisements*, C112. f. 9, 9.

21 *Collection of 231 Advertisements*, 551. a, 32, 98.

22 *Ibid.*, 551. a. 32, 171.

23 *Collection of 185 Advertisements*, C112. f. 9, 34.

24 *Ibid.*, C112. f. 9, 67.

25 *Ibid.*, C112. f. 9, 60.

26 De Beer (ed.), *Correspondence of John Locke*, letter 918, 14 March 1687.

27 *Collection of 185 Advertisements*, C112. f. 9, 140.

28 *Ibid.*,C112.f.9,78.

Chapter four

1 Fielding, *History of Tom Jones*, p.347.

2 There is a fine collection of Graham's newspaper advertisements in the Library of the Wellcome Institute for the History of Medicine, MS 73143; some are reproduced in Grose, *Guide to Health*. For a contextual approach to Graham, see Porter, 'The sexual politics of James Graham'; Thompson, *Mysteries of History*, pp.259-77; Whitwell, 'James Graham'.

3 Ward, *London Spy*, pp.131-2.

4 Thompson, *Quacks of Old London*, pp.214-15.

5 See the title-page of his autobiography: *History of the Travels of Adventures of the Chevalier John Taylor*.

6 *Collection of 185 Advertisements*, C112, f.9, 2.

7 *Ibid.*, C112. f.9, 57.

8 *Ibid.*, C112. f.9, 13.

9 *Ibid.*, C112. f.9, 17.

10 Thompson, *Quacks of Old London*, p.343.

11 *Collection of 185 Advertisements*, C112. f. 9, 173.

12 *Ibid.*, C112. f.9, 84.

13 *Ibid.*

14 *Ibid.*, C112. f.9, 58.

15 *Ibid.*

16 Thompson, *Quacks of Old London*, p.188. 'Frenchify'd' meant poxed.

42 [Turner], *Modern Quacks*, p.11.

18 Thompson, *Quacks of Old London*, p.142.

19 Hone, *Radcliffe*, p.71.

20 Thompson, *Quacks of Old London*, p.223.

21 Adair, *Essays on Fashionable Disorders*, p.193.

22 Thompson, *Quacks of Old London*, p.329.

23 *Ibid.*, p.29.

24 *Collection of 185 Advertisements*, C112. f.9, 92.

25 [Turner], *Modern Quacks*, pp.14-15.

26 Thomas, *Religion and the Decline of Magic*.

27 Quoted in Nicolson, 'Ward's Pill', p.132.

28 *Collection of 185 Advertisements*, C112. f.9, 10.

29 Thompson, *Quacks of Old London*, p.170.

30 *Ibid.*, p.168.

31 *Tatler*, 21 October 1710.

32 [Turner], *Modern Quacks*, p.7.

33 Ward, *London Spy*, 134-5.

34 Goldsmith, *Citizen of the World*, p.189.

35 Porter, *Mind Forg'd Manacles*, p.165.

36 Black, *English Press*, p.52 [22 May 1725].

37 Thompson, *Quacks of Old London*, p.100.

38 *Collection of 185 Advertisements*, C112. a. 32, 17.

39 *Bath Herald*, 21 January 1798.

41 *Bath Journal*.

42 Anstey, *New Bath Guide*.

43 Black, *English Press*, p.64.

44 Sheridan, *Works*, p.450.

45 *Bath Herald*, 3 March and 10 March 1798.

46 All these were variously advertised in Bath newspapers. For sharing with me their expertise and materials on Yorkshire and Wiltshire newspapers respectively, I am deeply indebted to Dr J.J. Looney and C.Y. Ferdinand. In the late stages of writing this book, I was also much helped by Ben Zuber Swanson's 'Methods and Media of Dental Advertising, ca. 1700-1921' (M.Phil. thesis, University College, London, 1987).

Chapter five

1 *Collection of 185 Advertisements*, C112. f.9, 77; cf. Brian, *Pisse-Prophet*; Murphey, 'Art of uroscopy'.

2 Barry, 'Piety and the patient'.

3 Percival, *Medical Ethics*.

4 *Collection of 185 Advertisements*, C112. f.9, 30.

5 *Collection of 231 Advertisements*, 551.a. 32, 12.

6 *Collection of 185 Advertisements*, C112. f.9, 75.

7 *Ibid.*, C112. f.9, 69.

8 *Ibid.*, C112. f.9, 9.

9 *Ibid.*, C112. f.9, 11.

10 *Ibid.*, C112. f.9, 24.

11 *Ibid.*, C112. f.9, 131.

12 *Ibid.*, C112. f.9, 8.

13 *Ibid.*, C112. f.9, 71.

14 *Ibid.*, C112. f.9, 2.

15 *Ibid.*, C112. f.9, 40.

16 *Ibid.*, C112. f.9, 10.

17 *Ibid.*, C112. f.9, 137; f.9, 35; f.9, 89.

18 *Ibid.*, C112. f.9, 8.

19 *Ibid.*, C112. f.9, 56.

20 *Ibid.*, C112. f.9, 89.

21 *Ibid.*, C112. f.9, 71A.

22 *Ibid.*, C112. f.9, 16.

23 *Ibid.*, C112. f.9, 29.

24 *Ibid.*, C112. f.9, 58.

25 *Ibid.*, C112. f.9, 73.

26 *Ibid.*, C112. f.9, 19.

27 *Ibid.*, C112. f.9, 17.

28 Porter, 'Introduction' to Trotter, *Essays on Drunkenness*.

29 *Collection of 185 Advertisements*, C112. f.9, 78.

30 Coleridge, *Table Talk*, p.83.

31 *Collection of 185 Advertisements*, C112. f.9, 15.

32 *Ibid.*, C112. f.9, 12.

33 *Ibid.*, C112. f.9, 19.

Chapter six

1 *Collection of 185 Advertisements*, C112. f.9, 156; f.9, 61.

2 *Ibid.*, C112. f.9, 2.

3 *Ibid.*, C112. f.9, 168, 2-3.

4 Solomon, *Account of the Balm of Gilead*, p.55.

5 *Collection of 185 Advertisements*, C112. f.9, 108; f.9, 86; f. 9, 89.

6 *Collection of 231 Advertisements*, 551.a. 32, 85.

7 *Collection of 185 Advertisements*, C112. f.9, 93; f.9, 103; f.9, 166; f.9, 116.

8 *Ibid.*, C112. f.9, 2.

9 *Ibid.*, C112. f.9, 46.

10 *Collection of 231 Advertisements*, 551.a. 32, 182

11 *Collection of 185 Advertisements*, C112. f.9, 45.

12 *Ibid.*, C112. f.9, 42.

13 *Collection of 231 Advertisements*, 551.a. 32, 14.

14 *Collection of 185 Advertisements*, C112. f.9, 59.

15 *Ibid.*, C112. f.9, 65; f.9, 7.

16 *Collection of 231 Advertisements*, 551.a. 32, 7.

17 *Collection of 185 Advertisements*, C112. f.9, 5.

18 *Ibid.*, C112. f.9, 81; f.9, 159.

19 *Ibid.*, C112. f.9, 91.

20 *Collection of 231 Advertisements*, 551.a. 32, 22.

21 *Collection of 185 Advertisements*, C112. f.9, 7.

22 Angelo, *Reminiscences*, 11, pp.61-62; quoted in Jameson, *Natural History of Quackery*.

23 Graham, *General State of Medical and Chirurgical Practice*.

24 Contemporary (1783) newspaper advertisement quoted in Grose, *Guide to Health*, pp.26-27.

25 Graham, *Sketch*, p.151.

26 *Ibid.*

27 *Ibid.*

28 Newspaper clipping, 'Collection of cuttings', 73143, Wellcome Institute for the History of Medicine, London.

29 Graham, *Lecture on… Generation*, p.3.

30 *Ibid.*, p.4.

31 *Ibid.*, p.19. Graham married at twenty-five.

32 *Ibid.*, p.19.

33 *Short Treatise on the All-Cleansing Earth*, p.4. For the idea of 'viriculture' see Easlea, *Science and Sexual Oppression*. On alternative male and female visions of nature see also Merchant, *Death of Nature*.

34 Graham, *New and Curious Treatise*, p.28.

35 Graham, *Lecture on Generation*, 20.

36 Brodum, *Guide to Old Age*.

37 Solomon, *Guide to Health*, p.49.

Chapter seven

1 Marlow (ed.), *Diary of Thomas Isham*, p.113.

2 *Collection of 185 Advertisements*, C112. f.9, p.27.

3 Irish, *Levamen infirmi*, p.32.

4 *Collection of 185 Advertisements*, C112. f.9, 179.

5 *Ibid.*, C112. f.9, 17.

6 *Ibid.*, C112.f.9, 146.

7 *Ibid.*, C112. f.9, 162.

8 *Ibid.*, C112. f.9, 79.

10 Adair, *Essays on Fashionable Disorders*.

11 Buchan, *Domestic Medicine*, p.471.

12 Heberden, *Medical Commentaries*, p.291.

13 Trotter, *View of the Nervous Temperament*, p.122.

14 Adair, *Essays on Fashionable Disorders*, p.232.

15 Beddoes, *Hygeia*, 1, p.259.

16 *Collection of 185 Advertisements*, C112. f.9, 150; f.9, 50.

17 *Collection of 231 Advertisements*, 551.a. 32, 63; 32, 131.

18 *Collection of 185 Advertisements*, C112. f.9, 78.

19 *Ibid.*, C112. f.9, 1.

20 Willich, *Lectures on Diet*, p.16.

21 *Collectionof 185 Advertisements*, C112. f.9, 14.

22 *Ibid.*, C112.f.9,70.

23 *Collection of 231 Advertisements*, 551.a. 32, 49.

24 *Collection of 185 Advertisements*, C112. f.9, 171; f.9, 47.

25 *Collection of 231 Advertisements*, 551 .a. 32, 91.

26 *Ibid.*, 551.a. 32, 9.

27 *Ibid.*, 551.a 32, 122.

28 *Collection of 185 Advertisements*, C112. f.9, 50.

29 *Ibid.*, C112. f.9, 52.

30 Beddoes, *Letter to Joseph Banks*.

31 King-Hele (ed.), *Letters of Erasmus Darwin*, pp.16-17.

32 Butterfield (ed.), *Letters of Benjamin Rush*, I, pp.284-5.

33 Adair, *Essays on Fashionable Disorders*, pp.7, 232.

34 *Ibid.*, p.13.

35 Little and Kahrl (eds), *Letters of David Garrick*, 11, p.1090. Myersbach's name was variously spelled at the time.

36 See *The New Method of Curing Diseases by Inspecting the Urine Examined*, London, J. Bew [?1776], p.2. One hint here is that Myersbach was also an abortionist.

37 *The Impostor Detected*, p.13.

38 This is reproduced in Lettsom, 'Fugitive Pieces', II, p.11.

39 *Gazetteer*, 2 October 1776.

40 Lettsom, 'Fugitive Pieces', III, MS note at beginning. For 'murdering empirics', see *Gazetteer*, 26 August 1776.

41 *New Method of Curing Disease*, p.22.

42 *The Impostor Detected*, p.3.

43 See Lettsom, 'Fugitive Pieces', II, p.69.

44 'London Spy', *Gazetteer*, 15 October 1776.

45 Lettsom, 'Fugitive Pieces, II, p.102.

46 *Public Ledger*, 30 September 1776. Cf. Lettsom, 'Fugitive Pieces', II, p.29ff.

47 *Gazetteer*, 3 January 1777 (Lettsom, 'Fugitive Pieces', 11, p.139). The identification is by Lettsom.

Chapter eight

1 *Lancet*, I, 1828-9, p.335.

2 *Ibid.*, I, 1837-8, p.630.

3 *Ibid.*, I, 1839-40, p.237.

4 *Ibid.*, p.683.

5 *Ibid.*, II, 1838-9, p.598.

6 *Ibid.*, II, 1835-6, p.57.

7 *Ibid.*

8 *Ibid.*, II, 1835-6, p.123.

9 *Ibid.*, II, 1838-9, p.823.

10 *Ibid.*, II, 1834-5, pp.712-13.

11 *Ibid.*, II, 1825-6, p.869.

12 *Ibid.*, I, 1836-7, p.948.

13 Harrison, 'Early Victorian radicals', p.46.

Bibliography

Abraham, J.J., *Lettsom, his Life, Times, Friends and Descendants*, London, Heinemann, 1933.

Adair, J.M., *Essays on Fashionable Disorders*, London, Bateman, 1790.

Agneau, J.P., *The Market and the Stage*, Cambridge, Cambridge University Press, 1987.

Agnew, L.R.C., 'Quackery', in C.D. O'Malley (ed.), *Medicine in Seventeenth Century England*, Berkeley, University of California Press, 1974.

Alcock, I., and Wilmot, J., *The Famous Pathologist or the Noble Mountebank* ed. by V. Da Sola Pinto, Nottingham, University of Nottingham Press, 1961.

Altick, R., *The Shows of London*, Cambridge, Mass., Belknap Press, 1978.

Andrews, C. B. (ed.), *The Torrington Diaries*, 4 vols, London, Eyre & Spottiswoode, 1954.

Anstey, C., *The New Bath Guide*, Bath, 1766.

Archenholtz, J.W.von, *Picture of England*, London, [for the booksellers], 1797.

Armstrong, D., *The Political Anatomy of the Body*, Cambridge, Cambridge University Press, 1983.

Arthos, J., *The Language of National Description in Eighteenth Century Poetry*, Ann Arbor, University of Michigan Press, 1949.

Bagley, J.J. (ed.), *The Great Diurnal of Nicholas Blundell*, transcr. and annot. by F. Tyrer, 3 vols, Record Society of Lancashire and Cheshire, 110 1968; 112 1970; 114 1972.

Balint, M., *The Doctor, the Patient and his Illness*, London, International Universities Press, 1957.

Barbeau, A., *Life and Letters at Bath in the Eighteenth Century*, ed. by A. Dobson, London, Heinemann, 1904.

Barker-Benfield, G.J., *The Horrors of the Half-Known Life*, New York, Harper & Row, 1976.

Barnum, P. Taylor, *The Humbugs of the World*, London, 1866.

Barrett, C.R.B., *The History of the Society of Apothecaries of London*, London, Elliot Stock, 1905.

Barrow, L., 'Anti-establishment healing: spiritualism in Britain', in W. Sheils (ed.), *The Church and Healing*, Oxford, Blackwell, 1982, pp.225-48.

————, *Independent Spirits: Spiritualism and English Plebeians, 1850-1910*, London, Routledge & Kegan Paul, 1986.

————, 'An imponderable liberator: J.J.Garth Wilkinson', in R. Cooter (ed.), *Studies in the History of Alternative Medicine*, London, Macmillan, 1988, pp.88-116.

Barry, Jonathan, 'The cultural life of Bristol, 1640 1775' Oxford University, D.Phil. thesis, 1986.

————, 'Piety and the patient: medicine and religion in eighteenth-century Bristol', in R. Porter (ed.), *Patients and Practitioners*, Cambridge, CUP, 1985.

————, 'Publicity and the public good: presenting medicine in eighteenth-century Bristol', in W.F. Bynum and R. Porter (eds), *Medical Fringe and Medical Orthodoxy*, 1750-1850, London, Croom Helm, 1987.

Barthes, R., *Mythologies*, London, Cape, 1972.

Bauman, R., and Sherzer, J., *Explorations in the Ethnography of Speaking*, Cambridge, CUP, 1974.

Beattie, J.M., The English Court in the Reign of George I, Cambridge, CUP, l967.

Beddoes, T., *Hygeia*, 3 vols, Bristol, Phillips, 1802-3.

————, *A Letter to the Right Honorable Joseph Banks*, London, Phillips, 1808.

Beier, L.M., *Sufferers and Healers. The Experience of Illness in Seventeenth-Century England*, London, Routledge & Kegan Paul, 1987.

Berg, M., *The Age of Manufactures 1700-1820*, London, Fontana, 1985.

Berman, Morris, *The Re-Enchantment of the World*, Ithaca, Cornell University Press, 1981.

Berridge, V., and Edwards, G., *Opium and the People*, London, Allen Lane, 1981.

Besant, H., *London in the Eighteenth Century*, London, Black, 1902.

Bessborough, Earl of, and Aspinall, A. (eds), *Lady Bessborough and her Family Circle*, London, Murray, 1940.

Bigsby, C.W.E. (ed.), *Approaches to Popular Culture*, London, Edward Arnold, 1976.

Billington, S., *A Social History of the Fool*, Brighton, Harvester Press, 1984.

Black, J., *The English Press in the Eighteenth Century*, London, Croom Helm, 1986.

Blackman, J., 'Popular theories of generation: the evolution of Aristotle's works. The study of an anachronism', in J. Woodward and D. Richards (eds), *Health Care and Popular Medicine in Nineteenth-Century England*, London, Croom Helm, 1977, pp.56-88.

Bloch, M., *The Royal Touch: Sacred Monarchy and Scrofula in England and France*, London, Routledge & Kegan Paul, 1973.

Bonnard, G.A. (ed.), *Edward Gibbon. Memoirs of My Life*, London, Nelson, 1966.

Bottomley, F., *Attitudes to the Body in Western Christendom*, London, Lepus, 1979.

Boucé, P.-G., 'Aspects of sexual tolerance and intolerance in eighteenth-century England', *British Journal for Eighteenth-Century Studies*, III, 1980, pp.173-89.

———— (ed.), *Sexuality in Eighteenth-Century England*, Manchester, Manchester University Press, 1982.

————, 'Some sexual beliefs and myths in eighteenth-century Britain', *British Journal for Eighteenth-Century Studies*, II, 1980, pp.28~6.

Brewster, P., 'Physicians and surgeons as represented in sixteenth and seventeenth century English literature', *Osiris*, XIV, 1962, pp.13-32.

Brian, T., *The Piss-Prophet Northridge*, Cal., Rilker Labs, 1968. Reprint of first edition, London, Thrale, 1637.

British Medical Association, *Secret Remedies*, London, 1909.

————, *Today's Drugs*, London, 1964.

Broadhurst, J., 'Peeps with Pepys at hygiene and medicine', *Annals of Medical History*, 1st Series, X, 1928, pp.165-72.

Brodum, W., *A Guide to Old Age or a Cure for the Indiscretions of Youth*, London, J.W. Myers, 1795.

Brody, H., *Stories of Sickness*, New Haven, Yale University Press, 1987.

Brook, C., *Battling Surgeon*, Glasgow, Strickland Press, 1945.

Brooks, E. St J., *Sir Hans Sloane*, London, Batchworth, 1954.

Brooks-Davies, D., 'The mythology of love: Venusean and related iconography in Pope, Fielding, Cleland and Sterne', in P.-G. Boucé (ed.), *Sexuality in Eighteenth-Century Britain*, Manchester, Manchester University Press, 1982, pp.176-97.

Brown, P.S., 'Female pills and the reputation of iron as an abortifacient', *Medical History*, XXI, 1977, pp.291-304.

————, 'Medicines advertised in eighteenth-century Bath newspapers', *Medical History*, XX, 1976, pp.152-68.

————, 'Social context and medical theory in the demarcation of nineteenth-century boundaries', in W.F. Bynum and R. Porter (eds)., *Medical Fringe and Medical Orthodoxy 1750-1850*, London, Croom Helm, 1987, pp.21~33.

————, 'The vendors of medicines advertised in eighteenth-century Bath newspapers', *Medical History*, XIX, 1975, pp.352-69.

Brown, T., 'The College of Physicians and the acceptance of iatromechanism in England 1665-1695', *Bulletin of the History of Medicine*, XLIV, 1970, pp.12-30.

Browne, Sir Thomas, *Works*, ed. by C. Sayle, 6 vols, Edinburgh, Grant, 1912.

Buchan, W., *Domestic Medicine, or a Treatise on the Prevention and Cure of Diseases by Regimen and Simple Medicines*, Edinburgh, Balfour, Auld & Smellie, 1769.

Buranelli, V., *The Wizard from Vienna*, New York, Coward, McGann, 1976.

Burger, H., 'The doctor, the quack and the appetite of the public for magic in medicine', *Proceedings of the Royal Society of Medicine*, XVII, 1933, pp.171-6.

Burke, P., *Historical Anthropology of Early Modern Italy*, Cambridge, CUP, 1987.

————, *Popular Culture in Early Modern Europe*, London, Temple Smith, 1978.

————, 'Popular culture in seventeenth century London', *London Journal*, III, 1977, pp.14~62.

Butterfield, L.H. (ed.), *The Letters of Benjamin Rush*, 2 vols, Princeton, Princeton University Press, 1951.

Bynum, W.F., 'Health, disease and medical care', in G.S. Rousseau and R. Porter (eds), *The Ferment of Knowledge*, Cambridge, CUP, 1980, pp.211-54.

————, 'Treating the wages of sin: venereal disease and specialism in eighteenth-century Britain', in W.F. Bynum and R. Porter (eds), *Medical Fringe and Medical Orthodoxy, 1750-1850*, London, Croom Helm, 1987, pp.5-28.

———— and Porter, R. (eds), *Medical Fringe and Medical Orthodoxy, 1750-1850*, London, Croom Helm, 1987.

Camp, J., *Magic, Myth and Medicine*, London, Priory Press, 1973.

Campbell, C., *The Romantic Ethic and the Spirit of Modern Consumerism*, Oxford, Basil Blackwell, 1987.

Campbell, R., *The English Tradesman*, London, David & Charles, 1969; 1st ed. 1747.

Campbell, W.A., 'Portrait of a quack: Joshua Ward 1685-1761', *University of Newcastle Medical Gazette*, 1964.

Cantor, G.N., and Hodge, M.J.S. (eds), *Conceptions of Ether*, Cambridge, CUP, 1982.

Carpenter, K.J., *The History of Scurvy and Vitamin C*, Cambridge, Cambridge University Press, 1986.

Cartwright, A., *Patients and their Doctors*, London, Tavistock, 1967.

Cassel, E.J., *Talking to Patients*, Cambridge, Mass., M.I.T.Press, 1985.

Chamberlain, M., *Old Wives' Tales: their History, Remedies and Spells*, London, Virago, 1981.

Chambers, J.D., *Population, Economy, and Society in Pre-Industrial England*, Oxford, OUP, 1972.

Chance, B., *Ophthalmology*, New York, Hafner, 1962.

Chapman, R.W. (ed.), *The Letters of Samuel Johnson*, 3 vols, Oxford, Clarendon Press, 1984.

Chapman, S., *Jesse Boot of Boots the Chemist*, London, Hodder & Stoughton, 1974.

Cheats of London Town Exposed, The, London, 1766.

Clark, G., *A History of the Royal College of Physicians of London*, 3 vols, Oxford, Clarendon Press, 1964-72.

Clark, S., 'French historians and early modern popular culture', *Past and Present*, 100, 1983, pp.62-99.

Clarkson, L., *Death, Disease and Famine in Pre-Industrial England*, Dublin, Gill & Macmillan, 1975.

Clowes, W., *A Brief and Necessarie Treatise*, London, East, 1585.

Coats, G., 'The Chevalier Taylor', in R. Rutson James (ed.), *Studies in the History of Ophthalmology in England Prior to the Year 1800*, Cambridge, CUP, 1933, pp.132-219.

————, 'Historical notes', in *ibid.*, pp.220-46.

Coleman, W., 'Health and hygiene: a medical doctrine for the bourgeoisie', *Journal of the History of Medicine*, XXIV, 1974, pp.399-421.

Coleridge, S.T., *Table Talk*, London, John Murray, 1835; G. Routledge, 1874.

Collins, K.E., 'Two Jewish quacks in eighteenth-century Glasgow and how they advertised their cures in the Glasgow Advertiser', *Jewish Echo*, 27 January 1984, p.5.

Coltheart, P., *The Quacks Unmasked*, London, [the author], 1727.

Comfort, A., *The Anxiety Makers*, London, Nelson, 1967.

Cook, H., *The Decline of the Old Medical Regime in Stuart England*, Ithaca, Cornell University Press, 1986.

————, 'The failure of the old medical order in seventeenth-century London. The College of Physicians, medical regulation, and the medical marketplace', unpublished paper, Harvard University, 1983.

Cook, R., *Sir Samuel Garth*, Boston, Twayne, 1980.

Cook, T.M., *Samuel Hahnemann*, Wellingborough, Thorson's, 1981.

Cooter, R., 'Bones of contention? Orthodox medicine and the mystery of the bone-setter's craft', in W.F. Bynum and R. Porter (eds), *Medical Fringe and Medical Orthodoxy, 1750-1850*, London, Croom Helm, 1987, pp.158-73.

————, 'Deploying "pseudo-science". Then and now', in M.P. Hanen, M.J. Osler, and R.C. Weyant (eds), *Science, Pseudo-Science and Society*, Waterloo, Ontario, Wilfred Laurier University, 1980.

————, 'Medicina e Cultura Alternativa', *Prometeo*, I, 1983.

———— (ed.), *Studies in the History of Alternative Medicine*, London, Macmillan, 1988.

————, 'Alternative medicine, alternative cosmology', in *ibid.*, pp.62-77.

Cope, Sir Z., *The History of the Royal College of Surgeons of London*, London, Anthony Blond, 1959.

Corry, John, *The Detector of Quackery*, London, Hurst, 1802.

————, *A Satirical View of London*, London, Ogle, 1803.

Corsini, A., *Medici Ciarlatani e Ciarlatani Medici*, Bologna, 1922.

Couliano, J., *Eros et Magie*, Paris, Flammarion, 1984.

Cozens-Hardy, B. (ed.), *The Diary of Sylas Neville 1767-1788*, London, Oxford University Press, 1950.

Crabtre, D.D., *The Funny Side of Physic*, Hartford, Burr, 1874.

Cranfield, G.A., *The Development of the Provincial Newspaper 1700-60*, Oxford, Clarendon Press, 1962.

Crawford, P., 'Printed advertisements for women medical practitioners in London, 1670-1710', *Society for the Social History of Medicine Bulletin*, XXXV, 1984, pp.66-70.

————, 'Attitudes to pregnancy from a woman's spiritual diary, 1687-88', *Local Population Studies*, XXI, 1978, pp.43-45.

————, '"The sucking child": adult attitudes to child care in the first year of life in seventeenth-century England', *Continuity and Change*, I, 1986, pp.23-51.

————— 'Attitudes to menstruation in seventeenth-century England', *Past and Present*, 91,1981, pp.47-73.

————— 'The construction and experience of maternity in seventeenth-century England', in V. Fildes (ed.), *Women as Mothers in Early Modern England*, London, Routledge, 1989.

Crawfurd, R.H.P., *The King's Evil*, Oxford, Clarendon Press, 1911.

Crellin, J., 'Dr James's Fever Powder', *Transactions of the British Society for the History of Pharmacy*, I, 1974, pp.136-43.

————— and Scott, J.R., 'Lionel Lockyer and his pills', *Proceedings of the XXIII International Congress of the History of Medicine*, 2 vols, London, Wellcome Institute for the History of Medicine, 1972, pp.1182-6.

Crocker, L.G., *An Age of Crisis: Man and World in Eighteenth-Century Thought*, Baltimore, Johns Hopkins University Press, 1959.

—————, *Nature and Culture: Ethical Thought in the French Enlightenment*, Baltimore, Johns Hopkins University Press, 1963.

Cunningham, H., *Leisure in the Industrial Revolution*, London, Croom Helm, 1980.

Cunnington, P., and Lucas, C., *Occupational Costume in England*, London, Black, 1967.

Curry, P., 'The decline of astrology in early modern England, 1642-1800', University of London, Ph.D. thesis, 1986.

————— (ed.), *Astrology, Science and Society: Historical Essays*, Woodbridge, Suffolk, 1987.

Darnton, R., *Mesmerism and the End of the Enlightenment in France*, Cambridge, Mass., Harvard University Press, 1968.

Darwin, F. (ed.), *The Life and Letters of Charles Darwin*, 3 vols, London, Murray, 1888.

Davie, D., *The Language of Science and the Language of Literature 1700-40*, London, Sheed & Ward, 1963.

Davies, H., *Worship and Theology in England*, Princeton University Press, 1975.

Davis, J.C., *Fear, Myth and History: the Ranters and the Historians*, Cambridge, CUP, 1986.

Day, R., 'Psalmanazar's "Formosa" and the British Reader' in G.S. Rousseau and R.Porter (eds), *Exoticism in the Enlightenment*, Manchester, Manchester University Press, 1989.

De Beer, E.S. (ed.), *The Diary of John Evelyn*, 6 vols, Oxford, OUP, 1955.

————— (ed.), *The Correspondence of John Locke*, 8 vols, Oxford, Clarendon Press, 1976-81.

Debus, A.G., 'Scientific truth and occult tradition: the medical world of Ebenezer Sibly 1751-99', *Medical History*, XXVI, 1982, pp.259-78.

Devlin, J., *The Superstitious Mind. French Peasants and the Supernatural in the Nineteenth Century*, New Haven, Yale University Press, 1987.

Dewhurst, K., *The Quicksilver Doctor. The Life and Times of Thomas Dover*, Bristol, John Wright, 1957.

Dingwall, R., and Lewis, P. (eds), *The Sociology of the Professions*, London, Macmillan, 1983.

Dittrick, H., 'Fees in medical history', *Annals of Medical History*, X, 1928, pp.90-101.

Dobson, M.J., 'Population, disease and mortality in southeast England, 1600-1800', University of Oxford, D.Phil. thesis, 1982.

—————, 'A chronology of epidemic disease and mortality in southeast England, 1601-1800', *Historical Research Series*, 19, 1987.

—————, *From Old England to New England: Changing Patterns of Mortality*, Oxford, University of Oxford School of Geography Research Paper 38, 1987.

Doherty, F., 'The anodyne necklace: A Quack Remedy and its Promotion', *Medical History*, xxxiv, 1990, pp.268-293

Doughty, O., 'The English malady of the eighteenth century', *Review of English Studies*, II, 1929, pp.257-69.

Dover, T., *The Ancient Physician's Legacy to his Country*, London, A. Bettesworth& C. Hitch etc., 1732.

Duden, B., *Geschichte unter der Haut. Ein Eisenacher Arzt und Seine Patientinnen um 1730*, Stuttgart, Klett-Cotta, 1987.

Dumas, F. Ribadeau, *Cagliostro*, London, George Allen & Unwin, 1967.

Durey, M., 'Medical elites, the general practitioner and patient power in Britain during the cholera epidemic of 1831-2', in I. Inkster and J.B. Morrell (eds), *Metropolis and Province. Science in British Culture 1780-1850*, London, Hutchinson, 1983.

Earle, P., *The Making of the English Middle Class*, London, Methuen, 1989.

Easlea, B., *Science and Sexual Oppression*, London, Weidenfeld & Nicolson, 1981.

————, *Witch-Hunting, Magic and the New Philosophy*, Hassocks, Sussex, Harvester, 1980.

Eccles, A., *Obstetrics and Gynaecology in Tudor and Stuart England*, London, Croom Helm, 1983.

Elliott, B.B., *A History of English Advertising*, London, Business Pubns, 1962.

Elliott, J., *The Old World and the New London*, Cambridge University Press, 1965.

Ellis, A., *The Penny Universities, a History of the Coffee Houses*, London, Secker & Warburg, 1956.

Essay on the Inspection of the Urine: Shewing the Impossibility of Being Acquainted with the Diseases Incident to the Human Body, by the Inspection Only, London, 1776.

Evans, R., *Rudolph II and his World*, Oxford, OUP, 1973.

Everitt, G., *Doctors and Doctors*, London, Sonnenschein, 1888.

Eversley, D.E.C., 'The home market and economic growth in England 1750-1800', in E.L. Jones and C.E. Mingay (eds), *Land, Labour and Population in the Industrial Revolution*, London, 1967, pp.206-59.

Farrer, W., *A Treatise on Onanism*, 3rd ed., London, 1773.

Fawcett, T., *The Rise of English Provincial Art*, Oxford, OUP, 1974.

Fellman, A.G., and Fellman, H., *Making Sense of Self*, Philadelphia, University of Pennsylvania Press, 1981.

Festoon, The: a Select Collection of Epigrams, 4th ed., London, 1744.

Fielding, Henry, *The History of Tom Jones*, Harmondsworth, Penguin, 1975.

Figlio, K., 'Chlorosis and chronic disease in nineteenth-century Britain: the social constitution of somatic illness in a capitalist society', *Social History*, III, 1978, pp.167-97.

Fischer-Homberger, E., 'Hypochondriasis of the eighteenth century – neurosis of the present century', *Bulletin of the History of Medicine*, XLIV, 1972, 391-401.

Fishbein, M., *Fads and Quackery in Healing*, New York, Covici Friede, 1932.

Fissell, M.E., 'The physic of charity: health and welfare in the West Country, 1690-1834', Philadelphia, University of Pennsylvania Ph.D. thesis, 1988.

Flinn, M., *The European Demographic System 1500-1820*, Brighton, Harvester Press, 1981.

————, 'The stabilization of mortality in pre-industrial western Europe', *Journal of European Economic History*, III, 1974, pp.285-318.

Foss, M., *The Age of Patronage. The Arts in Society 1660-1750*, London, Hamish Hamilton, 1971.

Foucault, M., *A History of Sexuality*. Vol 1: Introduction, London, Tavistock,.1979.

Foxon, D., *Libertine Literature in England 1660-1745*, London, 1964.

Francesco, Grete de, *Die Macht des Charlatans*, Basle, Schwabe, 1937.

Francis, Anne, *A Guinea a Box*, London, Hale, 1968.

Freidson, E., *Profession of Medicine*, New York, Dodd, Mead, 1970.

Friedli, L., '"Passing women": a study of gender boundaries in the eighteenth century', in G.S. Rousseau and R. Porter (eds), *Sexual Underworlds of the Enlightenment*, Manchester, Manchester University Press, 1988, pp.234-60.

Galt, J., *Annals of the Parish*, ed. by J. Kinsley, Oxford, OUP, 1986.

Garlick, K., and Macintyre, A. (eds), *The Diary of Joseph Farington*, vols I-VI, New Haven, Yale University Press, 1978-9.

Gasking, E.B., *Investigations into Generation* 1651-1828, London, Hutchinson, 1964.

Gay, P., 'The Enlightenment as medicine and as cure', in W.H. Barber (ed.), *The Age of the Enlightenment. Studies Presented to Theodore Besterman*, Edinburgh, St Andrews University Publications, 1967, pp.375 86.

George, D.F., *Blake and Freud*, Ithaca, Cornell University Press, 1980.

Giglioni, P.P. (ed.), *Language and Social Context*, Harmondsworth, Penguin, 1975.

Gilman, S., *Difference and Pathology*, Ithaca and London, Cornell University Press, 1985.

Ginzburg, C., *The Cheese and the Worms: the Cosmos of a Sixteenth-Century Miller*, London, Routledge, 1980.

Glyster, G., [pseud.], *A Dose for the Doctors; or the Aesculapian Labyrinth Explored*, London, Kearsley, 1789.

Goellnicht, D.C., *The Poet-Physician. Keats and Medical Science*, Pittsburgh, University of Pittsburgh Press, 1984.

Golby, J.M., and Purdue, A.W., *The Civilization of the Crowd: Popular Culture in England, 1750-1900*, London, Batsford, 1984.

Goldsmith, O., *A Citizen of the World*, London, Everyman, 1934.

Gorin, G., *History of Ophthalmology*, New York, Publish or Perish Press, 1982.

Gosse, P., *Dr. Viper. The Querulous Life of Philip Thicknesse*, London, Cassell, 1952.

Graham, James, *Address to the Public in General* (handbill).

————, *The General State of Medical and Chirurgical Practice Exhibited*, London, Almon, 1779.

————, *Lecture on the Generation, Increase and Improvement of the Human Species*, London, [for the author], 1780.

————, *A New and Curious Treatise*, London and Bath, Cruttwell, 1780.

————, *A Sketch, or Short Description of Dr Graham's Medical Apparatus*, London, Almon, 1780.

————, *Proposals for the Establishment of a New and True Christian Church*, Bath, Cruttwell, 1788.

————, *A Discourse Delivered in Edinburgh…*, Hull, Briggs, 1787.

————, *A Short Treatise on the All Cleansing Earth*, Newcastle, Hall, 1790.

Griggs, B., *Green Pharmacy. A History of Herbal Medicine*, London, Jill Norman & Hobhouse, 1981.

Grose, F., *A Guide to Health, Beauty, Riches and Honour*, London, 1796.

Hagstrum, J.H., *Sex and Sensibility: Erotic Ideal and Erotic Love from Milton to Mozart*, London and Chicago, University of Chicago Press, 1980.

Hambridge, R., 'Empiricomany, or an infatuation in favour of empiricism or quackery. The socio-economics of eighteenth-century quackery', in S. Soupel and R. Hambridge, *Literature and Science and Medicine*, Los Angeles, Clark Memorial Library, University of California Press, 1982, pp.47-102.

Hand, W.O., 'The folk healer; calling and endowment', *Journal of the History of Medicine*, XXVI, 1971, pp.263-75.

Hanen, M.P., Osler, M.J. and Weyant, R.G. (eds)., *Science, Pseudo-Science and Society*, Waterloo, Ontario, Wilfred Laurier University, 1980.

Hare, E.H., 'Masturbatory insanity: the history of an idea', *Journal of Mental Science*, 108, 1962, 1-25.

Harley, D., 'Honour and property: the structure of professional disputes in eighteenth-century English medicine', unpublished paper, 1987.

Harris, L., and Knowles, L., 'The golden days of Dr Quack', *History of Medicine*, VI, 1975, pp.76-81.

Harris, M., *London Newspapers in the Age of Walpole: A Study of the Origins of the Modern English Press*, Madison, Wisc., Fairleigh Dickinson University, 1987.

Harrison, J.F.C., 'Early Victorian radicals and the medical fringe', in W.F. Bynum and R. Porter (eds)., *Medical Fringe and Medical Orthodoxy 1750-1850*, London, Croom Helm, 1987, pp.198-215.

Hartsthorne, A. (ed.), *Memoirs of a Royal Chaplain, 1729-63. The Correspondence of Edmund Pyle, D.D. Chaplain in Ordinary to George II, with Samuel Kerrich D.D., Vicar of Dersingham, Rector of West Newton*, London, John Lane: Bodley Head, 1905.

Hatfield, G., 'Quacks, pettifoggers and parsons: Fielding's case against the learned professions', *Texas Studies in Literature and Language*, IX, 1967, 69-83.

Heathcote, R., *Sylva*, London, Payne, 1786.

Heberden, W., *Medical Commentaries*, London, T. Payne, 1802.

Heilbron, J., *Electricity in the Seventeenth and Eighteenth Centuries*, Berkeley, University of California Press, 1979.

Helfand, W.H., 'James Morison and his pills', *Transactions of the British Society of the History of Pharmacy*, I, 1974, pp.101-35.

Hill, B., 'Medical impostors', *History of Medicine*, II, 1970, pp.7-11.

————, 'Scavenger of the Faculty. Joshua Ward 1658-1761', *Practitioner*, CCIII, 1969, pp.820-5.

Hillam, F.C., 'The development of dental practice in the provinces from the late eighteenth century to 1855' University of Liverpool, PhD. thesis, 1986.

————, 'James Blair 1747-1817, provincial dentist', *Medical History*, XXII, 1978, pp.44-70.

Himes, Norman E., *Medical History of Contraception*, Baltimore, Williams & Wilkins, 1936.

Holbrook, S.H., *The Golden Age of Quackery*, New York, Macmillan, 1959.

Holmes, G., *Augustan England. Professions, State and Society 1680-1730*, London, Allen & Unwin, 1982.

Hone, C.R., *The Life of Dr. John Raddiffe 1652-1714. Benefactor of the University of Oxford*, London, Faber & Faber, 1950.

Hopkins, D., *Princes and Peasants: Smallpox in History*, London and Chicago, University of Chicago Press, 1983.

Howe, G.M., *Man, Environment and Disease in Britain. A Medical Geography Through the Ages*, New York, Barnes & Noble, 1972.

Hultin, N.C., 'Medicine and magic in the eighteenth century: the diaries of James Woodforde', *Journal of the History of Medicine*, XXX, 1975, pp.349 66.

Hunter R., and Macalpine, I., *Three Hundred Years of Psychiatry*, 1535-1860, London, OUP, 1963.

Illich, I., *Limits to Medicine. The Expropriation of Health*, Harmondsworth, Penguin, 1977.

Impostor Detected; or The Physician the Greater Cheat: Being a Candid Enquiry Concerning the Practice of Dr. Myersbach… And Shewing his Practice to be Defensible upon Natural and Philosophical Principles, London, [n.d.].

Inglis, B., *Fringe Medicine*, London, Faber & Faber, 1964.

————, *Natural Medicine*, London, Fontana, 1979.

Inkster, I., 'Introduction: aspects of the history of science and science culture in Britain 1780-1850 and beyond', in I. Inkster and J.B. Morrell (eds), *Metropolis and Province. Science in British Culture 1780-1850*, London, Hutchinson, 1983.

————, 'Marginal men: aspects of the social role of the medical community in Sheffield, 1790-1850', in J. Woodward and D. Richards (eds), *Health Care and Popular Medicine in Nineteenth Century England*, London, Croom Helm, 1977.

Irish, D., *Levamen Infirmi*, London, [the author], 1700.

Isaac, R., *The Transformation of Virginia 1740-1790*, Chapel Hill, University of North Carolina Press, 1982.

Jackson, D.M., 'Bach, Handel and the Chevalier Taylor', *Medical History*, XII, 1968, pp.385-93.

Jameson, E., *The Natural History of Quackery*, London, Michael Joseph, 1971.

Jarrett, Derek, *England in the Age of Hogarth*, London, Hart Davis, 1974.

————, *The Ingenious Mr Hogarth*, London, Joseph, 1976.

Jenkins, J., *Observations on the Present State of the Profession and Trade of Medicine*, London, [for the author], 1810.

Jewson, N., 'The disappearance of the sick man from medical cosmology 1770-1870', *Sociology*, X, 1976, pp.225-44.

————, 'Medical knowledge and the patronage system in eighteenth-century England', *Sociology*, VIII, 1974, 369-85.

Johnson, T.J., *Professions and Power*, New Jersey, Humanities Press, 1972.

Jones, E.L., 'The fashion manipulators: consumer tastes and British industries 1660-1800', in L.P. Cain and P.J. Uselding (eds), *Business Enterprise and Economic Change*, Kent, Ohio, Kent State University Press, 1973, pp.217-20.

Jones, G.W., 'A relic of the golden age of quackery: what Read wrote', *Bulletin of the History of Medicine*, XXXVII, 1963, pp.226-38.

Jones, R.F., *Ancients and Moderns*, St Louis, Washington University Press, 1936.

Jonson, Ben, *Volpone*, ed. by P. Brockbank, London, 1908.

Jordanova, L.J., 'Natural facts: a historical perspective on science and sexuality', in C. MacCormack and M. Strathern (eds), *Nature, Culture and Gender*, Cambridge, CUP, 1980, pp.42-69.

————, 'Policing public health in France 1780-1815', in T. Ogawa (ed.), *Public Health*, Tokyo, Taniguchi Foundation, 1981, pp.12-32.

————, 'The social sciences and history of science and medicine', in P. Corsi and P. Weindling (eds), *Information Sources in the History of Science and Medicine*, London, Butterworth, 1983, pp.81-98.

Kaplan, S.L. (ed.), *Understanding Popular Culture: Europe from the Middle Ages to the Nineteenth Century*, New York, Mouton, 1984.

Kass, A.M., and Kass, E.H., *Perfecting the World. The Life and Times of Dr Thomas Hodgkin 1798-1866*, Boston, Harcourt, Brace, Jovanovich, 1988.

Keevil, J.J., 'Coffee house cures', *Journal of the History of Medicine*, IX, 1954, pp.17-29.

Kett, J.F., 'Provincial medical practice in England, 1730-1815', *Journal of the History of Medicine*, XXIX, 1964, pp.17-29.

Kiefer, J.H., 'Uroscopy, the artists' portrayal of the physician', *Bulletin of the New York Academy of Medicine*, XXIX, 1964, pp.759-66.

————, 'Uroscopy: The clinical laboratory of the past', *Transactions of the American Association of Genito-Urinary Surgeons*, XL, 1958, pp.161-72.

King, L.S., *The Medical World of the Eighteenth Century*, Chicago, University of Chicago Press, 1958.

————, *The Road to Medical Enlightenment, 1650-95*, London, Macdonald, 1970.

King, W., *Political and Literary Anecdotes of his own Time*, 2nd ed., London, 1819.

King-Hele, D. (ed.), *The Essential Writings of Erasmus Darwin*, London, MacGibbon & Kee, 1968.

————, *Doctor of Revolution: the Life and Genius of Erasmus Darwin*, London, Faber & Faber, 1977.

———— (ed.), *The Letters of Erasmus Darwin*, Cambridge, CUP, 1981.

Kleinman, A., *The Illness Narratives: Suffering, Healing, and the Human Condition*, New York, Basic Books, 1988.

Knox, R., *Enthusiasm*, London, OUP, 1950.

Kramer, J.C., 'Opium rampant: medical use, misuse and abuse in Britain and the west in the seventeenth and eighteenth centuries', *British Journal of Addiction*, LXXIV, 1979, pp.377-89.

LaCasce, S., 'Swift on medical extremism', *Journal of the History of Ideas*, XXXI, 1970, 599-606.

Lain Entralgo, P., The Therapy of the Word in Classical Antiquity, New Haven, Yale University Press, 1970.

Lane, J., 'The medical practitioners of provincial England in 1783', *Medical History*, XXVIII, 1984, 353-71.

————, 'The provincial practitioner and his services to the poor 1750-1800', *Society for the Social History of Medicine Bulletin*, 28, 1981, pp.10-14.

————, 'The role of apprenticeship in eighteenth-century medical education in England', in W.F. Bynum and R. Porter (eds), *William Hunter and the Eighteenth-Century Medical World*, Cambridge, CUP, 1985, pp.57-104.

Larner, C., *Witchcraft and Religion: the Politics of Popular Belief*, Oxford, Basil Blackwell, 1984.

Larson, M.S., *The Rise of Professionalism*, Berkeley, California University Press, 1977.

Latham, R., and Matthews, W. (eds), *The Diary of Samuel Pepys*, 11 vols, London, Bell & Hyman, 1970-83.

Lawrence, C., 'William Buchan: medicine laid open', *Medical History*, XIX, 1975, pp.20-35.

————, 'Incommunicable knowledge: science, technology and the clinical art in Britain, 1850-1914', *Journal of Contemporary History*, XX, 1985, pp.503-20.

————, 'The nervous system and society in the Scottish enlightenment', in B. Barnes and S. Shapin (eds), *Natural Order*, Beverly Hills and London, Sage Publications, 1980, pp.19-40.

Leith, D., *A Social History of English*, London, Methuen, 1983.

Lettsom, J.C., 'Fugitive Pieces' MS in the Wellcome Institute for the History of Medicine, London.

————, *Observations Preparatory to the Use of Dr. Myersbach's Medicines: in which the Efficacy of Certain German Prescriptions given in English is Ascertained by Facts… with Cases Tending to Shew the Impossibility of Acquiring a Knowledge of Disease by Urine*, London, 1776.

Leventhal, H., *In the Shadow of the Enlightenment: Occultism and Renaissance Science in Eighteenth-Century America*, New York, New York University Press, 1976.

Levine, J., *Dr Woodward's Shield*, Berkeley, University of California Press, 1977.

Liebenau, J., *Medical Science and Medical Industry*, London, Macmillan, 1987.

Lillywhite, B., *London Signs*, London, Allen & Unwin, 1972.

Little, D., and Kahrl, G. (eds), *The Letters of David Garrick*, 3 vols, London, OUP, 1963.

Locker, D., *Symptoms and Illness. The Cognitive Organization of Disorder*, London, Tavistock, 1981.

Looney, J.J., 'Advertising and society in England, 1720-1820: a statistical analysis of Yorkshire newspaper advertisements', Princeton University, Ph.D. thesis, 1983.

Loudon, I.S.L., 'Chlorosis, anaemia and anorexia nervosa', *Journal of the Royal College of General Practitioners*, 30, 1980, pp.1669-87.

————, 'The nature of provincial medical practice in eighteenth-century England', *Medical History*, XXIX, 1985, pp.1-32.

————, *Medical Care and the General Practitioner 1750-1850*, Oxford, Clarendon Press, 1986.

————, 'The vile race of quacks with which this country is infested', in W.F. Bynum, and R. Porter (eds), *Medical Fringe and Medical Orthodoxy, 1750-1850*, London, Croom Helm, 1987, pp.106-28.

Lowe, D., *History of Bourgeois Perception*, Brighton, Harvester, 1982.

Lustig, J.S., and Pottle, F.A. (eds), *Boswell: the Applause of the Jury, 1782-85*, London, Heinemann, 1982.

Macalpine, I., and Hunter, R., *George III and the Mad Business*, London, Allen Lane, 1969.

McCabe, C. (ed.), *The Talking Cure*, London, Macmillan, 1981.

Maccubbin, R. (ed.), *'Tis Nature's Fault. Unauthorized Sexual Behaviour in the Enlightenment*, Cambridge, Cambridge University Press, 1987.

MacDonald, M., 'Anthropological perspectives on the history of science and medicine', in P. Corsi and P. Weindling (eds), *Information Sources in the History of Science and Medicine*, London, Butterworth, 1983.

MacDonald, R.H., 'The frightful consequences of onanism', *Journal of the History of Ideas*, XXVIII, 1967, pp.423-41.

Macfarlane, A., *The Origins of English Individualism*, Oxford, Basil Blackwell, 1978.

MacGregor, H., 'Eighteenth-century V.D. publicity', *British Journal of Venereal Disease*, XXXI, 1955, pp.117-18.

Mackay, C., *Memoirs of Extraordinary Popular Delusions*, London, National Illustrated Library, 1851.

McKendrick, N., 'The consumer revolution of eighteenth-century England', in N. McKendrick, J. Brewer, and J.H. Plumb, *The Birth of a Consumer Society: the Commercialization of Eighteenth Century England*, London, Europa, 1982, pp.9-33.

————, 'George Packwood and the commercialization of shaving: the art of eighteenth century advertising, or "The Way to Get Money and be Happy"', in *ibid.*, pp.149-56.

————, Brewer, J., and Plumb, J.H., *The Birth of a Consumer Society: the Commercialization of Eighteenth Century England London*, Europa, 1982.

McLaren, A., 'The pleasures of procreation' in W.F. Bynum and R. Porter (eds), *William Hunter and the Eighteenth Century Medical World*, Cambridge, CUP, 1985, pp.323-42.

————, *Reproductive Rituals*, London, Methuen, 1984.

MacLeod, C., 'Patents for invention and technical change in England, 1660-1753' Cambridge University, PhD thesis, 1983.

————, *Inventing the Industrial Revolution. The English Patent System 1660-1800*, Cambridge, CUP, 1988.

Macmichael, W., *The Gold-Headed Cane*, London, Longman, 1854.

MacPherson, C.B., *The Political Theory of Possessive Individualism*, Oxford, OUP, 1962.

Malcolmson, R.M., *Popular Recreations in English Society 1700-1850*, Cambridge, CUP, 1973.

Maple, E., *Magic, Medicine and Quackery*, London, Hale, 1968.

Marchand, L.A. (ed.), *Byron's Letters and Journals*, 12 vols, London, John Murray, 1973-81.

Marcovich, A., 'Concerning the continuity between the image of society and the image of the human body. An examination of the work of the English physician, J.C.Lettsom 1746-1815', in P. Wright and A. Treacher (eds), *The Problem of Medical Knowledge*, Edinburgh, Edinburgh University Press, 1982, pp.69-86.

Marcuse, H., *One Dimensional Man*, London, Abacus, 1972.

————, *Eros and Civilization*, London, Abacus, 1972.

Marland, H., *Medicine and Society in Wakefield and Huddersfield, 1780-1870*, Cambridge, CUP, 1987.

Marlow, N. (ed.), *The Diary of Thomas Isham of Lamport*, London, Gregg, 1971.

Marshall, P.J., and Williams, G., *The Great Map of Mankind*, London, Heinemann, 1982.

Marten, J., *A Treatise of all the Degrees and Symptoms of the Venereal Disease*, 6th ed., London, S. Crouch, 1708.

Martin, J., *Animal Magnetism Examined*, London, Stockdale, 1790.

Matthews, L.G., 'Licensed mountebanks in Britain', *Journal of the History of Medicine*, XIX, 1964, pp.26-45.

————, *History of Pharmacy in Britain*, Edinburgh and London, E. & S. Livingstone, 1962.

Matthews, W. (ed.), *The Diary of Dudley Ryder 1715-16*, London, Methuen, 1939.

Mayer, H., *Outsiders: a Study in Life and Letters*, Cambridge, Mass., M.I.T. Press, 1984.

Mechanic, D., *Medical Sociology: A Selective View*, New York, Free Press, 1968.

Medical Anecdotes, London, 1816.

Medical Advertisements, British Library.

Medicina Flagellata; or, The Doctor Scarify'd, London, J. Bateman & J. Nicks, 1721.

Merchant, C., *The Death of Nature: Women, Ecology, and the Scientific Revolution*, San Francisco, Harper & Row, 1980.

Michaels, L., and Ricks, C. (eds), *The State of the Language*, Berkeley, University of California Press, 1980.

Miley, U., and Pickstone, J.V., 'Medical botany around 1850: American medicine in industrial Britain', in R. Cooter (ed.), *Studies in the History of Alternative Medicine*, London, Macmillan, 1988, pp.139-153.

Miliburn, J.R., *Benjamin Martin, Author, Instrument Maker and 'Country-Showman'*, Leiden, Noordhoff, 1976.

Miller, Genevieve, *The Adoption of Inoculation for Smallpox in England and France*, London, Oxford University Press, 1957.

Mills, H. (ed.), *George Crabbe, Tales, 1812, and Other Poems*, Cambridge, CUP, 1967.

Money, J., *Experience and Identity: Birmingham and the West Midlands, 1760-1800*, Manchester, Manchester University Press, 1977.

Moore, C.A., 'The English malady', in C.A. Moore (ed.), *Backgrounds of English Literature 1700-60*, Minneapolis, University of Minnesota Press, 1953, pp.179-235.

Moravia, S., 'The Enlightenment and the sciences of man', *History of Science*, XVIII, 1980, 247-68.

————, *Il Pensiero Degli Ideologues*, Florence, La Nuova Italia, 1974.

Morrell, J.B., 'Individualism and the structure of British science in 1830', *Historical Studies in the Physical Sciences*, III, 1971, pp.18~204.

Murphey, L.J.T., 'The art of uroscopy', *Medical Journal of Australia*, 1967, pp.879-86.

Needham, J., *A History of Embryology*, 2nd ed., Cambridge, CUP, 1959.

Neve, M., 'Natural philosophy, medicine and the culture of science in provincial England: the cases of Bristol, 1796-1850, and Bath, 1750-1820' University of London, PhD thesis, 1984.

————, 'Orthodoxy and fringe: medicine in late Georgian Bristol', in W.F. Bynum and R. Porter (eds), *Medical Fringe and Medical Orthodoxy, 1750-1850*, London, Croom Helm, 1987, pp.40-55.

Nevett, N., *Advertising in Britain. A History*, London, Heinemann, 1982.

New Method of Curing Diseases by Inspecting the Urine Explained: as practised by the German Doctor. Intended for the Serious Perusal of Physicians, Surgeons, Apothecaries, and the Public in General, London, [n.d.].

Nicholls, P.A., *Homoeopathy and the Medical Profession*, London, Croom Helm, 1988.

Nichols, J., *Literary Anecdotes of the Eighteenth Century*, 9 vols, London, Nichols, 1812-15.

Nicolson, M.H. (ed.), *The Conway Letters*, New Haven, Yale University Press, 1930.

————, *Science and Imagination*, Hamden, Conn., Archon Books, 1976.

————, *Newton Demands the Muse*, Princeton, Princeton University Press, 1966.

————, 'Ward's pill and drop and men of letters', *Journal of the History of Ideas*, XXIX, 1968, pp.173-96.

———— and Rousseau, G.S., 'Bishop Berkeley and tar water', in H.K. Miller, T. Rothstein, and G.S. Rousseau (eds), *The Augustan Milieu*, Oxford, Clarendon Press, 1970, pp.102-37.

Norton, J.E. (ed.), *The Letters of Edward Gibbon*, 3 vols, London, Cassell, 1956.

Obelkevitch, J., *Religion and Rural Society: South Lindsey, 1826-1875*, Oxford, Clarendon Press, 1976.

Ober, W.B., *Boswell's Clap and other Essays: Medical Analyses of Literary Men's Afflictions*, Carbondale, Southern Illinois University Press; London and Amsterdam, Feffer & Simons, 1979.

————, 'Bach, Handel and 'Chevalier' John Taylor, M.D., ophthalmiator', *New York State Journal of Medicine*, LXIX, 1969, pp.1797-1806.

————, 'Noble quacksalver: the Earl of Rochester's merry prank', *History of Medicine*, V, 1973, pp.24-6.

Opie, I., and Opie, P., *The Lore and Language of Schoolchildren*, Oxford, OUP, 1959.

Outram, D., 'The language of natural power: the eloges of George Cuvier and the public language of nineteenth century science', *History of Science*, XVI, 1978, pp.153-78.

Paget, S., *John Hunter*, London, Unwin, 1897.

Pagliaro, H.E. (ed.), *Irrationalism in the Eighteenth Century: Studies in Eighteenth Century Culture*, vol.2., Cleveland, 1972.

Parry, N., and Parry, J., *The Rise of the Medical Profession: A Study of Collective Mobility*, London, Croom Helm, 1976.

Pattison, F.L.M., *Granville Sharp Pattison, Anatomist and Antagonist 1791-1851*, Edinburgh, Canongate, 1987.

Paulson, R., *Literary Landscape, Turner and Constable*, New Haven, Yale University Press, 1982.

————, *Popular and Polite Art in the Age of Hogarth and Fielding*, Notre Dame, University of Notre Dame Press, 1979.

Payne, H.C., 'Elite vs. popular mentality in the eighteenth century', *Studies in Eighteenth Century Culture*, VIII, 1979, pp.3-32.

Pelling, M., 'Medical practice in early modern England: trade or profession?', in W. Prest (ed.), *The Professions in Early Modern England*, London, Croom Helm, 1987, pp.90-128.

————, 'Medicine since 1500', in P. Corsi and P. Weindling (eds), *Information Sources in the History of Science and Medicine*, London, Butterworth, 1983, pp.379-410.

———— and Webster, C., 'Medical practitioners', in C. Webster (ed.), *Health, Medicine and Mortality in the Sixteenth Century*, Cambridge, CUP, 1979, pp.165-235.

————, 'Appearance and reality: Barber-surgeons, the body and disease', in A.L. Beier and R. Finlay (eds), *London 1500-1700: the Making of the Metropolis*, New York, Longman, 1986, pp.82-112.

Pendleton, D., and Hasler, J. (eds), *Doctor-Patient Communication*, London, Academic Press, 1983.

Percival, T., *Medical Ethics*, Manchester, Johnson & Bickerstaff, 1803.

Perkin, H., *The Origins of Modern English Society*, London, Routledge & Kegan Paul, 1969.

Petersen, J., *The Medical Profession in mid-Victorian London*, Berkeley, University of Califomia Press, 1978.

Pettigrew, T.J., *Memoirs of the Life and Writings of the Late John Coakley Lettsom*, London, Longman, 1817.

Pickstone, J.V., 'Establishment and dissent in nineteenth-century medicine', in W.J.Sheils (ed.), *The Church and Healing*, Oxford, Basil Blackwell, 1982.

Pinder, Peter, *Physic and Delusion*, London, [n.d.].

'Piss-Pot Science', *Journal of the History of Medicine*, X, 1955, pp.121-3.

Plumb, J.H, *The Commercialization of Leisure in Eighteenth-Century England*, Reading, University of Reading Press, 1973.

————, *Georgian Delights*, London, Weidenfeld & Nicolson, 1980.

Pocock, J.G.A., *Politics, Language and Time*, London, Methuen, 1972.

Pollock, L.A., 'Embarking on a rough passage: the experience of pregnancy in early modern society', in V. Fildes (ed.), *Women as Mothers in Early Modern England*, London, Routledge, 1989.

Porter, D., and Porter, R., *Patient's Progress*, Cambridge, Polity Press, 1989.

————, 'The politics of prevention: anti-vaccinationism and public health in nineteenth-century England', *Medical History*, XXXII, 1988, pp.231-52.

Porter, R., 'Science, provincial culture and public opinion in Enlightenment England', *British Journal for Eighteenth Century Studies*, III, 1980, pp.20-46.

————, 'The Enlightenment in England', in R. Porter and M. Teich (eds), *The Enlightenment in National Context*, Cambridge, CUP, 1981, pp.1-18.

————and Teich, M. (eds), *The Enlightenment in National Context*, Cambridge, CUP, 1981.

————, *English Society in the Eighteenth Century*, Harmondsworth, Penguin, 1982.

————, 'Mixed feelings: the Enlightenment and sexuality in eighteenth-century Britain', in P.-G. Boucé (ed.), *Sexuality in Eighteenth-Century Britain*, Manchester, Manchester University Press, 1982, pp.1-28.

————, 'The sexual politics of James Graham', *British Journal for Eighteenth-Century Studies*, V, 1982, pp.201-6.

————, 'The doctor and the word', *Medical Sociology News*, IX, 1983.

————, 'The rage of party: a glorious revolution in English psychiatry?', *Medical History*, XXVII, 1983, pp.35-50.

————, 'Sex and the singular man: the seminal ideas of James Graham', *Studies on Voltaire and the Eighteenth Century*, 228, 1984, pp.1-24.

————, 'Spreading carnal knowledge or selling dirt cheap? Nicholas Venette's Conjugal Love in the eighteenth century', *Journal of European Studies*, XIV, 1984, pp.233-55.

————, 'Lay medical knowledge in the eighteenth century: the evidence of the Gentleman's Magazine', *Medical History*, XXIX, 1985, pp.138-68.

————, 'Laymen, doctors and medical knowledge in the eighteenth century: the evidence of the Gentleman's Magazine', in R. Porter (ed.) *Patients and Practitioners: Lay Perceptions of Medicine in Pre-industrial Society*, Cambridge, CUP, 1985, pp.283-314.

————, 'Making faces: physiognomy and fashion in eighteenth-century England', *Etudes Anglaises*, XXXVIII, 1985, pp.385-96.

————, 'The patient's view: doing medical history from below', *Theory and Society*, 14, 1985, pp.175-98.

———— (ed.), *Patients and Practitioners: Lay Perceptions of Medicine in Pre-Industrial Society*, Cambridge, CUP, 1985.

————, '"Under the influence": mesmerism in England', *History Today*, September 1985, pp.22-9.

————, 'William Hunter: a surgeon and a gentleman', in W.F. Bynum and R. Porter (eds), *William Hunter and the Eighteenth Century Medical World*, Cambridge, CUP, 1985, pp.7-34.

————, 'The language of quackery in England 1660-1800', in P. Burke and R. Porter (eds), *The Social History of Language*, Cambridge, CUP, 1986, pp.73-103.

————, 'Love, sex and madness in eighteenth-century England', *Social Research*, LIII, 1986, pp.212-42.

————, 'Medicine and the decline of magic', *Strawberry Fayre*, autumn, 1986, pp.88-94.

————, '"I think ye both quacks": the controversy between Dr Theodor Myersbach and Dr John Coakley Lettsom', in W.F. Bynum and R. Porter (eds), *Medical Fringe and Medical Orthodoxy 1750-1850*, London, Croom Helm, 1987, pp.56-78.

————, 'Medicine and religion in eighteenth-century England: a case of conflict?', *Ideas and Production*, VII, 1987, pp.4-17.

————, '"The secrets of generation display'd": Aristotle's Master-piece in eighteenth-century England', in R.P. Maccubbin (ed.), *'Tis Nature's fault. Unauthorized Sexuality During the Enlightenment*, Cambridge, CUP, 1987, pp.7-21.

————, 'Before the fringe', in Cooter, R. (ed.), *Studies in the History of Alternative Medicine*, London, Macmillan, 1988, pp.1-27.

————, 'A touch of danger: the man-midwife as sexual predator', in G.S. Rousseau and R. Porter (eds), *Sexual Underworlds of the Enlightenment*, Manchester, Manchester University Press, 1988, pp.206-32.

————, 'Introduction' to Thomas Trotter, *An Essay on Drunkenness*, London, Routledge Reprint, 1988 (1st ed. 1804).

————, 'Libertinism and Promiscuity', in J. Miller (ed.), *The Don Giovanni Book: Myths of Seduction and Betrayal*, London, Faber, 1990, pp.1-19

————, 'The Rise of Physical Examination', in W.F. Bynum and R. Porter (eds), *Medicine and the Five Senses*, Cambridge, CUP, 1992, pp.179-97

————, 'Introduction' to George Cheyne, *The English Malady*, London, Routledge Reprint, 1989 (1st ed. 1734).

———— and Porter D., *In Sickness and In Health: the English Experience, 1650-1850*, London, Fourth Estate, 1988.

———— and Porter D., 'The rise of the English Drugs Industry: The Role of Thomas Corbyn', *Medical History*, xxxiii, 1989, pp.297-95. Reprinted in Jonathan Liebenau, Gregory J. Higby and Elaine C. Stroud (eds), *Bill Peddlers. Essays on the History of the Pharmaceutical Industry, Madison*, Wisc., American Institute of the History of Pharmacy, 1990, pp.5-28

Poynter, F.N.L. (ed.), *The Evolution of Pharmacy in Britain*, London, Pitman, 1965.

Prestbury, F., *The History and Development of Advertising*, New York, 1929.

Price, C., *Theatre in the Age of Garrick*, Oxford, Basil Blackwell, 1973.

Price, Rees, *Critical Inquiry into the Nature and Treatment of the Princess Charlotte*, London, 1817.

Price, Robin, 'Hydropathy in England 1840-70', *Medical History*, XXV, 1981, pp.269-80.

Pride, J.B., and Holmes, J. (eds), *Socio-Linguistics*, Harmondsworth, Penguin, 1972.

Probyn, C., 'Swift and the physicians', *Medical History*, XVII, 1974, pp.249-61.

Quackery, its Danger, Irrationality and Injustice: the Causes of its Success, the Best Means for its Suppression, London, Gibbs, 1836.

Quackery of the Medical Profession, The, London, Westley, 1844.

'Quacks and Quackery', *British Medical Journal*, I, 1911.

Quacks and Quackery by a Medical Practitioner, London, 1844.

Quennell, P. (ed.), *The Private Letters of Princess Lieven to Prince Metternich, 1820-26*, London, John Murray, 1937.

Raeff, M., *The Well-Ordered Police State*, New Haven, Yale University Press, 1983.

Ramsey, M., *Professional and Popular Medicine in France, 1770-1830. The Social World of Medical Practice*, Cambridge, CUP, 1988.

————, 'Property rights and the right to health: the regulation of secret remedies in France, 1789-1815', in W.F. Bynum and R. Porter (eds), *, 1750-1850*, London, Croom Helm, 1987, pp.79-105.

———— 'The repression of unauthorized medical practice in eighteenth-century France', *Eighteenth-Century Life*, VII, 1982.

Rankin, G., 'Professional organization and the development of medical knowledge: two interpretations of homeopathy', in R. Cooter (ed.), *Studies in the History of Alternative Medicine*, London, Macmillan, 1988, pp.45-61.

Reay, B. (ed.), *Popular Culture in Seventeenth-Century England*, London, Croom Helm, 1985.

Redwood, J., *Reason, Ridicule and Religion, the Age of Enlightenment in England, 1660-1750*, London, Thames & Hudson, 1976.

Rees, K., 'Hydropathy in Matlock', in R. Cooter (ed.), *Studies in the History of Alternative Medicine*, London, Macmillan, 1988, pp.27-44.

Reynolds, F., *The Life and Times of Frederick Reynolds*, London, Colburn, 1826.

Risse, G. (ed.), *Medicine without Doctors*, New York, Science History Publications, 1977.

Ritterbush, P.G., *Overtures to Biology*, New Haven, Yale University Press, 1964.

Rivers, I. (ed.), *Books and their Readers in Eighteenth-Century England*, Leicester, Leicester University Press, 1982.

Roberts, R.S., 'The personnel and practice of medicine in Tudor and Stuart England', *Medical History*, VI, 1962, pp.363-82.

Robinson, H.W., and Adams, W. (eds), *The Diary of Robert Hooke 1672-80*, London, Taylor & Francis, 1935.

Robinson, N., *The Theory of Physick*, London, Betteworth, 1729.

Roe, S.A., *Matter, Life and Generation*, Cambridge, CUP, 1984.

Rogers, N., 'Aristocratic clientage, trade and independency: popular politics in pre-radical Westminster', *Past and Present*, 61, 1973, pp.70-106.

Rogers, P., *Grub Street*, London, Methuen, 1972.

Rosen, G., 'Enthusiasm', *Bulletin of the History of Medicine*, XLII, 1968, pp.393~21.

————, *A History of Public Health*, New York, MD Publications, 1958.

————, *From Medical Police to Social Medicine*, New York, Science History Publications, 1974.

Rosenberg, C., 'Medical text and medical context; explaining William Buchan's Domestic Medicine', *Bulletin of the History of Medicine*, LVII, 1983, pp.22-24.

Rosenfeld, S., *The Theatre of the London Fairs in the Eighteenth Century*, Cambridge, CUP, 1960.

Rousseau, G.S., 'Literature and medicine; the state of the field', *Isis*, LXXII, 1981, pp.406-24.

————, 'Nerves, spirits and fibres: towards defining the origins of sensibility with a postscript 1976', *The Blue Guitar*, III, 1976, pp.125-33.

————, 'Psychology', in G.S. Rousseau and R. Porter (eds), *The Ferment of Knowledge*, Cambridge, CUP, 1980.

————, 'Science and the discovery of the imagination in Enlightenment England', *Eighteenth-Century Studies*, III, 1969, pp.108-35.

————, Tobias Smollett, *Essays of Two Decades*, Edinburgh, Clark, 1982.

———— and Porter, R. (eds), *Sexual Underworlds of the Enlightenment*, Manchester, Manchester University Press, 1988.

———— and Porter, R. (eds), *Exoticism in the Enlightenment*, Manchester, Manchester University Press, 1989.

Rowbotham, S., *Hidden from History*, London, Pluto, 1973.

Rowe, H., *The Sham Doctor* [n.p., n.d., late eighteenth century].

Rowse, A.L., *Simon Forman, Sex and Society in Shakespeare's Age*, London, Weidenfeld & Nicolson, 1974.

Sampson, H., *A History of Advertising*, London, Chatto & Windus, 1874.

Saunders, J.W., *The Profession of Letters*, London, 1964.

Schaffer, S., 'Natural philosophy and public spectacle in the eighteenth century', *History of Science*, XXI, 1983, pp.1-43.

————, 'Natural philosophy', in G.S. Rousseau and R. Porter (eds), *The Ferment of Knowledge*, Cambridge, CUP, 1980.

Schnorrenberg, B.B., 'Medical men of Bath', *Studies in Eighteenth-Century Culture*, XIII, 1984, pp.189-203.

Schupbach, W, 'Sequah: an English American medicine-man in 1890', *Medical History*, XXIX, 1985, pp.272-317.

Sedgwick, R. (ed.), *Lord Harvey's Memoirs*, London, Kimber, 1952.

Seligman, S.A., 'Mary Toft the rabbit breeder', *Medical History*, V, 1961, pp.349-60.

Senate, E., *The Medical Monitor*, London, [the author], 1810.

Sennett, R., *The Fall of Public Man*, Cambridge, CUP, 1974.

Shapiro, B., *Probability and Certainty in Seventeenth-Century England*, Princeton, Princeton University Press, 1983.

Shastid, T.H., *An Outline History of Ophthalmology*, Southbridge, Mass., American Optical Company, 1927.

Sheils, W. (ed.), *The Church and Healing*, Oxford, Basil Blackwell, 1982.

Shorter, E., *Bedside Manners: the Troubled History of Doctors and Patients*, New York, Simon & Schuster, 1986.

Shortland, M., 'The body in question; some perceptions, problems and perspectives of the body in relation to character, c.1750-1850' University of Leeds, Ph.D. thesis, 1985.

————, 'The figure of the hypocrite: some contours of an historical problem', *Studies in the History of Psychology and the Social Sciences*, IV, 1987, pp.256-74.

Sibly, E., *The Medical Mirror; or, Treatise on the Impregnation of the Human Female. Shewing the Origin of Diseases, and the Principles of Life and Death*, London, Champante, 1796.

Silvette, H., *The Doctor on the Stage*, Knoxville, Tenn., University of Tennessee Press, 1967.

————, 'On quacks and quackery in seventeenth-century England', *Annals of Medical History*, 3rd series, I, 1939.

Slack, P., 'Mirrors of health and treasures of poor men: uses of the vernacular medical literature of Tudor England', in C. Webster (ed.), *Health, Medicine and Mortality in the Sixteenth Century*, Cambridge, CUP, 1979, pp.237-74.

Smith, F.B., *The People's Health 1830-1910*, London, Croom Helm, 1979.

Smith, V.S., 'Prescribing the rules of health: self-help and advice in the late eighteenth-century England', in R. Porter (ed.), *Patients and Practitioners*, Cambridge, CUP, 1985, pp.249-82.

————, 'Cleanliness: the development of an idea and practice in Britain 1770-1850', University of London, Ph.D. thesis, 1985.

————, 'Physical puritanism and sanitary science: material and immaterial beliefs in popular physiology 1650-1840', in W.F. Bynum and R. Porter (eds), *Medical Fringe and Medical Orthodoxy, 1750-1850*, London, Croom Helm, 1987, pp.174-97.

Smollett, T., *Ferdinand Count Fathom*, ed. by D. Grant, London, OUP, 1971.

————, *Launcelot Greaves*, ed. by P. Evans, Oxford, OUP, 1977.

Snorrason, E., *C.G. Kratzenstein and his Studies on Electricity During the Eighteenth Century*, Odense, Odense University Press, 1974.

Snyder, C., 'Johann Sebastian Bach and Chevalier Taylor', in *Our Ophthalmic Heritage*, London, Chisholm, 1967, pp.77-9.

Solomon, S., *Account of the Balm of Gilead*, London, Clarke, 1801.

————, *A Guide to Health, or, Advice to Both Sexes in a Variety of Complaints*, 56th ed., London, [the author], *c*.1800.

Sorsby, A., *A Short History of Ophthalmology*, London, Bale, 1948.

Southey, R., *Letters from England*, London, Cresset, 1951.

Spillane, J., *The Doctrine of the Nerves*, London, OUP, 1981.

Spilsbury, F.B., *Free Thoughts on Quacks and their Medicines*, London, J. Wilkie, 1776.

Spinke, J., *Quackery Unmask'd; or Reflections on the Sixth Edition of Mr Martin's Treatise on the Venereal Disease; ...and the Pamphlet [by T.C.Surgeon] Call'd the Charitable Surgeon, Containing a Detection and Refutation of Some Gross Errors etc of those Authors*, London, D.Brown, 1709.

————, *Venus's Botcher: or the Seventh Edition of Mr Martin's Comical Treatise on the Venereal Disease... Examin'd and Expos'd*, London, S. Popping, 1711.

Sprott, D. (ed.), *1784*, London, Allen & Unwin, 1984.

Stansfield, D.A., *Thomas Beddoes M.D. 1760-1808, Chemist, Physician, Democrat*, Leiden, Reidel, 1984.

Starobinski, J., 'Moliere and the doctors', *Ciba Symposium*, XIV, 1966, pp.143-8.

Stedmanlones, G., *Languages of Class. Studies in English Working Class History 1832-1982*, Cambridge, CUP, 1983.

Steneck, N., 'Greatrakes the Stroker: The interpretations of historians', *Isis*, LXXIII, 1982, pp.160-77.

Stengers, J., and Van Neck. A., *Histoire d'une Grande Peur: La Masturbation*, Brussels, University of Brussels Press, 1984.

Stern, P., *Medical Advice to the Consumptive and Asthmatic People of England… And a New Easy Method of Cure*, London, J. Almon, 1767.

Stone, L., *The Family, Sex and Marriage in England, 1500-1800*, London, Weidenfeld & Nicolson, 1977.

Strachey, C. (ed.), *The Letters of the Earl of Chesterfield to his Son*, 2 vols, London, Methuen, 1901.

Straus, R., *The Unspeakable Curll*, New York, Kelley, 1970.

Strong, L.A.G., *Dr Quicksilver 1660-1742*, London, Melrose, 1955.

Strong, P.M., *The Ceremonial Order of the Clinic*, London, Routledge, 1979.

Sutton, G., 'Electrical medicine and mesmerism', *Isis*, LXXII, 1981, pp.375-92.

Swainson, I., *Direction for the Use of Velno's Vegetable Syrup*, London, Ridgeway, 1790.

Szasz, T., *The Myth of Mental Illness*, New York, Paladin, 1961.

Taylor, John 'Chevalier', *The History of the Travels and Adventures of the Chevalier John Taylor*, London, Williams, 1760.

————, *An Account of the Mechanism of the Eye. Wherin its Power of Refracting the Rays of Light, and Causing them to Converge at the Retina, is consider'd: With an Endeavour to ascertain the true Place of a Cataract, and to Shew the Good or Ill Consequences of a Judicious Removal of it. By John Taylor, Surgeon in Norwich*, London and Norwich, 1727.

————, *A New Treatise on the Diseases of the Chrystalline Humour of a Human Eye; Or, of the Cataract and Glaucoma*, Paris, 1735.

Thackray, A., 'Natural knowledge in cultural context: the Manchester model', *American Historical Review*, LXXIX, 1974, pp.672-709.

Thirsk, J., *Economic Policy and Projects*, Oxford, Clarendon Press, 1978.

Thomas, K.V., 'An anthropology of religion and magic', *Journal of Interdisciplinary History*, VI, 1975, pp.91-110.

————, *Man and the Natural World*, London, Allen Lane, 1983.

————, *Religion and the Decline of Magic: Studies in Popular Beliefs in Sixteenth and Seventeenth-Century England*, London, Weidenfeld & Nicolson, 1971; reprinted, Harmondsworth/New York, Penguin, 1978.

Thompson, C.J.S., *Mysteries of History*, London, Faber & Gwyer, 1928.

————, *The Quacks of Old London*, London, Brentano, 1928.

Thompson, E.P., 'Patrician society, plebeian culture', *Journal of Social History*, 8, 1974, pp.382-405.

Thompson, R., *Unfit for Modest Ears*, London, Macmillan, 1979.

Thompson, S. (ed.), *Stedman's Journal, 1744-1797*, London, Mitre Press, 1962.

Thomson, A., *The Family Physician*, 2nd ed., London, R. Phillips, 1807.

Tibble, J.W., and Tibble, A. (eds), *The Prose of John Clare*, London, Routledge & Kegan Paul, 1951.

Tissot, S.-A.A.D., *Onanism or a Treatise Upon the Disorders Produced by Masturbation*, trans. A.Hume, London, [n.p.], 1766.

Toynbee, Mrs Paget (ed.), *The Letters of Horace Walpole*, 16 vols, Oxford, Clarendon Press, 1903-25.

Trimmer, E.J., 'Medical folklore and quackery', *Folklore*, XX, 1965, pp.161-75.

Tring, F.C., 'The influence of Victorian "patent medicines" on the development of early twentieth-century medical practice', University of Sheffield, Ph.D. thesis, 1982.

Trotter, T., *A View of the Nervous Temperament*, London, Longman, Hurst, Rees & Owen, 1807.

Tucker, S., *Protean Shape*, London, Athlone Press, 1967.

[Turner, D.], *The Modern Quacks*, London, Roberts, 1718.

————, *Vindication of the Noble Art of Chirurgery*, London, Whitlock, 1695 .

Turner, E.S., *The Shocking History of Advertising*, Harmondsworth, Penguin, 1965.

————, *Call the Doctor. A Social History of Medical Men*, London, Michael Joseph, 1958.

Tytler, G., *Physiognomy in the European Novel*, Princeton, Princeton University Press, 1982.

Vaisey, D. (ed.), *The Diary of Thomas Turner*, Oxford, OUP, 1984.

Vestergard, T., and Schroder, K., *The Language of Advertising*, Oxford, Basil Blackwell, 1985.

Viseltear, A., 'Joanna Stephens and eighteenth-century lithontriptics; a misplaced chapter', *Bulletin of the History of Medicine*, XLII, 1968, pp.199-220.

Wadd, W., *Mems., Maxims and Memoirs*, London, Callow & Wilson, 1872.

Waddington, I., 'General practitioners and consultants in early nineteenth-century England: the sociology of an intra-professional conflict', in J. Woodward and D. Richards (eds), *Health Care and Popular Medicine in Nineteenth-Century England*, London, Croom Helm, 1977, pp.164-88.

————, *The Medical Profession in the Industrial Revolution*, Dublin, Gill & Macmillan, 1984.

Wagner, P., *Eros Revived: Erotica of the Enlightenment in England and America*, London, Secker & Warburg, 1988.

————, 'The veil of science and morality: some pornographic aspects to the ONANIA', *British Journal for Eighteenth-Century Studies*, IV, 1983, pp.179-84.

Wallis, R., and Morley, P. (eds), *Marginal Medicine*, London, Owen, 1976.

Walpole, H., *Memoirs of George II 1751-1754*, ed. by J. Brooke, New Haven, Yale University Press, 1985.

Ward, N., *The London Spy*, ed. by K. Fenwick, London, Folio Society, 1955.

Warner, J .H., *The Therapeutic Perspective: Medical Practice, Knowledge and Id entity in America, 1820-1885*, Cambridge, Mass., Harvard University Press, 1986.

Watt, I., *The Rise of the Novel*, Harmondsworth, Penguin, 1957.

Wear, Andrew, 'Puritan perceptions of illness', in R. Porter (ed.), *Patients and Practitioners: Lay Perceptions of Medicine in Pre-Industrial Society*, Cambridge, CUP, 1985, pp.55-99.

Weatherill, L., *Consumer Behaviour and Material Culture in Britain, 1660-1760*, London, Routledge, 1988.

Webster, C., 'Alchemical and Paracelsian medicine', in C. Webster (ed.) *Health, Medicine and Mortality in the Sixteenth Century*, Cambridge, CUP, 1979, pp.301-34.

————, *The Great Instauration, Science, Medicine and Reform 1626-1660*, London, Duckworth, 1975.

————, *Health, Medicine and Mortality in the Sixteenth Century*, Cambridge, CUP, 1979.

————, 'The historiography of medicine', in P. Corsi and P. Weindling (eds), *Information Sources in the History of Science and Medicine*, London, Butterworth, 1983.

Weeks, J., *Sex, Politics and Society*, London, Longman, 1981.

Welsh, C., *A Bookseller of the Last Century, being Some Account of John Newbery and the Books he Published*, London, Griffin, 1903.

————— (ed.), *Goody Two-Shoes*, London, 1881.

Wheatley, H.B., 'The Company of Undertakers', in *Hogarth's London*, London, Constable, 1909.

Whitbread, H. (ed.), *I Know my Own Heart. The Diaries of Anne Lister, 1791-1840*, London, Virago, 1988.

Whitwell, H.I., 'James Graham, masterquack', *Eighteenth-Century Life*, IV, 1977-8.

Whorton, J.C., *Crusaders for Fitness: the History of American Health Reformers*, Princeton, Princeton University Press, 1982.

Wiles, R.McK., *Freshest Advices*, Columbus, Ohio, Ohio State University Press, 1965.

Willey, B., *The Seventeenth-Century Background*, London, Chatto & Windus, 1934.

Williams, G., *The Age of Agony*, London, Constable, 1975.

Williams, J.B., 'The early history of London advertising', *Nineteenth Century and After*, LXII, 1907.

Williams, N., *Powder and Paint*, London, Longmans, 1957.

Willich, A.F.M., *Lectures on Diet and Regimen*, London, Longman & Rees, 1799.

Wimsatt, W.R., *Philosophical Words*, New Haven, Yale University Press, 1948.

Wood Playstead, James, *The Story of Advertising*, New York, Ronald, 1958.

Woodward, J., and Richards, D., 'Towards a social history of medicine', in *idem* (eds), *Health Care and Popular Medicine in Nineteenth Century England*, London, Croom Helm, 1977.

Wright, A.D., 'The quacks of John Hunter's time', *Transactions of the Hunterian Society*, XI, 1952-53.

Wrigley, E.A., and Schofield, R.S., *The Population History of England 1541-1971: a Reconstruction*, London, Edward Arnold, 1981.

Wyman, A.L., 'The surgeoness. The female practitioner of surgery, 1400-1800', *Medical History*, XXVII, 1984, pp.22-41.

Yearsley, M., *Doctors in Elizabethan Drama*, London, Bale, 1933.

Young, J.H., *The Medical Messiahs*, Princeton, Princeton University Press, 1967.

—————, *The Toadstool Millionaires*, Princeton, Princeton University Press, 1961.

Zwanenberg, D. van, 'The Suttons and the business of inoculation', *Medical History*, XXII, 1978, pp.71-82.

Index

Numbers in bold refer to illustrations, **C** denoting a colour plate